Dutch Newspapers on War Victims and Their LSD-treatment by Jan Bastiaans

Dutch Newspapers on War Victims and Their LSD-treatment by Jan Bastiaans:

From KZ-syndrome to PTSD

By

Leo van Bergen

Cambridge Scholars Publishing

Dutch Newspapers on War Victims and Their LSD-treatment by Jan Bastiaans: From KZ-syndrome to PTSD

By Leo van Bergen

This book first published 2023

Cambridge Scholars Publishing

Lady Stephenson Library, Newcastle upon Tyne, NE6 2PA, UK

British Library Cataloguing in Publication Data
A catalogue record for this book is available from the British Library

ISBN (10): 1-5275-0120-5
ISBN (13): 978-1-5275-0120-1

For this publication a grant has been received from the Dutch foundations Historia Medicinae and Research Fund Medical Polemology.

"I've never felt really liberated."
—Berthe Meijer, Bergen-Belsen survivor and author of *Life after Anne Frank.*[1]

"The people who continued to suffer their entire lives have never been liberated."
—Eddie Jaku, Auschwitz survivor and author of *The Happiest Man in the* World.[2]

"A trauma victim can be liberated through treatment methods such as psychedelic drugs."
—Bessel van der Kolk, psychiatrist and author of *The Body Keeps the Score.*[3]

"The KZ syndrome can be an expression of both external and internal lack of freedom."
—Jan Bastiaans in 'The KZ syndrome and human freedom'.[4]

TABLE OF CONTENTS

Introduction 1

1. The first reports about the KZ syndrome and Bastiaans' thesis 21

2. Attention is increasing 29

3. The psychoanalytic conference in Amsterdam in July 1965 33

4. About LSD and the reverse burden of proof... 38

5. The movie *Do you now understand why I cry...* 44

6. The Working Group Camp Syndrome.. 57

7. The advent of the post concentration camp syndrome clinic................ 64

8. The Breda Three 67

9. The TV broadcast of *Do you now understand why I cry...* 80

10. The influence of the Breda Three discussion...................................... 89

11. The construction of the Post Concentration Camp Syndrome Clinic.... 95

12. The opening of Centre '45 108

13. The war syndrome and LSD's medical use both criticised
and praised... 124

14. The first Moluccan hostage-takings: Wijster and Amsterdam.......... 132

15. A first dent in the image 141

16. 4 May 1977: commemorating the dead 147

17. Two more Moluccan hijackings: Bovensmilde and De Punt............ 150

18. Right and wrong 162

19. The *Holocaust* TV Series 172

20. The caregiving criticised 188

21. The story continues... 196

22. The East Indies camp syndrome... 204

23. The aftercare under fire and the hostage-taking in Tehran 211

24. Financial and medical worries 220

25. The book *People at Hostage-takings*.. 223

26. The endgame 229

Closing remarks.. 246

Words of gratitude.. 258

Literature 259

Abbreviations 303

Endnotes 305

Index of persons 354

INTRODUCTION

> A tree lined road evokes memories of long rows of gallows with dangling bodies, and someone raising her arms evokes associations of fellow inmates who were hung by their arms. Children playing suddenly reminds her of other children in those days, starved, abused, murdered.[1]

That is how the newspaper article by the Jewish (or declared Jewish by the Nazis) physician Joseph Kater entitled "Concentration Camp syndrome" started on 30 May 1964. These were only a few of the distorted images – that could hardly be shared with third parties – the Norwegian Jewish doctor Leo Eitinger described at the annual meeting of the World Organisation for Mental Health in 1961. He was a camp survivor himself. Together with other symptoms, such as constant fatigue, persistent anxiety or difficulty to concentrate, they formed the concentration camp syndrome, the KZ syndrome (*KonZentrationslager* syndrome; KL was the official abbreviation, KZ the one used by the *Häftlinge*, the prisoners). It has been described as "the complex of mental and physical phenomena, that is characteristic of people who have experienced a long and severe psychological war trauma". In the *Nieuw Israëlietisch Weekblad NIW* (New Israelite Weekly*)*, it was defined more succinctly: "A collection of physical and mental illnesses as a result of staying in a camp."[2] Kater himself described it as "a series of disorders of a physical and mental nature which are observed in all countries where former camp inmates live".[3] The word syndrome here stands for the disease symptoms that are associated with a disease and are to be regarded as a unit.

Just like psychiatrist Jan Bastiaans, in an article entitled "The KZ syndrome and human freedom",[4] the Dutch historian Stephen Snelders rightly pointed out that the description 'syndrome' in KZ syndrome is somewhat misleading. It wasn't so much a series of disorders as a four-stage process: shock accompanied by powerlessness, alarm with intense emotions, adaptation with flight or fight reactions, and finally exhaustion.[5] Partly due to the lack of clarity about the KZ syndrome and the multiplicity of the definition,[6] combined with the failure to diagnose the problems arising from the concentration camps using known (war) neuroses like *soldier's heart*, *nostalgia* or *shell shock*, the door was opened to a focus on the symptoms rather than the cause. This shift was a worldwide phenomenon and in this book it will be highlighted for the Netherlands, the country where 107,000 Jewish people were deported, 75 percent of the pre-war number of Jews, of whom only 5000 returned. As a result of that shift, as time progressed, more and more groups were pulled or withdrew into the concentration camp syndrome, who, in fact, only had mental problems attributed to past events in common. Furthermore, they differed from each other in many respects, such as in their experiences both during and after the war (was surviving family to be expected or not, for example), and in the reasons for persecution (if there was persecution at all). As a result, the meaning of the term concentration camp syndrome was diluted, and more general terms emerged. References to the war and the camps were omitted, so even more people could take shelter under the terms.[7]

Kater's article is a good example of how the Dutch were informed about the problems a stay in a concentration camp could still cause after the war, and the way in which the medical profession dealt with and looked at them. How, in other words, the Dutch population became familiar with terms like KZ syndrome, psychological trauma, and later PTSD (post-traumatic stress disorder), at a time when the newspaper was still generally seen as an honourable gentleman and not as a deeply untrustworthy disseminator of fake news. It isn't for nothing that the Letter to the editor column in the former resistance newspaper *Het Parool* (The Parole) was called "But sir".

According to Kater, who himself escaped death by going into hiding, the KZ syndrome made it difficult to function socially because "the family, the environment, and society" simply asked for "a whole, sane person". And all this while the war was already over for twenty years, even though the Auschwitz trials, such as the one against Adolf Eichmann in 1961, "revived the horrors of the concentration camps and even a layman will doubtlessly understand that even the most powerful personality couldn't have survived them undamaged".[8] At some point every one of us will collapse, as military psychiatrist Thomas Arthur Ross stated in his *Lectures on War Neuroses*, as early as 1941. It only happens sooner to the one person and a little later to the other.[9]

But therein lies the crux of the matter. Laymen, and not just them, but also and above all doctors, denied this for decades. And even if in their hearts they did know, the politico-military setting they had to work in made it impossible to get this out there and/or act according to this conviction. Many doctors – of course there were exceptions – believed a psychological trauma after experiencing a shocking event was due more to character weakness, inherited or not. At most, the event itself was the trigger that brought out the already present weakness. This, for example, was what many of the troubled soldiers in the trenches of World War I came to hear. Traumatic neurosis, the psychological damage caused by experiencing serious events, was even declared dead by psychiatrists in Germany in 1916, and the German psychiatrists and neurologists were far from alone in this.[10]

This was also the story of the Netherlands after 1945: *pack up your troubles in your old kit bag and smile, smile, smile*, exactly what those same World War I soldiers were already told in a song written in 1915. Military psychiatrists, at the time of the decolonisation war (1946-1949), said that it didn't explain the neurotic problems of soldiers.[11] Indulgence had to be avoided. When they talked about mental war damage, they meant general moral decay, not individual psychological problems. The Netherlands had to reconnect with West Germany because of the communist danger. War criminals were pardoned. The need to celebrate Commemoration Day and Liberation Day, on respectively 4 and 5 May, was under discussion. The myth that in the Netherlands – a country in which every religion and ideology had its own 'pillar', its own political party, musical bands, and football clubs – the population resisted the Nazis on a large scale and had hidden the Jewish people en masse, prevented a reflection on matters that conflicted with this sunny view of the past. It wasn't helpful to focus on the war years too much, for instance by paying attention to the large number of Jewish people who had not survived the war and the problems the survivors experienced as a result. There was only limited interest in the concentration camps.[12]

This changed in the 1960s. The war became visible again. The related psychological problems were discussed and now the war was declared as their cause. The time to just move on and not look back was over. The social changes – depillarisation, secularisation, democratisation, emancipation – resulted in a diminishing stigma on psychological problems. The culture of silence changed into a culture of talking. The history of ordinary men and women became interesting, including their personal troubles. Victims began to organise. Emotions were emancipated. They were allowed to be shown, privately and publicly. The shame that was felt if an experience couldn't be mentally processed decreased. The *old kit bag* was unpacked. This had consequences in just about every area of society, and it translated into an explosion of war pension applications and complaints about physical and psychological problems associated with war experiences, especially in the 1970s.[13]

Therefore, that Kater, following Ross' lead, wrote in the mid-1960s that even a layman could understand that everyone had a breaking point – a statement, by the way, that can neither be proved nor invalidated –, and that shocking experiences could have a psychological and physical effect for a long time, wasn't obvious at all. It was a relatively new insight that many patients wanted to know little about for a long time. If anything was wrong, then physically. "It's not me head, it's me heart."[14]

Jan Bastiaans

That this slowly but surely changed was, from a medical point of view, the result of preparatory movements such as pre-war phenomenology and post-war psychosomatics. Together with the increasing attention for the war itself from the late 1950s, this led in fits and starts, with intervals and flare-ups to a greater attention for mental war problems. A first sign of this was a 1957 thesis, *Psychosomatische Gevolgen van Onderdrukking en Verzet* (Psychosomatic Consequences of Oppression and Resistance), written by the already briefly mentioned Jan Bastiaans. However, it took a while before outside the narrow psychiatric circle it was recognised that the problems described in it could take off. In his dissertation, he briefly pointed out three factors that caused the trauma, in addition to the war experiences themselves of course. Those were a troubled childhood, the stress resulting from it and the lack of care immediately after the war, including the difficulties in determining disability percentages. The bigger the youth problem, the greater the chance of war trauma, even with mild experiences. The more pleasant childhood experiences were, the more one could handle. Due to lack or even absence of treatment, the trauma was often ingrained and that made it difficult to treat later in life.[15]

We will see that Bastiaans certainly wasn't the first to publish about the post-war problems of resistance fighters and camp survivors. According to Kater, however, Bastiaans did have the honour of demonstrating that the stress the resistance fighters, his research group, endured in the concentration camps "not only caused, but clearly promoted psychoneurotic disorders ten years after the liberation". Examples were asthma, high blood pressure and joint pain. According to Kater, following up on Bastiaans, diseases such as tuberculosis were also more common among camp survivors than among others.[16]

Bastiaans was appointed professor of psychiatry in Leiden at the end of 1963,[17] just at the beginning of a period that can be characterised by the words medical secularisation. A professor of medicine was a god in his own department, and to a lesser extent, so were practicing physicians in the 1950s and 1960s. They decided on their own what therapy and combined drugs were prescribed and administered to their patients. If a doctor wanted to use a certain drug in the 1950s and early 1960s, even if it was controversial, there was nothing and no one that could stop him. He – female doctors were still a rarity, let alone female professors of medicine – weighed and decided. When Bastiaans left the university in the mid-eighties, there was little left of this supreme position.[18] Social democratisation put an end to it. Gradually doctors became less 'men who'll know best'. Physicians changed from infallible supreme beings to normal, and therefore, fallible human beings, and in the case of the professors among them, from sole rulers in their own department to one of many in a larger medical care and decision-making chain.

Bastiaans, who himself went into hiding at the end of the war, looked upon the treatment of traumatised camp survivors and resistance members as "a matter of honour for nations, governments and researchers, to be done out of respect for those who were denied the chance to witness the transition from fascism to democracy".[19] He did so in an article entitled 'Vom Menschen im KZ und vom KZ im Menschen' (About human beings in a concentration camp and the concentration camp in human beings), that was included in a collection of articles coedited by, dedicated to and intended to financially support the Jewish Austrian war crime investigator and Nazi hunter, Simon Wiesenthal.[20] He also treated soldiers who suffered from psychological problems caused, or thought to be caused, by the war, for example by taking them back to the place where they had fought.[21] That makes him the father of the nowadays popular return pilgrimage. To their satisfaction, it was a method he also used for concentration camp survivors.[22] Willem Wilbrink, for example, survivor of Dachau, who spent two years in therapy with Bastiaans to his great satisfaction, said: "At first I didn't want to hear anything about it, but I have profited from it greatly."[23]

Bastiaans stated several times that his past in the student resistance was of great importance for his efforts on behalf of war victims. It was also of great importance that this involvement in the Dutch resistance was nipped in the bud by (probably) a wrong injection in one of his legs after it was injured,[24] a medical mistake that plagued him throughout his life. As a result, he came out of the war relatively unscathed. At least: according to himself. Others say that because of this he too suffered from *survivor's guilt,* also called *survival syndrome.*[25] It was the result of feeling guilty for having survived, a syndrome that often tormented the camp survivors he treated (also because there could be a relationship between surviving and not surviving). It was articulated by the psychiatrist and Auschwitz survivor Eddy (Eliazar) de Wind. At the end of his *Eindstation… Auschwitz* (Final Destination… Auschwitz), probably the only novel written in that camp, he wrote:

> More people were killed in this place than anywhere else in the world. Here a destruction system of perfection without comparison reigned. But still not completely perfect. Otherwise, he wouldn't be able to stand here, he wouldn't be alive either. Why was he alive? What gave him the right to live? In what way had he been better than all those millions who had perished? It seemed an unfathomable wickedness to him that he hadn't shared the fate of all those others.[26]

Bastiaans himself never linked his work to the survival syndrome. He stated that he could sense the misery of those who were badly damaged because of his initial resistance. By having to stop doing that early, he was able to keep the medically necessary distance during treatment.[27] A best of both worlds.

Bastiaans – mentally and physically an impressive figure in every way – was a man who didn't shy away from the media, to say the least. His face was frequently seen in the newspapers and, from the late 1960s, on television. It was through these newspaper reports and TV appearances that the Dutch identified him with the psychological war problems, although he was anything but the only psychiatrist treating people suffering from KZ syndrome. He became, so to speak, the superhero of the syndromes that were associated with war experiences and developed into a national and international celebrity. He became a man whose word was taken into account from top to bottom and who was appointed Commander in the Order of Orange-Nassau for his work on behalf of war victims in 1988. He held a position in the field of psychotraumatology in the 1970s that certainly transcended that of people like Anthony Fauci at the time of the COVID-19 pandemic. He was a source of information and oracle in one. It isn't for nothing that the Dutch history tv programme *Andere Tijden* (Other Times) devoted one of its first episodes to him and his – by that time highly controversial – methods of treatment, in 2000, just three years after his death.[28]

Bastiaans used his fame to have his say in all kinds of areas. He was regularly asked for an opinion, that he always had and was willing to give. This could concern related subjects, including his advice, widely shared in the media and adopted by the court in September 1962, to hospitalise and discharge a woman who had murdered her two children, because of childhood psychiatric problems.[29] Also related to the KZ problem is the point of view he gave in 1965 that in the upbringing of the older generation too much emphasis was placed on control. This led to a disturbed emotional life and hence to psychosomatic complaints.[30]

To a certain extent this also applied to the opinion Bastiaans made public in early 1974, that many physicians gave sedatives to patients with suicidal tendencies instead of looking for the cause of their unrest and depression.[31] Or that asthma was a physical reaction to a psychosocial conflict situation, as he, for example, put forward at a conference on the psychosomatic aspects of that lung condition in 1978.[32] Or that victims of traffic accidents often become psychiatric patients because, on the one hand, settling financial claims took too long and, on the other hand, both the insurance and the treating physicians made mistake after mistake, as he stated in 1981 and 1983.[33]

And then there was his heavily criticised psychosomatic opinion in 1983 as well, that people who bottled up their emotions had a fair chance of developing cancer. He experienced that especially the *silent* war victims died of this disease.[34] This led to the controversial term 'cancer personality': according to Bastiaans they were usually people, "who hadn't learned to stand up for themselves in their childhood". Psychotherapy could therefore play an important role in treating cancer patients and in preventing cancer. In addition to a lot of television attention, this opinion received a variety of disapproving comments from people as diverse as a columnist, a psychologist, a cardiologist, and a professor of medical history.[35]

But he also didn't shy away from giving his opinion on matters that had little to do with psychological trauma, such as his view, noted in 1960, that the man played a subordinate role in birth control and how disastrous that was.[36] Or that modern society was rotten because of people's increasingly egocentric behaviour, also because they were given a lot more information on television than they could handle, as Bastiaans said at the end of 1969.[37] Or that, in 1970, the societal protests of the younger generation didn't make him happy.[38] These newspaper articles with opinions that weren't related to war trauma also contributed to his fame. And this is even more true of his frequent television appearances, that weren't always about the psychological effects of war and other forms of violence either.[39]

These frequent media appearances brought about a transformation. From a psychiatrist affiliated with the *Wilhelmina Gasthuis* (Wilhelmina Hospital) in Amsterdam, he simply became 'Bastiaans'.[40] There were more people called Bastiaans in the news from the sixties to the eighties: from a writer of books about the Netherlands East Indies via a frequent contributor of political left-wing letters to the papers, to a tennis champion and two brothers playing futsal. But after the discussion of the possible release of the Breda Three, three war criminals imprisoned in the town of Breda, in 1972, and certainly after the hostage-takings by Moluccan youth in the mid-seventies, that one word was enough to make it clear to everyone who was meant. There were a lot of people who were called Bastiaans, but there was only one who *was* Bastiaans. And with the growing fame of the leading medical expert on the KZ syndrome, the general acceptance grew of what some call a timeless fact and others a social construct: that experiencing a shocking event (let alone multiple events) leads to psychological problems, not only immediately after the event(s), but many years later as well.

Narcoanalysis and LSD

Bastiaans was one of the few physicians who partially used the increasingly controversial hallucinogenic drug LSD (Lyserg-Säure-Diäthylamid), more specifically LSD-25. Now these treatments are in the spotlights once again, due to research into possible positive effects of using MDMA (Methylene-Dioxy-Meth-Amphetamine), the active ingredient of the drug XTC, when treating PTSD.[41] Psychiatrist Bessel van der Kolk, who worked for Bastiaans in 1966, discusses this as well in his worldwide bestseller *The Body Keeps the Score.* He explains the benefits and the positive, according to him even astonishing, results achieved so far, but nevertheless concludes with words of caution:

> Psychedelic substances are powerful agents with a troubled history. They can easily be misused through careless administration and poor maintenance of therapeutic boundaries. It's to be hoped that MDMA will not be another magic cure released from Pandora's box.[42]

LSD was synthesised in 1943, right on time for the post-war psychopharmacological revolution. It was very usable as an aid to psychoanalysis, the treatment that dominated the psychiatric field at that time. By using LSD and other narcotic drugs (a treatment called narcoanalysis or psycholysis) the psychiatrists believed they had their hands on a sharp and precise scalpel to mark out and heal abnormalities in the mind and brain.[43] Narcoanalysis was already in use at Leiden University before the arrival of Bastiaans,[44] who experimented with mind-altering drugs on his patients since 1946. He started to use them more specifically when treating war victims however, and he introduced LSD, which he started to use at the University of Amsterdam in 1961, in Leiden. According to him, LSD would release all the suppressed emotions and feelings like fear and anger far better than the previously used narcotics did, and furthermore preserve the memory of the reliving. This was problematic and led to rather disappointing results up to that moment. Reliving traumatic events became easier when using LSD and this led to a substantial reduction of complaints such as the frequency and severity of nightmares.[45]

The drug, though only used by a minority of his patients, became his double-edged sword. Historian Bram Enning noted in his dissertation *De Oorlog van Bastiaans* (Bastiaans' War) that its use confirmed the seriousness of the syndrome, and the healing process was proof of the power of the drug.[46] LSD, as newspaper *De Telegraaf* (The Telegraph) wrote in 1994, had turned Bastiaans, "this giant in person and thought", into the "liberator from the inner camp" of "desperate patients".[47]

However, LSD was anything but undisputed, neither socially nor scientifically.[48] The drug was viewed with suspicion by the government, by parts of the medical establishment and by large parts of society in general from the mid-1960s on. From a medical point of view, for example, there were suspicions of chromosome damage, doubts about the reported results, or the critique that by using LSD doctors intervened in and altered the essence of the individual human being.[49] There were also doubts whether it was indeed LSD that was responsible for any improvement in the patient's condition. In his thesis *LSD en Psychiatrie in Nederland* (LSD and Psychiatry in the Netherlands) Snelders pointed out the importance of drug, set and setting. In other words: for the success of the use of a psychopharmacon, not only the drug itself is of the utmost importance, but also the setting (the physical environment, the atmosphere, the attitude of other people present), and the set (the expectation of what the drug will do).[50]

Snelders also made it clear that the government and large parts of society also mistrusted the use of LSD by doctors, was mainly the result of the psychedelic revolution. This involved the increasing non-medical use of psychedelics, especially LSD, mainly focused on pleasure and self-liberation, by members of the so-called counterculture in the 1960s,[51] although it was certainly used outside of this as well. For example, actor Cary Grant who could certainly be called an anti-hippy in terms of appearance and image, used the drug on a weekly basis. It helped him fight the demons arising from his poor childhood and the contradiction between his real self and the characters he usually had to play.[52]

It was this personal use that led to the inclusion of the drug in the Opium Act in 1966, not entirely coincidentally after the provos, anarchist activists in the Netherlands, threatened to use it to disrupt the marriage between crown princess Beatrix and Claus von Amsberg. This ban also made medical use more problematic, although the psychiatrists used the drug in much lower doses than the flower children of this world consumed. In other words, it wasn't medical critique that stopped the LSD treatment. Social developments were the cause of this.[53] Although some of the internal medical criticism predated this, the often conservative, religiously inspired, aversion to the use of drugs just for pleasure reinforced the critique. That can be seen clearly in an advisory report by the Dutch Health Council published in 1985, about a request from Bastiaans to be allowed to continue using LSD. Continuation of the drug's medical use, because of "seemingly therapeutic uses", detracted the "work to contain the massive drug problem".[54]

Method

Snelders' and Enning's theses prove that already quite some historical scientific material has been published about war trauma and the rise of psychotrauma in the Netherlands, and certainly about Bastiaans and his treatment methods.[55] The problem is that these works are often based on internal documents or articles from medical magazines that aren't intended for the general public, such as the *Maandblad Geestelijke Volksgezondheid* (Public Mental Health Monthly). The effect was that certainly *Bastiaans' War* was so critical that the unsuspecting reader would have wondered how the man could ever have become that popular and managed to achieve such status. Consequently, in addition to a lot of praise, Enning also received a lot of criticism. It was said that he had looked back with nowadays morals and insights to condemn the Bastiaans of that time and he would only have used information from interviews that strengthened his criticism.[56]

Enning wondered how it was possible that Bastiaans could continue to use a treatment method considered controversial by various doctors for so long. As an explanation, he pointed out the almost unconditional, and not always purely peacefully expressed, support of his patients, who for the most part were former resistance fighters.[57] However, this doesn't explain his popularity with the general public, that also played a role in the perseverance of his method. To explain this popularity, one has to look at information that was available to everyone, in other words the newspaper coverage. After all: people don't act and think and judge according to scientific truth, they do so according to what they think is the truth. And that is based on the information they take in. These public reports form the basis of the story presented here, a story that will largely follow the chronology in which it was released.

To outline this process, I collected about 1,100 articles from the period 1954, the year that the first reports on psychological problems linked to camp experiences appeared, until December 31, 1987. At that point Bastiaans took his leave from the hospital *Centrum '45* (Centre '45) in Oegstgeest near Leiden, where he treated his patients at the end of his university career. Because this more or less coincided with the adoption of the term PTSD, this farewell also marks the end of the period that will be covered in this book. In this period many names of psychological traumas are mentioned, just like all kinds of events directly related to them, such as the opening of that same Centre '45 in 1973. Among these are Dutch national events (the already mentioned discussion about the Breda Three and the Moluccan hostage-takings, but also the broadcast of the Holocaust series), as well as international events (the Vietnam War, the treatment of dissidents by psychiatrists in the Soviet Union, the hostage-taking of Americans in Tehran).

I have (almost) limited myself to newspaper articles. If weekly or monthly magazines are mentioned, for example *Panorama* or *Vrij Nederland* (Free Netherlands) this is because attention has been paid to them in general reporting or in sections such as 'Uit de Weekbladen' (From the Weekly's). The only exception I've made is the already mentioned *NIW*. This weekly can be characterised as the mouthpiece of the Jewish survivors during the period I examined, and given the theme of this book, that isn't a group to be neglected.

Of course, not all newspaper articles presented in this book have been read by everyone. Between 1950 and 1990, many Dutch people lived in a bubble as well. The chance that someone read both the reports in the protestant *Nederlands Dagblad* (Dutch Daily) and the communist former resistance newspaper *De Waarheid* (The Truth) is quite small and the number of inhabitants of Maastricht, in the far south, who read *Het Nieuwsblad van het Noorden* (The News of the North) at breakfast, will have been negligible. In addition, the content will often have been forgotten, immediately or over time. This doesn't alter that through these articles (and, as said, various broadcasts on the subjects on television, that quickly grew from almost non-existent to a mass medium during this period) knowledge about endured misery and its effects, delayed or not, trickled into the living rooms.

The first result of this search was tangible evidence of the transience of psychiatric terminology. While the term 'camp syndrome' yielded 70, 76, 95, and 150 articles from the 1960s up to and including the 1990s, the figures for the 'KZ syndrome', that was certainly more established in the 1970s, were: 11, 191, 97 and 10. No surprise there. The letters KZ are riveted to the German camps. Meanwhile, problems were also reported by survivors of the Japanese internment camps – in the Netherlands usually, and, intentionally or unintentionally, rather racist, called 'Jap camps'. That, in spite of their different experiences, both groups were brought together under the same heading is indicative of the story that will be told here.

The differences in war experience, their equalisation, and the expansion of the diagnosis

That in the years of the Third Reich about six million times a Jewish person was murdered, is the result of a system explicitly aimed at destroying the Jewish people. In other words, Jewish people were persecuted for what they *were*. As a result, the war experiences of Jewish survivors, not only in but also outside the camps, differed in principle from those of other people, such as former resistance fighters. They were imprisoned for what they *did*. According to some, this gave the latter group a psychological advantage that increased their chances of survival,[58] however small these chances were for them, as they paid for their resistance with a trip to one of the camps. Because of this difference between being and doing, part of the resistance, especially the communists, didn't want to be seen as victims for a long time. The dehumanising persecution that the Jewish people faced has been put forward as *the* cause of the KZ syndrome, but it obviously lost importance as the number of groups that also received this diagnosis expanded further and further.

Those who were persecuted purely because of birth and those who were persecuted purely because of resistance – with the further consequence that, unlike the resistance members, the surviving Jewish people hardly had any relatives left –[59] form the two extremes of a weave of different, interrelated cross-linked groups. For example, there were Jews who were persecuted both for who they were and for the resistance they put up.[60] Despite the fact that they lived through the same period, they all had different stories to tell, due to individual experiences before, during, and after the war. Consequently, their traumatising experiences differed from individual to individual as well. To name just a few examples. Even if we pass by the reasons for being brought to a camp, one camp wasn't the same as the other. Jewish children who survived the war by going into hiding were told to be grateful instead of mourning the loss of their parents. Upon their return and unlike former resistance fighters, Jewish people, to put it mildly, weren't always welcomed with open arms. After the war, communist resistance fighters quickly changed from acclaimed heroes to reviled enemies. A consequence of the latter was that, in their eyes, fascism and capitalism became even more linked than they already were, which in fact means that, according to them, the Jewish people had fallen victim, not so much to a racist ideology, but to an economic system.[61]

One of the things the many articles made clear is that all the problems arising from all those different experiences were placed more and more under one diagnostic heading. Gradually the word 'victim' became the decisive factor. Whether someone had been in a camp, in the resistance or in hiding: "We are all victims after all". It was the psychological slogan with which previously politically exclusive and opposing groups gathered in 1972 to protest against the possible release of the three war criminals staying in the Breda prison: Franz Fischer, Joseph Kotalla and Ferdinand aus der Fünten.[62] The discussion of this can therefore be seen as a key moment in the paradigm shift, analysed by historians Jolande Withuis and Annet Mooij and which can be observed in the ways the war was remembered: from a fierce struggle against totalitarianism to a cause of trauma. This change is typical for the Netherlands. The general acceptance of the idea in the 1970s that psychological problems can arise many years after the traumatising event, caused an enormous growth in the number of traumatised people and a considerable growth of their financial rights.[63]

In the year following the Breda Three discussion, the *Maandblad Geestelijke Volksgezondheid,* which paid no attention whatsoever to war as a source of mental suffering in the 1950s and 1960s,[64] published a special issue about the KZ syndrome. In it one of the psychiatrists of Centre '45, A. Hustinx, criticised the explicit reference in both KZ syndrome and camp syndrome to concentration camp experiences. Firstly, according to him, the syndrome not only occurred after having been in a camp, but also after experiencing other traumatic events. In other words, the syndrome was seen more broadly, or at least had to be diagnosed more broadly, than only in former camp inmates. It therefore also had to be given a broader, more general name. The stress caused by an event was more important for the psychological problems experienced after the event, than the event itself. And secondly, he said many associated the letters KZ with '*K*rank-*Z*innig', the Dutch word for 'insane'. The alternative he proposed, the existential emotional stress syndrome (EESS), has never become established, although it did find some following.[65] The importance of stress itself as a cause of psychological problems, however, found massive following. A book by psychiatrist Mardi J. Horowitz, entitled *Stress Response Syndromes,* was published some years after Hustinx's article, and is seen as a trailblazer for the post-traumatic stress disorder of today.[66]

Like Bastiaans, Hustinx not only looked at traumatising events as a cause of psychological problems, but also at predisposing circumstances like the importance of personality and, in particular, a strict moralising, religious and/or political upbringing. That, according to him, such an upbringing would lead to all kinds of negative character traits and manners, sincerely shocked the psychiatrist André de Leeuw, who was also a Member of Parliament for the *Communistische Partij Nederland* CPN (Dutch Communist Party). He lashed out against Hustinx and in the same blow also against the entire Dutch mental health system, West Germany and the Dutch Minister of Justice, the catholic Dries van Agt who, at the time, was busy preparing the release of the already mentioned Breda Three. Resistance fighters, like many members of the CPN had been, weren't neurotics and, in fact, the derogatory word 'war victim' shouldn't be used for any of them. And what about the troubled Jewish people who survived? Had all of them enjoyed a restrictive upbringing leading to anal tendencies, he asked rhetorically.

It's one of the reasons why Withuis, in her book on the road from war trauma to a culture of complaint, with the short but apt title *Erkenning* (Acknowledgement), wrote that until the 1970s, when it dawned upon them that war trauma could be used as a political weapon, the Dutch communists didn't want to know anything about psychological war traumas, also because they believed they themselves were immune to it. They benefited from having ended up in a camp because of their anti-fascist views and actions. In other words, the camp was the consequence of who they wanted to be, not what they were at birth. But for this their faith in the socialist utopia had to remain intact. When the safe haven the communist pillar provided vanished into thin air, the war demons still dived into the open wound many times, for if the faith was gone, all the trials, all the struggles, all the suffering endured in the name of their ideal was in vain.[68]

That EESS didn't become a psychiatric success story is certainly partly the result of the publication of the third *Diagnostic and Statistical Manual of Mental Disorders* (DSM) almost a decade later. It started the worldwide advance of the equally multi-usable and substantially comparable term PTSD that appeared for the first time in a Dutch newspaper in 1985, more specific in an article about a Vietnam nurse. It isn't surprising that, according to Hans Binneveld, the Dutch historian of psychiatry, it's a "little imaginative, colourless concept". The term was a compromise agreed upon after lengthy discussions.[69] It's inclusive instead of exclusive (as the KZ syndrome was), it makes clear that even the strongest among us can get psychological problems after an event that is experienced as traumatic (*post*-trauma) and it's seen as a real disease for which no one has to feel ashamed. After all, the final word 'disorder' stands for an abnormality in the body or the mind or in its functioning, for an absent or defective function or specific structure. It was the only disorder in the DSM-III in which not only symptoms, but also the cause, in casu a shocking event, was one of the criteria for diagnosis. The disorder follows the event and the event is seen as the cause of the disorder. It does make a difference to the seriousness and nature of the disorder whether it concerns one event (single trauma or type I) or multiple events (multiple trauma or type II). This wasn't the case with other disorders mentioned in the manual that also (possibly) arose from traumatic events. This has contributed to the fact that, despite of or thanks to the far from clear or unambiguous definition criteria,[70] PTSD is the term that springs to everyone's mind nowadays when trauma is discussed, and that research into this surpassed other research into the possibility of trauma as a cause of other problems.[71]

Characteristic of both EESS and PTSD is that an external factor causing stress has to be at the root of the experienced problems. Because of their comprehensiveness, they can be seen as the psychiatric translation of the general broadening and generalisation, if not trivialisation, of words like disaster and trauma that has occurred since the 1950s, just as PTSD itself has been trivialised since the 1980s. The term trauma had an almost entirely physical meaning not so long ago, although the first time it was used in the psychological sense of the word dates back to 1878.[72] It got associated more and more with psychological suffering during the past half century up to the point that the word 'trauma' is mentioned when a favourite football club suffers a painful defeat (when the word 'disaster' is also never far away). In this way trauma has become a term that is already used when pointing out setbacks that happen in everyday life. All this has little to do with the suffering endured in concentration camps, and it's also far removed from definitions of traumatic events in the psychiatric literature, including phrases such as "actual or threatened death or serious injury" and "threat to physical integrity".[73]

This doesn't alter, but rather confirms, the fact that character and/or political-economic, cultural context, both before, during and after the event, no longer play a role in labelling an event as traumatic. And this also applies to pointing out the objective seriousness of the event itself, because this inevitably leads to what many consider to be a reprehensible hierarchy of suffering. It's sufficient if the person who experienced the event characterises it as traumatic and stressful, and if the problems felt, have arisen after it. Whether they also occurred *as a result* of the event simply has to be assumed, because this can hardly be proved.[74]

Without this process of inclusion, the emergence of the term PTSD in the 1980s can't be explained. It can be called the accumulation of the tendency, outlined more fully below, to draw the troubles life sometimes has in store for all of us into the world of war trauma.[75] Devoid of any reference to the cause of the symptoms other than that it must have been traumatising, this generic name reflects that, unlike words like shell shock, *combat fatigue*, Vietnam syndrome or KZ syndrome, trauma was no longer associated with war, let alone some specific facet of war.

This generalisation of terminology hasn't gone unchallenged. According to various critics, it's highly unjustified. They point out, for example, that it isn't correct to say, 'Shell shock, what we now call PTSD', or 'PTSD, what we used to call shell shock'. The symptoms differ, the diagnosis differs, the time of manifestation differs, and perhaps above all, the context in which the problems occurred differs. According to these critics the military medical saying: "Show me the wounds and I reveal to you the nature of the war", not only applies to the physical, but also to the mental damages done. In short: every war, every traumatic event, has its own madness.[76]

Generalisation of trauma has the opposite effect: not containment, but expansion of the number of people suffering from it. The vaguer the term, the sooner someone falls under it. On the other hand, however, it must be said that if a term did refer explicitly to war, for example with words like shell or concentration camp, this didn't guarantee that the number of people who were diagnosed to suffer from it, didn't increase. Even then this happened. Even soldiers who were never near any exploding shells were diagnosed with shell shock after a while. This resulted in an unsuccessful attempt by the military medics to see it replaced by the general *Not Yet Diagnosed (Nervous).* The abbreviation GOK was also used informally, expressing the desperation of the doctors: God only knows.[77]

PTSD became the generally accepted term for psychological problems after experiencing, undergoing, or even causing events seen or felt as traumatic, certainly in the public discourse. It may range from barely surviving genocide or other forms of mass murder, such as in the war of 1939-1945 or in former Yugoslavia or Rwanda in the 1990s, to witnessing a car accident, or from helplessly having to watch your family and friends being massacred to taking part in acts of violence oneself. We will come back to this again and again with regard to the KZ syndrome, but it can already be said that one of the greatest quantitative additions to the camp syndrome consisted of those who were imprisoned in the Japanese internment camps in the Netherlands East Indies in the years 1942 to 1945. According to many former residents of the Netherlands East Indies, these were just as bad as the German ones, which is indicative of the feelings of frustration arising from feeling disregarded that was prevalent within this group.

This equalisation was a stumbling block for someone like the writer Rudy Kousbroek, who himself was interned in a Japanese camp as a teenager. Without even in the slightest wishing to downplay the sufferings and horrors in these camps, he insisted that the major differences with the German concentration and extermination camps couldn't be denied. In a column, called 'The camp syndrome', he left little intact of the above view.

While, in his 1952 dissertation *Het Duitse Concentratiekamp* (The German Concentration Camp), the Jewish psychiatrist Elie Aron Cohen had just soberly pointed out the differences in death rates, both in absolute and relative terms,[78] Kousbroek practically cried out:

> For God's sake, we were *interned.* Those people have been *exterminated,* they have been reduced to nothing, to less than lice. The survivors (of the German camps) have been somewhere we have never been, they had to give up something that we have never lost. Anyone who wants to claim that for themselves has lost all sense of proportion.[79]

To his surprise, in the years that passed since then, the camp syndrome grew into something that affected the most diverse groups, including groups made up of people who hadn't been in any camp, be it German or Japanese, as he wrote in 1991. We'll see that it's less strange than it seems, and then it seemed to him, that among them even were women who had undergone an abortion. He also observed this automatism with regard to the Japanese camps. Not only the people who actually were there now suffered from it, nor even "people whose *parents* were interned". "Even children that were born more than thirty years after the war, with one or more *grandparents* who were in a Japanese camp, say they suffer from it." And then there were the veterans from the decolonisation war who, according to him, were hiding behind trauma so they didn't have to discuss the severe violence they themselves committed.[80]

Kousbroek thought that the psychological, social and material benefits the label 'victim' delivered in the meantime, were part of the explanation. The more victim one was, or said one was, the greater those benefits were. Though it was sympathetic that he himself belonged to the group that in his eyes had suffered *less,* by doing so he pointed out a hierarchy of suffering many didn't agree to. After all, such a hierarchy also implies a hierarchy of victimhood. Not to mention whether one person's suffering is indeed worse or can be called worse, than the sufferings of someone else, it's striking that on the one hand this hierarchy of victimhood was denied, while on the other hand it was an undeniable fact. Not only from a general social point of view, but also within the groups that labelled themselves as victims, one person was seen by the other as less of a victim than he or she him or herself was – or even not recognised at all.[81]

The psychiatrists weren't entirely blameless, at least according to Kousbroek. They were guilty of "a certain enthusiasm, a kind of proselytism". Their word as physicians, as psychiatrists, as experts in psychological distress could not be doubted or changed. Those who did, had no knowledge of the matter and, moreover, left the victims, their patients, in the lurch with all the psychological consequences that entailed. Just like the well-known and feared Dutch columnist Gerrit Komrij in the 1980s, he argued that without them there probably wouldn't even have been a KZ syndrome. First you have the psychiatrists who name a syndrome they have identified, and then the people who suffer from it will follow. This certainly applied to someone like Bastiaans, of whom, according to Komrij, "half the Netherlands thought he even treated everyone who was locked in a public bathroom for some time".[82]

Komrij made his comments on the KZ syndrome in the secular and liberal *NRC Handelsblad* (NRC Trade Journal) in early 1983. Bastiaans was given ample opportunity in that newspaper to show his side of a conflict with the Leiden University (of which there have been many) shortly before. Komrij closed his comments by writing:

> Because of him, some war victims began to deeply immerse themselves in their suffering. Because of him, thirty years after the war, there even are war victims who had long forgotten that they had ever been war victims. A masterpiece of psychiatry.[83]

It must be said, however, that a psychotherapist such as Bastiaans aroused suspicion in advance in self-proclaimed rationalists such as Kousbroek and Komrij. And if people like Bastiaans were also members of the Advisory Board of an organisation such as IATROS (doctor), interested in psychic stuff, all warning signals jumped to red. Certainly Komrij would in such cases use his entire, not insignificant language virtuosity with sardonic pleasure to reduce his victim to an insignificant blob with his poisonous pen.[84]

The Age of War Trauma

The automatism with which differing groups were brought under one and the same diagnosis, the inkblot effect criticised by Kousbroek and Komrij, certainly contributed to the fact that *de Volkskrant* (the People's Paper) proclaimed the twentieth century to be the century of war trauma in 1999.[85] This effect can't be separated from what has been called the process of proto-professionalisation. Concerning this: laypersons and professionals alike have been permeated by complaints resulting from the war, and they then see them in others and start talking about them using the terminology previously only used by experts. This proto-professionalisation was part of the trap consisting of three chambers that Enning described: awareness of the war past, acceleration of the suspicion that complaints were related to that past, and finally going to the doctor who confirmed this suspicion. As an example, he points out Eibert Meester, who will be discussed extensively later on. He wound up in hospital with heart complaints and was sent to a psychiatrist because he said he had experienced a thing or two during the war. This could well be related to his symptoms. Please note: Meester was 57 years old at the time and smoked two packs of cigarettes a day.[86]

Kousbroek spotted the inkblot effect during the 1980s, but actually it already occurred much earlier. It will certainly have been partly caused by the fact that even medics, in this case psychiatrists, can't always suppress the tendency to demonstrate their indispensability. Designating more and more people who depend on help is an effective means of achieving this. A, probably even more important, cause is that the same effect can be seen with diagnoses as with medication. While at first medication is often only intended for a small specific group, it gradually gets prescribed to more and more people. The less severely affected will also demand the use of a drug of which they have heard it has benefited others. In healthcare as well, supply isn't solely dictated by demand. Demand can't be separated from supply, although of course there has to be something that created the supply – as professor of sociology and psychotherapist, Abram de Swaan, once said: "The supply creates the demand, not the misery."[87]

Medical diagnoses are subject to the same effect, as Komrij already stated. If, for instance, a term has been found for the psychological suffering as a result of certain experiences, other groups will quickly want to be labelled as such. This is irrespective of whether the experience and the suffering that ensued from it or was ascribed to it have been similar or entirely different – to leave words like 'worse', 'just as bad', or 'less bad' for what they are, though objectively they could and should be used. This effect has been seen in this double aspect, for example, with Prozac, the drug that was given against depression, and with Ritalin for ADHD.[88]

With terms like KZ syndrome or PTSD something more is added. Withholding such psychiatric, diagnostic terms from groups other than those originally intended is seen as withholding acknowledgement. Acknowledgement of the presence of an external stressor. Acknowledgement of what was done to them, in the war or afterwards. Acknowledgement of the negligent care and shelter after the traumatic event. In short, even if an external circumstance is rarely the sole, exclusive cause of psychological problems,[89] withholding acknowledgement of that external circumstance as the cause, and therefore withholding the psychiatric term used in others, is equivalent to withholding the acknowledgement that the patient wasn't crazy from the start. Withholding acknowledgement, of which receiving benefits became a symbol, was often seen as the decisive step on the road to a disorder or syndrome, certainly from the 1970s on.[90] Until … Until someone says: “Okay. I’ve been through something bad. Who hasn’t? Join the club. Shit happens. This doesn’t mean I’ve gone crazy. This doesn’t mean I got some DSM abbreviation in my head and have to go to a psychiatrist.” After this one can only hope that the denial will not be seen by psychiatrists as an obvious symptom of exactly the syndrome or disorder that was denied.

Leo van Bergen, October 2021

1. THE FIRST REPORTS ON THE KZ SYNDROME AND BASTIAANS' THESIS

For the Dutch, Kater's article certainly wasn't the first introduction to the concentration camp syndrome. This even goes for Bastiaans' dissertation. Without giving it a name, psychiatrist Jacques Tas, survivor of Bergen-Belsen, already indicated, in 1946, it had to be seriously taken into account that as time went by war victims could start suffering from psychological disturbances. These would manifest themselves only after a while because it could take some time before the emotions, suppressed in the camps, found a way out.[1]

In his research, Tas was able to build on publications that appeared in the years before. Merinus Vroom obtained his doctorate in Utrecht in 1942 for a thesis about psychological problems resulting from the war in Den Helder, the town in which he was a general practitioner. It was withdrawn from the market by the German occupier and re-released in 1946.[2] Psychoanalyst and general practitioner Joost Meerloo already "in one rage" conceived a book about "the psychology of war and peace in man" during the time of mobilisation, late in 1939 and the first months of 1940. After participating in resistance activities, he fled to England, became head of the psychology department of the War Office and secretary of the Inter-Allied Psychological Study Group. In that capacity, he wrote a number of articles about foreseeable and lasting problems occurring after war's end, which indeed occurred, for example in the form of psychoses.[3]

Cohen also survived the camps, more specifically: Auschwitz, and the so-called death marches following the Russian advance. His dissertation, *The German Concentration Camp*, was partly based on his own experiences. It dealt with the medical and psychological effects of Auschwitz during, not after the war. His supervisor was psychiatrist Henricus Cornelius Rümke, who a year earlier as well published on the effects of KZ-captivity. One of Cohen's conclusions was the camps had proved that "man's adaptability, both physically and mentally, was very great", much bigger than he thought possible.[4] However, that his dissertation didn't deal with post-war problems doesn't mean he kept silent on this altogether.

> In many former prisoners this black phase of their lives is repressed, which will have its consequences. This phase, in which they have been wounded, mortified, humiliated, and tortured, cannot be erased; it still lives in them. They feel misunderstood and on a daily basis experience that society doesn't want to take into account their enormous concentration camp sufferings. Although not calculated in advance, I would consider it a great gain if my publication results in a better understanding of my fellow sufferers.[5]

He would explain his ideas about the concentration camp syndrome in more detail in the *Nederlands Tijdschrift voor Geneeskunde NTvG* (Dutch Medical Journal) in 1969 and 1972.[6] And he hailed the arrival of Claude Lanzmann's film *Shoah* in 1986. "It must have been a liberation for a lot of people taking part in it to give witness about all they had been through."[7]

In addition to the already mentioned De Wind, psychiatrist Andries van Dantzig must be mentioned, as well as Andries Kaas, author of the chapter on the concentration camps in the four-part *Onderdrukking en Verzet* (Oppression and Resistance).[8] De Wind, Van Dantzig and Kaas had survived Auschwitz, Neuengamme, and Buchenwald respectively. In the first post-war years they too published about their experiences and the problems these already had caused or could cause. At the time publications about the camps enjoyed a great deal of interest, but this only lasted a couple of years.

Kaas was the son of a Jewish father and a non-Jewish mother. He was arrested for assisting Jews early in 1944 and was told that because of this henceforth he too would be treated as a Jew. Having first, in 1946, written a detached article about the problems of political prisoners in the camps, he published a more personal account of camp life in 1968: *Buchenwald. Conclusies na twintig jaar* (Conclusions twenty years later). He indicated that for him the change of personality and character occurring in and resulting from camp life was the major cause of post-war problems, for disappointments experienced after returning home could no longer be overcome.[9]

De Wind, who set up the Foundation for Research on Psychological War Consequences in 1984, continued to write about the camp until his death in 1987. In *Final Destination... Auschwitz* it becomes clear that he already intended to do so immediately after his liberation. "He thought of this girl's words in 'No pasaran': 'I have to live to tell, to tell everyone about this, to convince the people this actually has happened…'"[10]

In an article written in 1949, entitled 'Confrontatie met de dood' (Confronting death), De Wind wrote about the mental problems caused by the camp. Because of the chronicity of the threat, problems of camp inmates really were of a different order as compared to those of civilians who had

had to endure a much shorter bombardment or of soldiers in battle who have the opportunity to fight back. As Kaas, he had witnessed a "profound personality change" resulting from the camps, which could only be overcome after great effort. For this reason he was amazed that so many people still lacked even basic knowledge of the camps, whereas in order to be able to provide help knowledge of how the different groups and individuals in the camps had related to each other and what effects the camps had had on the minds and bodies of the former prisoners was of the utmost importance.[11]

The article 'Directe en late gevolgen van extreme belastingsituaties' (Immediate and late effects of extreme burden situations) followed in 1966. In it, De Wind for the first time used the term trauma in a psychological sense for adult survivors of extermination camps. Previously, and only in the years immediately after the war, in this sense the term had been reserved for Jewish war foster children. On the occasion of the fortieth anniversary of the February Strike – a strike in February 1941, as protest against the treatment of Jewish Dutchmen – he wrote a long piece about the way he ended up in Auschwitz (mistakes on his part) and how he survived (a combination of Nazi blunders, coincidence, and sheer luck). In conclusion, he wrote some words on the KZ syndrome.

> For years the psychological effects of the war have been neglected. But now – late and for many too late! – they are recognised, and help is taken in hand. Unfortunately, this assistance is needed more by the day. Every swastika somewhere on a wall anywhere in the world, every overt or cryptic fascist slogan represents a new trauma for the survivors and after bomb attacks and other acts of terror they again lie awake at night. But here and there also the fight against fascism is started once more, giving the survivors that elated feeling: "they stand beside us in solidarity …", as it was during the February strike.[12]

Bastiaans thus certainly was not the first to draw attention to the development of psychological problems caused by war experiences. He wasn't in the Netherlands and he certainly wasn't internationally. There had already been several conferences on post concentration camp suffering before 1957, such as in Copenhagen in 1954. Conferences in Paris, Brussels, Moscow and Oslo followed. In Copenhagen, alongside illnesses such as typhoid fever, stress-related issues such as hunger stress or camp stress were identified as the main causes.[13]

This indicates that Annet Mooij's observation that the regularly heard view that in early post-war years no attention was paid to the psychological problems of war victims, was unfounded, is correct. However, she rightly went on stating this didn't say much about the impact this attention had, including in newspapers. Hence, this misconception didn't come out of the blue. It was based on a lack of interest for the existing attention, also from many psychiatrists. They often had a keener eye for the well-being of society as a whole than for individual camp survivors.[14]

The silence was broken, albeit softly, in 1954, the year of the Copenhagen conference. At the time, a single newspaper reported on the life of a man who survived concentration camps, developed mental health problems, and started embezzling money. The question was, did the embezzling result from his problems and were these problems a result of camp life? Before the war, he and his wife had earned a good income from the pharmacy she ran. However, it had been dismantled during the war and the compensation for it had only amounted to *f*3000.- (€1365.-). According to a psychiatric report, this disappointment had made him loose his sense of right and wrong. However, his lawyer pointed out during the trial that there were indications, endorsed by other psychiatrists, that "mental disorders in concentration camps and after returning sometimes occur years later, because aspiration in the camps had been impossible". The court was requested to take this into account.[15]

This article was followed by another one in the *Algemeen Dagblad* (General Daily) entitled 'Concentratiekampziekte tastte de hersenen aan' (Concentration camp disease affected the brain). This article was written because of the publication of the results of an official French investigation, ordered three years earlier, "into the consequences of the deportation to and time in the concentration camps during the last world war". These results were compared with a similar Danish study among 1,300 Danish deportees. It prompted some Danish psychiatrists, including Neuengamme survivor Paul Thygesen, to coin the term KZ syndrome.[16]

It was clear that in addition to those already ill or injured before they arrived in the camp – who mostly died there –, and those suffering at the time from the widespread disease tuberculosis, there was a third and, according to the *Algemeen Dagblad,* most interesting group to be distinguished. It consisted of people "showing certain physical and mental abnormalities after returning home from the camp", which were entirely due to "the poor conditions in the concentration camp". The cause was not unequivocal. Reference was made to "the great emotions, the constant attitude of defence and the intense tension", to which the persistent lack of food could be added. Since, it had been shown that prolonged starvation could lead to severe brain damage. The conclusion was that the French report "would undoubtedly contribute to a better understanding of the concentration camp victims and therefore to improving aid giving as well".[17] Bastiaans was credited for the fact that his dissertation broadened knowledge about concentration camp disease resulting from these studies, and made it applicable to those who had been traumatised by other forms of violence, such as hostage-takings and disasters.[18] If this is correct, it means that there is a direct line from Bastiaans' dissertation to PTSD.

Hunger continued to attract attention. Psychiatrist Johannes Barnhoorn presented a report on "starvation as possible cause of nervous, psychological and psychosomatic problems" early in 1955. It was drawn up at the request of the extraordinary pension council, called into being to investigate war victims' pensions. Barnhoorn, the man who introduced electroshock in the Netherlands in 1939 and published the book *Psychopathie, Misdadigheid en Rechtspraak* (Psychopathy, Crime and Justice) in 1940, concluded that more attention should be paid during inspection to problems possibly linked to a prolonged period of starvation. In his introduction the medical adviser of the pension council, the internist Willem Frederik (Pim) Noordhoek Hegt, who had been one of the driving forces behind the Dutch medical resistance *Medisch Contact* (Medical Contact) during the war,[19] stated that time and again the belated consequences of time in a concentration camp were ascertained during the examinations. He added that, unlike for example in Denmark, the Dutch had experienced starvation at first hand. As a result, it was probable that hunger received less attention during these examinations than "psychological experiences which the examinee must have had resulting from his resistance work, stay in concentration camps or prison".[20]

Barnhoorn's report led to a full-page article in *Het Parool* written by Frank Peter Wibaut, the medical employee of the magazine. He was a general practitioner and sexologist in Amsterdam, and, as a sexologist, one of the few already advocating the use of contraception. Wibaut as well had taken part in the resistance, and, consequently, ended up in prison more than once. After the war he married Tineke Guillonard. She had been deported to Ravensbrück after her resistance group had been betrayed. Wibaut outlined the difficulty a pension council traditionally has in distinguishing between the ones still able to work – and thus not entitled to benefits – and those who are really no longer – and thus entitled to them. Moreover, he wrote, it could be questioned very much whether the decision taken – work or pension – was indeed the right one. All these considerations were by far the most problematic when assessing the psyche, and especially resistance fighters' psyche, the group Barnhoorn's report focused on. Many of them showed "deviations about which it can be said that regular work is the best physician". Many. Not all. The Danish, French and German studies showed that hunger can lead to years of persistent mental problems, which in turn severely reduced the ability to work. Therefore, this had to be taken into consideration when deciding whether to proceed to benefits. However, this could not mean that everyone who, after time in a camp, "didn't feel himself anymore and whose nervous system is somewhat shaken", automatically was entitled to receive a pension. Medically, this would be entirely mistaken. On the other hand, the opposite view was unjustified as well, to argue that time in a concentration camp was no ground for benefits. According to Wibaut, thanks to Barnhoorn's clear report the danger "that people were deprived of something they were fully entitled to" decreased significantly.[21]

The problems Barnhoorn and Noordhoek Hegt touched upon, the physical and mental troubles of resistance members resulting from having been in a camp, formed the basis of Bastiaans' dissertation, which was defended at the University of Amsterdam on 31 January 1957.[22] At the time, Bastiaans was a 39-year-old psychiatrist.[23] Like several other psychiatrists publishing on war issues, for instance Herman Musaph or Paul Theodoor Hugenholtz, he was a member of the psychosomatic working group of social physician Joannes Juda Groen in the Wilhelmina Hospital. Groen was appointed Professor in the Methodology of Psychobiological Research in Leiden in 1968 and thus became a colleague of Bastiaans.[24]

Bastiaans' dissertation was based on his own research among some forty former resistance members and files from the Extraordinary Pension Council. He didn't want to speak of a 'resistance-disease' because of the unclarity regarding who exactly could be seen as having participated in the resistance. Its detail would not be matched until fifteen years later by the German *Die Konzentrationslagerhaft und ihre Folgen* (The Concentration Camp and its Consequences) by Paul Matussek, head of the department for psychopathology and psychotherapy at the Max Planck Institute in Munich.[25]

Psychoanalyst Toon Westerman Holstijn informed his readers in *Het Parool* that Bastiaans' concluded that, apart from their camp experiences, almost all the people he studied had experienced traumatic events in their youth as well. The war had torn open these old wounds which sooner or later could have led to psychological problems anyway, depending on the shelter received and new problems they came across in their post-war life. The major problem remained demonstrating a relationship between the past war and present psychological troubles, a problem which, obviously, increased as the time span between war and present grew. Westerman Holstijn could not help but conclude that Bastiaans gave an excellent synthesis of the "medical, psychosomatic, psycho-analytical, psychological and anthropological approaches to these issues".[26]

This compliment was shared by the *NRC*,[27] and by Musaph in the *NIW* as well. The latter emphasised that the endured suffering and the seriousness of the psychological problems were anything but directly proportional. Previously endured problems – the childhood traumas popular with psychoanalysts – and the individual constellation certainly had as much to do with it. However, together with some others, Bastiaans had to be given credit that his work, written from a modern psychoanalytic point of view, made clear that even those who thought they endured their suffering unscathed and were mentally and/or physically in good shape, could still become damaged. Although he emphasised that it was indeed 'can' and not 'will', Musaph argued that this wouldn't only exert a hefty influence on psychiatric science. Moreover, it could become of great practical importance "for possible payments from Pension Councils and other funds".[28]

The attention the dissertation received, was used to provide readers with an insight into psychosomatics, a new medical specialism.[29] In the social-democratic *Het Vrije Volk* (The Free People) the Jewish psychologist Manuel van Loggem – who survived the war by not registering as a Jew and, unlike his parents, nor wearing the yellow star – wrote that these "victims of their ideal suffered from illnesses that today belong to the psychosomatic deviations". He pointed to things like asthma,[30] hypertension, adiposis or stomach ulcers. Therefore, Bastiaans' book could be read as an attempt to restore medical-scientific unity in a time of far-reaching specialisation. It was of great significance to this new branch of medical science since it provided insight into the causes of "the intricate psychological mechanisms contributing to the physical abnormalities."[31]

In *De Waarheid* – which had been the second-largest daily newspaper in the Netherlands after the war, rapidly saw the number of subscribers decline during the Cold War, and vanished immediately afterwards – general practitioner and former fighter in the Spanish Civil War, Theo van Reemst, wrote that psychosomatics was the doctrine concerned with the immediate or delayed translation of psychological tensions into physical problems. It was the doctrine which "considers physical and mental phenomena of a corporeal nature and those of the nervous system as a whole".[32] Van Reemst, who for years helped people trying to obtain a war pension with their application,[33] emphasised to his communist readers that Bastiaans hadn't limited himself to a curative account. In his "important work", in which one could constantly read between the lines how much he cared for his patients, he indicated as well how it could be prevented that problems occurred or intensified. And he entered the political field. In the Netherlands, in contrast to, for example, France, where ex-members of the illegality could count on psychological assistance, there were insufficient options for treatment also in comparison with the options offered to former soldiers. An example of soldiers' care was the convalescent home Austerlitz, near the former village of the same name near Utrecht, which in its turn was named after the Battle of the Three Emperors in 1805.[34]

Van Reemst also made it personal. "Many of us have been examined, helped with occupational issues or treated by Dr. Bastiaans too." What emerged from these issues was that illness symptoms of former resistance fighters and concentration camp inmates "were a source of widely differing assessments by the various physicians". In his dissertation Bastiaans stood up for "more well-founded and scientific assessments through psychosomatics". It also went into a lot of problems that were provided with solutions, benefiting the aid to resistance fighters. And therein lay its greatest value: the practical results for all who had suffered from hardship during the war years, including the positive influence the thesis would have on the quality of the examinations and treatments.[35]

Bastiaans personally committed himself to these consequences described by Van Reemst. He for instance joined the Compensation Commission Nazi Victims,[36] a committee trying to erect a Ravensbrück museum monument – an attempt crowned with success in September 1959 – and the Protest Committee against the Release of War Criminals, established late in 1959.[37] In a press release, this last committee called on all Dutch people to protest against the possible release of three national socialists, sentenced to life imprisonment: Willy Lages, Kotalla, and Aus der Fünten. The signatories wrote they had taken notice of the intention of the Dutch government to set them free with "dismay and deep indignation".[38] At that time there was no question of pardon for Fischer, the fourth man in the Breda prison. He was added to the list five years later, causing a renewed discussion on the subject,[39] and not for the last time.

2. Attention is Increasing

When the attention for Bastiaans' dissertation had died down, for several years the interest in mental problems resulting from war experiences disappeared from the public eye, despite the fuss about the possible release of three of the then Breda Four. An international conference in The Hague on 'The Belated Consequences of Imprisonment and Deportation' organised by the *World Veterans Federation* in November 1961, put the subject back on the Dutch agenda. In its article on the conference, *De Waarheid* emphasised that many had overcome the misery of the camps. This had to do with, first, the fact that circumstances differed from camp to camp, and second, that people from the resistance had been better prepared for it than those who had been arrested for what they were, as were those who already in the nineteen thirties had seen the Nazi terror coming and possessed a fixed ideology. The remarks on resistance and ideology of course refer to communists, although it was stated that this held for some religious groups as well, "albeit to a completely different degree". And finally, as always, it had to do with the fact that one person simply could endure more than another. Of course, the "vigorous short-lived emotions caused by the violently shocking events" camp life had been full of, could cause mental problems. In general, these problems were mastered.[1]

The really serious problems were caused by the life in a camp itself and the timespan this life had to be endured. Coupled with such things as hunger and torture (whether seen or experienced), the constant tension this life brought about often didn't fail to have its effect on the mental life of former captives. New Norwegian, psychiatric research again proved the connection between physical deprivation in the past and psychological problems in the present. This phenomenon had been demonstrated in 65 of hundred war victims studied and according to *De Waarheid* was called KZ syndrome for some time already.[2]

Added to this was the transition to post war life; a transition that to many had not come lightly. The hardships had been endured, but the alternative wasn't without its thorns too. Some of the camp survivors finally made it, some still struggled with adjustment issues. These could, *De Waarheid* said, not be separated from recent political events such as German rearmament, the granting of high positions in NATO to the German war criminals Hans Speidel and Adolf Heusinger, or the pardoning of other war criminals. All these events would never have happened in the first years after the war. It couldn't be denied that at the conference far too little attention had been paid to these disappointing political developments and the impact they had on former resistance fighters. It was up to the Dutch government to fill this gap, which was of far greater importance than granting war criminals their freedom.[3]

Meanwhile, Bastiaans was on his way to becoming a psychiatrist whose name rang a bell outside medical or resistance circles as well. Not for nothing the news that he would be appointed professor of psychiatry in Leiden received quite a bit of media attention in November 1963. Former resistance newspaper *Het Parool* explicitly recalled his war past, although this past had had nothing to do with the appointment. It was recalled that, shortly after the start of the German occupation, he founded the University Health Care Foundation in cooperation with people like Gerard Carel Heringa, the medical professor at the University of Amsterdam (UvA) who was dismissed on political grounds in 1942. It was also pointed out that due to an accident late in 1942 he had no longer been able to participate actively in the resistance.[4] As if to confirm the importance of this past, one of his first public acts after his appointment was to join the group pleading for an annual commemoration of the February strike at the monument 'The Dockworker' in Amsterdam.[5]

But Bastiaans wasn't the only one who had become well-known. The same holds for the KZ syndrome, which brings us to Kater's almost full-page article in the *Algemeen Handelsblad* (General Trade Journal) late in May 1964, quoted at the beginning of the introduction. Kater mentioned and praised Bastiaans as a trailblazer, but not after first praising other doctors who reported on the syndrome scientifically, such as Tas and Cohen.[6]

A year later, Kater was one of the organisers of a radio broadcast about the syndrome in which, according to Cohen in the *NIW,* "a number of ex-inmates confirmed the phenomenon". The broadcast was fairly positively discussed by him. He did point out, however, that in Germany there was even more attention for the subject than in the Netherlands. This was no coincidence. In the Netherlands only resistance fighters received compensation, whereas in Germany everyone who had suffered from persecution received it, including the "sick Jews" neglected in the Netherlands. He further wondered if the syndrome could have been prevented, a question he answered affirmative.

> My own experience has taught me that by writing about it you are applying an auto-analysis, as it were. And those who can't write about it, should have the opportunity to talk about it. A former resistance member said that talking to a psychiatrist had done him much good. (Unfortunately, after the war, many

were left to their own devices by the Jewish as well as the non-Jewish society, whereas they were convinced that the suffering endured gave them a right to extra care, extra devotion.)[7]

Cohen's main criticism was that all the good that had come from the personal suffering lavishly dished up in the broadcast, should have been mentioned as well. Among it, precisely because of that suffering, a high appreciation of all the niceties like freedom post-war Netherlands had to offer. Moreover, the opportunity could have been used to encourage all those Jewish survivors who hadn't been able to find their way back into society, to start a new life in Israel, the country that had emerged from the war.[8]

Cohen, chairman of the Dutch Zionist Association, would return to this theme in 1970. Referring to Eitinger's research among former resistance fighters living in Norway or Israel, he said that crippling physical and psychological effects of camp life appeared less or were even absent among those who had decided to emigrate to Israel. "They were welcome, they returned!" For this, in particular the kibbutz system was of great importance. In a kibbutz they received so much support that they were able to survive despite their problems.[9]

By the way, in his dissertation, Cohen also pointed to his Zionist convictions as an explanation for why, in his own words, he coped with the suffering in the camps better than many others. Before the war, he had preferred the comfortable, intellectual life of a doctor in the Netherlands over a hard, physical existence in Palestine, although his convictions should have forced him to choose the latter option. Because of this decision he was forced to lead a hard, physical life for nearly three years, a fate which undeniably had "a certain justice".[10]

Because of his appointment as professor at Leiden University, Bastiaans also became head of the Jelgersma Clinic for psychiatric patients in the nearby village of Oegstgeest, named after psychoanalyst Gerbrandus Jelgersma, one of his predecessors at Leiden. It was in these capacities that the Dutch public really got to know him. It soon became clear that a man had been appointed who knew how to find the media, and vice versa, and who moreover wasn't afraid to give his opinions outside his direct field of expertise. Shortly after the Leiden dean had done the same, he, for example, and perhaps bearing in mind the words of the German nineteenth-century social physician Rudolf Virchow that politics is medicine on a large scale, vehemently protested, at the start of a lecture for psychiatry students in December 1964, against the government's intention to declare a construction stop of new university buildings. According to Bastiaans, this proved that "deep reaching currents are active directed against the university and linked to a hatred of the intellectual elite". The government plans constituted an "assault on the universities' foundations" and "our country's highest values". It was immediately clear that Bastiaans was not a man shying away from big words. One of the articles on his outburst was entitled, "Professor of Psychiatry: Government Policy on University Extension is Political Madness." And another: "'Madness', says Leiden professor".[11]

3. THE PSYCHOANALYTIC CONFERENCE IN AMSTERDAM IN JULY 1965

In June 1965, the *NIW* noted that the international medical literature on and research into late psychological effects of wartime suffering was rapidly expanding. The newspaper pointed to an article in *The Canadian Medical Association Journal* by Wulf 'Wally' Grobin of *Mount Sinai Hospital* in Toronto. Based on a survey among a hundred concentration camp survivors he concluded that, although in general physical problems were rare, some of them had developed physical and mental problems after a period of rest in the years after liberation. It further pointed at some of the Dutch working on this issue, medically but also by trying to create financial security: Kater, Cohen, Tas, De Wind, and of course Bastiaans. The *NIW* concluded with a call to join forces quickly and set up a working group involving all those interested in the matter, at short notice examining what had to be done. "Otherwise, it probably won't be necessary anymore."[1]

That it was by no means exaggerated that the KZ syndrome increasingly came into the spotlight nationally as well as internationally, was proved a month later in Amsterdam. On the occasion of their 24th International Conference 900 psychoanalysts gathered in the Dutch capitol. The subject of the conference? The late psychological consequences of concentration camp survival. The *Algemeen Dagblad* said there rarely had been a conference of greater significance "for problems affecting all of humanity". One of the conclusions was that a mild form of compulsion had "frighteningly spread throughout our present society", crippling mental health. Many of those affected were concentration camp survivors. They often suffered from conditions similar to those seen in obsessive-compulsive neurotic patients. For a long time, it remained unclear what had caused these complaints. However, this slowly changed, not in the least because the German government had instituted an indemnity payment. This meant that the opinion of doctors had to be invoked.[2]

In an article devoted to the conference, entitled 'Suffering from camp life continues', *de Volkskrant* also pointed at the importance of the German decision to proceed with compensation. It forced the medical world to face facts. In the mid-1950s, it believed the problems would be solved automatically. War victims seemed to overcome them, and those who had developed problems after the war had been shown to have had problems before it as well. However, in recent years it became clear that even after so many years former inmates could become psychologically entangled. Nevertheless, it remained of the utmost importance to keep in mind continuously that there was no such thing as a stereotype reaction. According to De Wind, besides the differences between camps themselves, it also made quite a difference if at the time of deportation people knew they were almost certainly doomed to die, like the Dutch Jews, or whether there was still a glimmer of hope to be cherished.[3] When treating those psychologically affected, they must be given "the opportunity to relive their spasmodic feelings of sadness and anger. In this way they can heal from the compulsion under which they have had to live all these years."[4]

The emphasis – for the first time ever at a psychoanalyst's conference – was on the somatic, and in particular on compulsive neurotic consequences. Not for nothing the title of an article about it was: 'Specialists spend hours working on psycho-somatic illnesses'. This article also made clear that the subject was no longer an unknown side-show for the average reader. "An asthma patient, who behaves like a completely normal adult, can nevertheless – unconsciously – suffer from psychological conflicts from his early childhood. After countless popular science publications, this claim will also sound familiar to the layman."[5]

Of course, this focus on (psycho-)somatic problems is not to say that it was unclear that the conference was a psychoanalytical one. Bastiaans noted that the meeting once again showed that psychoanalysis evolved "into a science covering all areas of human behaviour".[6] He furthermore stated during a meeting with the press that, among other things, it indeed had been concluded that the psychosomatic symptoms could fall under compulsive neurotic behaviour, "with which the patient responded to childhood conflicts such as unconscious fear and feelings of insecurity". It was a remark remembering some people of an earlier remark made by Bastiaans in Brussels in the spring of 1965. A heart attack, he said, wasn't a psychosomatic illness in the direct sense of the word. Those who got one had a typical character often seen in resistance circles: the hard worker who thought his work was more important than his personal life, who did not participate in sports, did not take (full) holidays and was bad at delegating.[7] It's unclear whether Bastiaans realised at the time that he was painting a nice self-portrait.[8]

Bastiaans' comment on childhood conflicts underlying the problems of former inmates or resistance fighters was entirely in line with the conclusions he had drawn in his dissertation. However, it also indicated that psychoanalysis had a problem in treating significant numbers of war victims. This was not, as professor of psychiatry Rümke said, because of difficulties in comforting them.[9] The problem was that a large proportion of those affected, whether they had had childhood experiences or not, were already adults at the time of the events that at least had given rise to their problems.[10]

These problems were not lessened by another comment from Bastiaans. At the conference he, probably for the first time, claimed that no one survived the concentration camp period unscathed. It was, he said, "seriously doubtful whether people saying, 'this has done nothing to me', are not indeed sick". According to him, the problems manifested themselves in nervousness, nightmares, and later on in life – despite Grobin's conclusions – in lung disease, heart disease or rheumatic abnormalities.

> In the last ten years we have noticed an increasing number of cases of former resistance members who suddenly die from heart disease. One may assume that this is a belated consequence of the suffering in the camps. One year in a camp is equivalent to four years of normal life.[11]

In other words: sick, until proved healthy. The denial as confirmation. But apart from the fact that nothing is known about a KZ syndrome in the Auschwitz-surviving psychiatrists Cohen and De Wind – in contrast, by the way, to Andries Kaas in whom Buchenwald had brought about irreversible, psychological, and physical changes –[12] it seems difficult to maintain that all those developing problems after surviving the camps had had a problematic childhood. Such critical comments, however, were absent at the conference, at least judging by the newspapers' coverage.

In Amsterdam not only the state of affairs was put on the table and discussed. One of the keynote speakers, the American psychoanalyst of German descent, Martin Wangh, a professor at the *Albert Einstein College of Medicine* and involved in the German *Wiedergutmachungsprozesse* (compensation lawsuits), called on the participants to collect case histories so that at the next conference, in 1967, they could delve even deeper into the subject. This was necessary because, Wangh said, combined Norwegian, French, and Dutch research determined that, as a result of the heavy, prolonged weight loss, a lot of concentration camp survivors suffered from brain diseases. On anyone who had lost more than thirty percent of his or her normal weight during the war "irreparable damage to the nervous system had been inflicted. They all are ill to a greater or lesser extent."[13]

Bastiaans talked about former resistance fighters, Wangh included all survivors in his paper. He also discussed the decreased life expectancy, generally with ten years, and the feelings of guilt many of them carried with them because they survived and others had not, or even: because they survived *because* others had not, for example as a consequence of steeling scarce food. However, the main point Wangh made was that in the entire literature just one case in which psychoanalysis was applied, was mentioned. First, this was the logical consequence of the fact that many didn't want to talk at all about what had happened to them. But second, it also had to do with psychoanalysis itself, even if the previously noted focus on childhood trauma is put aside. According to Wangh, patient's distrust was severe. The psychiatrist could never ever understand him (or her, but the psychiatrists, almost all men themselves, mostly only talked of 'him'). In addition, and as a result, the psychiatrist himself was hesitant. Often, he was strongly identified by the patient with former guardians or even torturers, making analysis almost impossible. Bastiaans agreed. The stories of survivors could be so intense that they overwhelmed the psychiatrist.[14] Twenty years later he would mobilise this argument when explaining why it was so hard to find a suitable successor for his treatment of war victims.

In a double interview with Wangh and Bastiaans by *Het Parool*, the latter talked about a film he made of patients talking with him whilst "under 'a sedative', in other words, under treatment". This film was *Kampsyndroom. Psychosomatische consequenties van de oorlog* (Camp syndrome. Psychosomatic consequences of the war) by the young filmmaker At van Praag. It was a 45-minute long, never fully completed documentary about Bastiaans' treatment method. The movie, described as shocking by the Catholic *De Tijd* (The Time), was banned from public display in the Netherlands, partly for privacy reasons, and, although a staunch defender of the use of narcoanalysis and LSD, partly at the instigation of Nico Speijer, professor of social psychiatry and Bastiaans' co-director of the Jelgersma clinic. It was only to be used by medical (wo)men and students for instructive purposes.[15]

In the film patients talked about their experiences as if they had happened yesterday, instead of twenty years ago. They therefore suffered from a large number of unprocessed emotions. They had never been able to vent their anger on guards who had tortured their comrades. Psychosomaticus Bastiaans concluded: "The organism can't process such a massive anger, which has been suppressed for so long. That impotent anger is then stored somewhere: in the heart, in asthma, in diabetes, in other organs."[16]

For a long time, the medical world failed to see, "had not *wanted* to see", that the trials and weight loss had irreparably damaged the brain and nerves. After the war the survivors had to adapt quickly, which resulted in even more tension. This, however, was denied, by insurance companies and social authorities as well. As a result, there hardly was any money for therapy. "Most doctors (no, not just GPs, not at all) said in 1956: Now it's time to put an end to that man's nonsense. He's just a neurotic weakling. And now – oh tragedy – we wake up."[17] Psychoanalytic treatment could help to cope with the misery, but this possibility was lost because the necessary apparatus, the human being, had been damaged itself. This is why so many analytical healing attempts ended in disappointment. Added to this were financial problems. "It's so sad that to get pensions etc. for resistance fighters is easy, for they are purely physically affected. As long as you're physically ill, you're a nice guy. But if you develop nervous symptoms, you receive the short straw."[18]

And then others came along. It wasn't just camp survivors – Jews, political prisoners, resistance fighters – who suffered from mental problems. Bastiaans predicted that these problems would also affect "the wives of the resistance members" (the resistance was still seen, even by Bastiaans, as entirely male, barring a few confirmatory exceptions). Moreover, their children wouldn't be exempt from this which means that he preluded in 1965 the second-generation problem that would receive so much attention in later years. "Do you now understand why it's extremely important that we do something about it?"[19]

Raising the hot topic of pensions, which was discussed at the conference also, did anything but harm Bastiaans' popularity among concentration camp survivors and former resistance members. On the contrary. Michel Steijns, himself a former prisoner of camp Vught and Mauthausen and the medical advisor of the *Stichting Vriendenkring Oud-Natzweilers* (Friends of Former Natzweiler-inmates Foundation), said that generally speaking the survivors of camp Natzweiler were quite satisfied with the help given. In some cases, however, it had proved to be insufficient. This had everything to do with the fact that in order to receive a pension, causality had to be proved. In the Netherlands this turned out to be much more difficult to demonstrate than elsewhere, where often the reversed burden of proof had already been introduced. Besides, benefits were more generous and awarded more swiftly. Camp survivors in France received a 100 percent benefit for a carcinoma. In the Netherlands this percentage was zero. Fortunately, Steijns said, the struggle for receiving benefits was made easier by the research and writings of people like De Wind, Cohen and Bastiaans.[20]

4. About LSD and the Reversed Burden of Proof

As said, Bastiaans' treatments were partly based on the administration of psychedelics, including LSD, a drug increasingly criticised because of the personal, non-medical use by members of the so-called counterculture in the 1960s.[1] It's striking that LSD was never mentioned in the articles about Bastiaans and the camp syndrome before 1966, the year in which it was included into the so-called Opium Act and consequently forbidden. The reason that it was finally written about, was that it was mentioned during a discussion that closed the last of five documentaries on German television about the occupation of the Netherlands. In newspaper articles reporting on it, the abbreviation was written down without any further explanation, which means it was assumed that readers were familiar with it. The discussion involved, besides Bastiaans, Lou de Jong and Jacques Presser. De Jong, a non-religious Jew who lost large parts of his family during the war, was the director of the *Nationaal Instituut voor Oorlogsdocumentatie* NIOD (National Institute for War Documentation) and the historian appointed to write the history of the Netherlands in the war years. Presser, descendant of a socialist, also non-religious Jewish family whose wife died in a concentration camp, was the author of the voluminous *Ondergang. De vernietiging en verdelging van het Nederlandse Jodendom 1940-1945* published in 1965. (Downfall. The persecution and extermination of Dutch Jewry 1940-1945. The English version is titled *Ashes in the Wind. The destruction of the Dutch Jews.*) For three minutes the discussion was punctuated with silent images from Van Praag's film. On display were three Dutch former internees who had given permission for broadcasting the images. It was the first time the Dutch public was confronted with the LSD treatment of psychiatric patients, although they had to tune in to German television, which in those days was not uncommon. Nevertheless, because the film was banned for public display in the Netherlands, the images would be cut out if the documentary was broadcast on Dutch television as well.[2]

According to *De Telegraaf,* the three had visited Bastiaans hoping he would free them "from their memories of their concentration camp experiences. The recordings illustrated that LSD took them back to the camps. They even mistook a handkerchief for a rubber bat."[3] *De Volkskrant* made no bones about it in the title of the article on the "impressive" television discussion: 'Children from hunger winter still disturbed. Nazi victims relived torture'. According to Bastiaans, Presser and De Jong, the reason that the war still had such a major impact on the lives of many Dutch people was that the misery of occupation and deportation had been new. In France and Belgium, the experiences of 1940-1944 were dealt with somewhat more easily for they already had been through the 1914-1918 war. Apparently one can grow accustomed to everything. The images of Bastiaans' treatments were the dramatic highlight of the broadcast.

> Many who experienced the worst the Germans had to offer still live in two worlds, the past and the present. The normal psychological methods of helping them prove to be hardly useful, because they not seldom refuse to talk about the horrors they experienced. That is why Prof. Bastiaans has tried it with hypnosis, narcotics and finally LSD. As a consequence of this drug the three patients relived their time in the camps. The woman, who had once been beaten in the neck, again felt the blow, the men crawled away hiding for the blows, shivering with cold and wallowing on their beds in despair.[4]

The extent of the images' impact is clearly apparent in the coverage of *Het Vrije Volk.* It simply called the article about the documentary 'Prof. Bastiaans' poignant LSD film'. It had been those three minutes that showed the German population that for many Dutch people the war still was reality.

> A Dutch woman, shrinking and groaning under the caning given to her – this was one of the most horrific images witnessed by German TV viewers. What made it so horrific was that there was no stick. No one was hitting her. But under the influence of LSD, the woman relived her worst experiences.[5]

According to Bastiaans, the reason why the images proved to be so moving was that they were new to most people. Images of the occupation were familiar because of books and magazines, "but this effect of LSD was unknown. It was curious to see how, in the studio, the German TV employees reacted when the film was shown. They were shy about it; they didn't know how to react."[6]

In the article in *Het Vrije Volk*, Bastiaans also explained why he had started using LSD. Unlike other narcotics, that put the patients in a kind of twilight state, just a very little amount of LSD was needed to bring camp survivors, who had held themselves upright for two decades, completely "back to the war, into a situation of misery and powerlessness". Moreover, afterwards the patients still were aware of what happened and what had been said. Linking back to and raising awareness about the misery endured, caused by LSD, were a necessary part of the healing process. Suppressing psychological distress led to inner tensions and thus to all kinds of physical suffering. Acute cardiac death, for example, could be seen as "a heroic attempt by the organism to escape from that miserable state of powerlessness". Those who become aware of their suppressed past, are able to master it.[7] Or, as one of the patients put it: "You are boss in your own house once again; the images of the war have been given a permanent place in my head now; they don't get mixed up anymore. They haven't been forgotten, but they don't bother me no longer."[8]

So, nothing but positive stories about LSD as a medical therapeutic. However, the drug was also used outside of the doctor's office. Bastiaans couldn't escape from giving his opinion on non-medical use, certainly not in 1966, the year in which discussions about whether or not LSD should be banned, were heated. He made perfectly clear that non-medical use was extremely dangerous. But it was very understandable too. After all, modern man was locked up inside himself.

> Our whole society is aimed at pushing human beings into a certain isolation. They want to get out of it, and they rather do that miraculously than by gradually working on themselves. But the ones using LSD without medical indication, run the risk of destroying the protective boundary we all have in our structure. That is the grave danger of the so-called LSD experience certain groups of young people long for.[9]

In other words, Bastiaans wasn't very distraught when LSD was included into the Opium Act, as long as he as a doctor could continue using it. It was a negative opinion that resonated in the media. In a discussion on the Dutch translation of a book about LSD early in 1967 – preface: J. Bastiaans –, Herman Louis Heijermans, then known from the book *Het Sexuele Leven van de Mens* (The Sexual Life of Man), did not turn his heart into a killing pit.

> It can be said that LSD almost never leads to aggression, as is common with alcohol. But these are about the only positive words I have in store for the drug, which has led to several suicides, especially among the emotionally disturbed. LSD does not stimulate greater artistic achievements, it only destroys the personality, which, as it were, disintegrates. Anyone who wants to make a serious attempt of becoming insane should use it.[10]

Bastiaans not only had the media on his side regarding his opinion on the non-medical, but also on the medical use of LSD. Its inclusion in the Opium Act had as yet no effect on how they looked at the treatment of war victims, nor on the increasing importance they attached to it. In March 1967, *De Tijd* reported that the psychological pressure resulting from resistance and camp life still led to new victims. No fewer than 160 new patients had asked for a benefit from the Extraordinary Pension Council in 1966. If they could demonstrate that their complaints could, in whole or partly, be traced back to their war experiences, they were entitled to a pension.[11]

As described earlier, this conversion hadn't been an easy matter, reason for the Dutch Red Cross, traditionally an organisation for aid to war victims, to donate *f*10,000 (€4550) to the *Nederlandse Vereniging voor Psychiatrie en Neurologie* (Dutch Association for Psychiatry and Neurology) to support research in this field. Bastiaans, board member of this association, was asked to come up with a suitable destination. He certainly wanted to do so, although he hastened to declare that the amount should be called almost symbolic; *f*100,000 (€45,500) was the bare minimum. Nevertheless, in itself research was of great importance, both from a scientific point of view and, because of the financial aspect, for the patients. According to Bastiaans, after the phase of the immediate consequences and the subsequent phase of psychosomatic problems, the third phase of the aftermath of war had arrived: "the period in which all those who so far were able to pull themselves together no longer can live up to their believe that the concentration camp had had little or no effect on them". They too could be helped by LSD. It could bring them into a state in which the suppression of feelings was suppressed itself.[12]

Noordhoek Hegt, at that time director of the Red Cross Hospital in The Hague, as well saw the benefit of such research. He was convinced that the war still caused a lot of psychological suffering. This was a view he and his colleagues hadn't had all the time. "When shortly before the liberation we doctors discussed plans how to welcome the sick after the war, we mainly focused on infectious diseases. We never thought about the psychological after-effects, not even for a moment."[13] Having said that, at the same time Noordhoek Hegt was convinced that scientifically proving a relationship between past and present misery was such a complex issue that from the outset any outcome would be questionable. As an internist, he was much less convinced than psychiatrist Bastiaans that a multitude of physical complaints were due to psychological tension. Or in his own blunt words: "Much of what is said about psychosomatic illnesses is nonsense." Unlike Bastiaans, he did not believe in a connection between past war misery and a present-day heart attack. He added that he would never have dared to say this out loud if not for the fact that many colleagues wholeheartedly agreed with him. Sure, there were concentration camp survivors with problems, but there were many without problems as well. According to Noordhoek Hegt, it was not as much the camp time itself that was important in this respect, but the way in which they had been welcomed back and cared for after the war. It was precisely the ones for whom this didn't go well and who in the post-war period came under great pressure once again, who had begun to experience problems. For example, they had perhaps experienced difficulties in finding work while others hadn't in spite of their much more dubious war past. Noordhoek Hegt also pointed out that the pension council already treated former resistance fighters and camp survivors with leniency. It was enough if an aggravating effect could be demonstrated, which wasn't that difficult. And its attitude would become even more lenient once "the new law, already passed by parliament, reversing the burden of proof, comes into force". In that case, the patient no longer had to demonstrate a connection, but the pension council had to demonstrate that there wasn't one.[14]

Shortly afterwards, on account of an extension of the State War Victims Group Regulations, dating from 1961, the reversed burden of proof indeed was introduced. These regulations replaced the 1940-1945 War Victims Assistance Regulation, introduced in 1950. However, the most important regulation at the time was the Extraordinary Pension Act (WBP) of 1947. It provided physically or psychologically affected members of the resistance or their widows (not: widowers) the right to receive a benefit. If someone's disability was estimated above sixty percent and that person had committed intensive and demonstrable resistance or had been imprisoned for at least three months, then there was no longer any need to demonstrate a relationship between the war history and physical and/or mental problems. The 1940-1945 Benefits for Persecution Victims Act (WUV), introduced in January 1973, would further remove the restrictions, and in addition allowed other victims of persecution – such as Jews and gypsies (as they were still commonly called at the time) – to apply for benefits.[15] More on that later.

These changes were looked upon with dismay by some former resistance members or by some providing medical assistance, including Cohen and the chairman of the Zeeland district of the Foundation 1940-1945, L. Beurkens. According to them, the adjustments would make it a lot easier, too easy, to use a war pension as a welcome addition to a normal pension. All that needed to be done was to make up a resistance history, after which fraudsters could tell their GP they had all the KZ syndrome symptoms, which were frequently mentioned in the press. Criticisms like these, however, were kept silent in that same press.[16]

With the reversed burden of proof – which basically meant that problems arising in later life were linked exclusively to war experiences – the KZ syndrome front went into a two year-period in which all was quiet, at least as far as the papers were concerned. The only ripple was the repetition of an appeal made three years earlier by the Auschwitz Committee. Emphasising that it was not a communist umbrella organisation, as for example Lou de Jong said,[17] nor from any other ideology, the appeal stated that, as for instance was the case in West Germany, the pension rights of concentration camp survivors should be equal to those of resistance fighters or other victims of Nazi rule like the widows of the deported men from the village of Putten most of whom had not returned. (They were deported in retaliation for the killing of a German officer.) The committee was supported by De Wind. He stated that no less than eighty percent of the survivors, who were 50 to 55 years old at the end of the sixties, were at best partially but often not at all able to work.[18]

5. THE MOVIE *DO YOU NOW UNDERSTAND WHY I CRY…*

This relative quiet was greatly disturbed on 14 May 1969, a historic day for both Dutch cinema as psychiatric education, according to neurologist Coen van Emde Boas. In the Metropole-Tuschinski theatre in The Hague and in a mainly medical and political closed circle, the new movie of filmmaker Louis van Gasteren was screened: *Begrijpt u nu waarom ik huil...* (Do you now understand why I cry…, or, as the English under titled version on YouTube not quite correctly is called, Do you now get it…).[1] The premiere took place amid great, including governmental interest. Among others, Prime Minister Piet de Jong, and the Ministers Marga Klompé, of Culture, Recreation and Social Work (CRM), and Bé Udink, Developmental Work, were present. However, the State Secretary for Social Affairs and Public Health, the physician and public health expert Roelof Kruisinga, was absent. His aversion to psychedelics was too great. Queen Juliana, on the other hand, attended. Following the subsequent press conference, including a discussion, she continued to chat with the makers of the film, Van Gasteren and Bastiaans, for another 45 minutes.[2]

Although the psychiatrist and chef de clinique of the Jelgersma clinic, Dick van Tol, mostly led the sessions, not Bastiaans himself, it was the latter who presented the introductory. After all, he was the professor, the mastermind behind the LSD therapy, the man who had pioneered the KZ syndrome. By treating his patients with his method-Bastiaans – LSD or other psychotropic drugs in combination with psychoanalysis in a setting tailored to the Nazi era, including, for example, showing Nazi propaganda – he had ensured that their suppressed war past "finally became a past in reality. In the 1950's, these people were told by everyone, even official authorities, that the past should be forgotten. People didn't believe they were sick and would remain sick if left untreated."[3]

It was for instance asked during the discussion whether public broadcasting of the film would exceed the limits of medical secrecy and whether this could lead to "psycho-hygienic damage in the case of an unprepared lay audience".[4] As Speijer had done in relation to the film of Van Praag in 1966, Bastiaans advised the responsible minister, Klompé, against public cinema broadcasting, let alone television broadcasting, at least for the time being. He was, however, in favour of a wider distribution than just among medical specialists and students. It had to be shown to the largest possible number of specific groups. He further advised to put the question whether, in the long run, a public broadcast could be considered, in the hands of a group of about three hundred former resistance fighters,[5] in other words: in the hands of a group at the least largely if not completely consisting of Bastiaans' supporters.

Van Emde Boas, who estimated that there were at least a couple of thousand people in the Netherlands suffering from KZ syndrome, didn't hide his admiration for Bastiaans' LSD treatment, however controversial it may be. It was a very effective drug that, at least in his opinion, was highly regarded in medical literature, although it could lead to incurable physical, mental, and perhaps even genetic damage if used privately. In the hands of a skilled psychotherapist like Bastiaans, however, it could "help a person who otherwise couldn't be 'opened up' by verbal therapy alone to 'break free' an up until then closed inner world".[6]

This admiration extended to the film, described by Van Emde Boas as a "masterful demonstration of the concentration camp syndrome". He found it difficult to indicate what he admired the most: "the medical-scientific, the cinematic, the didactic, the political or (last but not least) the general human aspect." Thus, he was very much in favour of a more general display, although, of course, this was primarily dependent on the consent of Bastiaans' patient. The title of his extensive article reflects this admiration: 'Van Gasteren films the KZ syndrome, and many must see it'. Possible mental damage should not be an argument to withhold the film from the general public, because the positive by far exceeded the negative "not in the least from a human and political point of view". 'Human', firstly because the patient and his wife as well exposed themselves so enormously, and secondly because the film showed that people are always and everywhere and even under the most terrible conditions able to survive. 'Political' because the premiere had taken place in May, a month in which, Van Emde Boas angrily wrote down, once again the liberation of 5 May 1945 passed almost without attention. Therefore, the film could be seen as "an admonition that what has happened arose from general human qualities, which, should circumstances again lead to it, will once again seize their destructive chance".[7]

These were not the only reasons to switch to a general screening, on television if need be.

> The general public isn't protected against the psycho-hygienic dangers posed by aggressive westerns and other "necrophiliac" movies and comic strips. After all, paternalistic censors simply accept that the public can take quite a

> beating, just as the TV news and current affairs programmes continue to show the most horrific images from Korea, Vietnam, Biafra. So, why not show the horrific consequences of the Nazi regime? The answer is clear: the current political situation (Van Emde Boas probably referred to the political-military friendship with West Germany. LvB) forces us to forget, although the KZ syndrome sufferers can't.[8]

In the film – as said, not for the first time, as is often thought – a patient of Bastiaans was followed during a therapeutic LSD session. Van Gasteren made a total of 6.5 hours of film from the first of five sessions. In the end, a bit over an hour remained. But it was an hour "that for a long time to come will haunt those who have watched it". *Do you now understand why I cry...* – a phrase the patient uttered regularly although not always in the same phrasing – was funded by Leiden University, the Foundation 1940-1945, Klompé's Ministry of CRM, and the National Federation for Mental Health. The latter was responsible for its distribution, although at the time it was generally thought that it probably would never be seen by a cinema audience, let alone shown on TV.[9]

The LSD sessions were necessary because, as *Tubantia*, a regional paper, wrote, the man was still suffering from the psychosomatic effects of four years of hardships endured at Buchenwald, Ravensbrück, Sachsenhausen, and Bergen-Belsen. And he wasn't the only one by far.

> Still, almost a quarter of a century after the war, there are many former concentration camp inmates who haven't been able to free themselves from the terrible torments they have experienced. Even in their own environment they often are misunderstood. Sometimes women and children blame them.[10]

This was the case with this man whose "liberation had never been completed" and whose return had been "a stupendous disillusion" to his wife too. He no longer was the man she knew. He was a man to whom it was impossible to talk and who, mentally, still lived in the camps, day and night.[11]

Tubantia's editorial board wrote that it was a pity and somewhat unsatisfactory that, due to lack of money, Van Gasteren had had to stop filming after the first session. But Bastiaans assured that after having gone through the entire treatment the man was relieved of his trauma.[12] It was an assurance Van Emde Boas also emphasised in his article, including that this, at least according to Bastiaans, had resulted in a considerable rejuvenation of the patient, "a man who had aged early".[13]

(Judging from a later film by Van Gasteren, *De Prijs van Overleven* (The Price of Survival) (2003), this positive assessment must, however, be questioned. In it the patient's further life was followed, and the impact his camp experiences had on his family discussed. In any case, the positive effect hadn't been lasting. One of his sons, who had decided not to have children because he wanted to be sure not to pass his father's problems on to yet another generation, said that in 1945 his father physically had indeed been liberated, but psychologically remained locked up behind barbed wire until his death.)[14]

The slight criticism of the film that could be distilled from the reaction of the *Tubantia* editors was completely absent in the article written by its anonymous medical contributor. He gave a description of the KZ syndrome, diagnosed in many countries, as well as of its symptoms and of the, in his view, many advantages and few and manageable disadvantages of the use of LSD in psychotherapy. To him, the film was "a medical document of the first order" which had to be seen by everyone involved in decisioning whether war crimes could be statute-barred. As we shall see, this was a prelude to a crucial stage in the relay of camp syndrome acceptance and in the change from 'psychiatrist J. Bastiaans' to simply 'Bastiaans'. *Do you now understand why I cry...* showed, the medical contributor continued, that through the development of psychosomatic medicine over the past decades it became clear that psychological distress is the cause of various physical illnesses or more severe psychiatric problems. Some of these were part of the KZ syndrome with its delayed mental health problems, early dementia, and premature death. That is, when the victims of national socialism are considered. "Those who had been in Japanese internment camps generally seem to have suffered less severe mental consequences." Within a decade this view would have changed radically. (By the way, in 1977 the Dutch Central Bureau for Statistics published a report stating that camp survivors lived *longer* than those not having stayed in the likes of Auschwitz. Bastiaans delivered two explanations. First, the camps had already taken care of some sort of natural selection absent in normal life, and second, they lived longer because, as a consequence of their KZ syndrome, they were under constant medical supervision. But all this put aside, he said, "where is the joy of a longer life if the mind lacks harmony. Quality of life is what they want.")[15]

In *Het Parool,* which devoted no less than two major articles to the film, reporter Klaas Peereboom, who in the years ahead would regularly publish on Bastiaans and his method, used the screening to refer to a discussion in the *NTvG* about LSD as a therapeutic agent. It was a discussion that questions the opinion of Van Emde Boas that LSD was highly appreciated in medical literature. The professor of pharmacology and neuro-biochemistry at the Free University Amsterdam, Jan Booij, launched an attack on LSD in the journal in 1968. Starting with the Hippocratic words

Primum Nil Nocere (above all, do no harm) he argued, among other things and certainly not as the first one,[16] that if a remedy had been used for so many years and its use was still not proved, the conclusion must be that this use is at best small or even nil.[17] He reacted to a positively tinted piece[18] and in turn received criticism himself.[19] But there was agreement as well, for example from Tas.[20] Notably absent in the entire discussion was Bastiaans. He didn't respond until two years later, following a negative review that relied heavily on the critical pieces by Booij and Tas in the *NTvG* on LSD, of the film *Do you now understand why I cry....* His reaction will not have convinced the critics. It came down to stating that the reviewer had understood nothing about the film and even less about the use of LSD.[21]

The death knell for medical-therapeutic LSD use Booij had predicted in the *NTvG* discussion had not yet sounded at the time of the film screening in the Metropole-Tuschinski theatre. On the contrary. The articles in *Het Parool* about Van Gasteren's film can serve as proof. Despite reference to the discussion, they were extremely positive about medical LSD use. Peereboom drew only one conclusion from the discussion which was that history turned out differently than Booij predicted. Not a word in itself about the validity or invalidity of Booij's arguments.[22]

The mixed Zeitgeist that, on the one hand, gave rise to Booij's criticism and which ensured that LSD was included in the Opium Act in 1966, apparently also ensured that, on the other hand, critique on it was not generally shared, and certainly not when doctors said it was an excellent drug if used for specific purposes. Bastiaans himself can be mentioned as a typical example, seen his outpouring in the press conference after the film screening, in which he said he had recently visited the musical *Hair* in London; less as a music lover, by the way, than as a psychotherapeutic observer. This observation again made clear that while he saw the musical as a typical expression of an era in which self-liberation was high on the agenda, his embrace of LSD and self-liberation did not automatically imply that he was completely devoted to the counterculture or the flower power of *Hair.*

> What in text and sound springs forward from a musical like this is that it's one great outcry for contact, what I would call the "routing" of the I, of who you really, in essence are. The locking of that ego is not infrequently threatened by our tendency to withdraw to islands of so-called certainty: think of tradition, ideology, religious or political conviction, or the rules of the game associated with them. In this sense, *Do you now understand why I cry...* also – at least I hope so – is a sign of our times, next to, for example, Veronica (a radio pirate, operating from a boat in the North Sea. LvB) that doesn't stop confronting us with love, with musical attempts to break free from loneliness and abandonment, *which at the same time give a false satisfaction.* Furthermore,

> the film is a contemporary signal, just like the conversations now taking place between students and teachers, like ecumenicism, and like so many other phenomena, which are in fact attempts at delimitation, delimitation of oneself and delimitation of the other.[23] (Ital.: LvB)

An interesting aspect of the discussion about the documentary is that it was made by a well-known filmmaker. As a result, it wasn't just medical or political newspaper journalists who wrote about it. Film critics did as well, including Peter van Bueren, then at the start of his career but who would later be called an "eminent film critic". In *De Tijd* he wrote that the film made such a great impression on him that he wants to start with a personal confidence.

> One of the most annoying comments the older generation can make to us young, is: "Oh, you didn't live through the war." A snarl that (certainly in our eyes) is simply used too often. A boy doesn't like his food. The parents: "Eat up, you can see that you were born after the war. In those days we had to eat flower bulbs." An unjustified imposition of guilt, as if it was the boy's fault his parents had run out of potatoes. And what the connection between that sad circumstance and his aversion to endive is, is by no means clear to him. The annual commemoration of the dead has fallen out of grace within a large part of the youth, because to them the Second World War is a thing from the past. The meaning of a commemoration is accepted, but only in a broader context: commemoration of all war victims, including those who fell or suffered after 1945.[24]

Van Bueren refers to the young, feminist, former Amsterdam councillor Irène van de Weetering. On 3 May, she commented on whether 4 May (Commemoration Day) and 5 May (Liberation Day) should still be celebrated, that 4 May's focus on that one particular war was meaningless. According to Van de Weetering, a commemoration of the dead should be dominated by the will to prevent as much as possible that new deaths had to be regretted continuously. However, after World War II they had fallen in ample numbers as well. She even didn't see the point of celebrating liberation day, for example because everyone kept on talking about the Americans and Canadians, but nobody about the Russians who had suffered the most. And: in Germany, hardly any action was taken against the extreme right, while demonstrations by anti-fascist youth were violently disrupted. What, then, were we liberated from?[25]

Do you now understand why I cry... was a movie dealing with one of the most dramatic consequences of the Second World War and therefore, according to Van Bueren, added a new aspect to opinions like these: its victims still were victims. This caused him to question the decision to distribute it among doctors and medical students only.

> Shouldn't everybody see it? But people don't seem to dare to run the risk of too great a shock (for example during a television broadcast). I can imagine this vividly. "Do you now understand why I cry…" is a slap in the face. "You didn't live through the war." One looks upon such remarks differently after having watched a movie like this one.[26]

It was a conclusion completely in line with the comments of the reviewer of the protestant newspaper *Trouw* (Faithful). To him this was reason enough to plead in favour of a much broader display. After all, the film was more than just medical education. It was "a living dramatic testimony concerning us all".[27]

Constant Wallagh, the film critic of the *Algemeen Dagblad,* asked completely different questions in his 'Impressive report by Van Gasteren'. To him, the film proved that the answer to the question how far one can go in recording and then disseminating other people's intimacies – a question that, according to Wallagh, was as old as photography and cinema, but in fact dates from the moment man discovered how to draw – varies and evolves, in time and place. In this film, this intimacy involved "the state of mind of a mentally disturbed man".[28]

Wallagh briefly discussed the history of the film. For some time Van Gasteren had been working on a feature film called *Een Wintermiddag* (A Winter's Afternoon). In that film, which was never completed, he wanted to include a short clip about an LSD session. This made him contact Bastiaans. Gradually, the plan matured into making a documentary as well. Wallagh described it as impressive, penetrating, and sober. Van Gasteren rightly stayed away from image effects or other cinematic gimmicks. Nevertheless, the screening of the film was limited to a select audience, a decision neither Bastiaans nor Van Gasteren was happy with. They wanted it to be distributed more widely, perhaps even on television, although Bastiaans wasn't entirely sure of that yet. Understandable, Wallagh said. "The answer to the question above is difficult to find both theoretically and practically. But television or not, it has been agreed upon that a lot of people should be able to see this film. Maybe tomorrow, because today we don't know yet.[29] So it happened, although 'tomorrow' should be read as 'in a few years'.

The only film critic who put some real question marks was Bob Bertina from *de Volkskrant.* According to him the only reason why *Do you now understand why I cry...* was shown to film critics as well was that LSD treatment of war victims would play a role in Van Gasteren's upcoming movie. He completely agreed with the decision to only give doctors or medical students a chance to watch it. It undoubtedly would be very instructive to them. But not to others.

> An average viewer will find it difficult to remain, for 62 minutes, interested in the fate of a difficult family man, with inhibited feelings and repressed fears and suspicions. Watching the ongoing treatment of the patient, you get, as an ordinary viewer, the feeling of being forced into indiscretion. You feel like you're somewhere you'd rather not be. By then every objective drama has of course since long gone.[30]

This already indicates that Bertina didn't so much question general screening because of the intense theme or the shocking images. He dismissed it as a bad documentary, making the subject discussed, the KZ syndrome, less rather than more accessible. Because the patient was suffering from this ailment, "an element having to do with war crimes slips in the viewer's perception". Therefore, a connection was quickly made between 'German atrocities' and 'poor victim'. And, Bertina wrote, it was precisely in the registration of this added element that Van Gasteren hadn't been completely honest. The viewer really didn't need to be a psychiatrist to see that the patient in question, "this victim", was in fact just a nagging man "who had a need to be looked up to by his next of kin, to be seen as more of a man than he actually is". He clearly had the urge to be seen as a hero or martyr by his wife and children. He now could conveniently explain away his neuroses by pointing at his life in the camps. However, he would have had difficulties without the camps as well, he only would have had to settle for "a less spectacular coat rack". According to Bastiaans, the man was now completely healed. Hopefully, Bertina concluded, he had "liberated him from his unreasonable urge to assert himself" as well.[31]

Comments like these didn't go down well with everyone, to say the least. Bertina had indeed spoken as a *film* critic, but the film he criticised was not just any film, but a film about a sick person, a patient, a victim, a war victim at that. As a result, criticising the film was interpreted as criticising war victims, which increasingly was seen as a disgrace. One should never question a war victim's word. For example, in one of the letters to the editor it was asked whether the editors were willing to apologise for the "incompetent and indelicate way" in which Bertina discussed the movie.[32] The medical employee of *Het Parool,* endocrinologist, toxicologist, and paediatrician, Otto de Vaal, shared Bertina's view that public display was not desirable. But it was not the movie itself, but precisely the reviewer's "infamous piece" that supported this opinion. It proved that only a few had the necessary basic knowledge of both the syndrome and the drug to form a well-considered opinion. Therefore, a wider distribution would only lead to more misunderstanding and incomprehension.[33]

Although there was at least one physician backing up Bertina,[34] the protest grew to such massive proportions that the editors of *de Volkskrant* saw themselves forced to write that Bertina hadn't recognised and appreciated the symptoms of the KZ syndrome displayed by the patient. It had to be put right in an interview with one of the critics, the Jewish sociologist Herman Milikowski, chairman of the politically committed, communist-minded Sachsenhausen Circle of Friends. Milikowski, at the time a teacher at the paediatrics department of Leiden University Hospital and thus indirectly a colleague of Bastiaans, had survived several camps but lost his wife in the war. In the 1960s and 1970s, he was known for his knowledge of helping people showing unsocial behaviour. As he wrote in his repeatedly reprinted book *Lof der Onaangepastheid* (Praising Improperness), the focus should be on the social factors causing this behaviour, and not so much on the individuals displaying it. In the tome of the protests against the possible release of the Breda Three, to be discussed later, he was the representative of the Sachsenhausen Committee in the confidential committee consulting Minister of Justice, Dries Van Agt, composed of representatives of the Central Organisation Former Resistance and Victims (COVVS).

Milikowski already criticised the review before he had seen the film itself; after that, his critique only became fiercer. In the days leading up to the interview, he talked a lot with his fellow survivors from Sachsenhausen about "the incomprehension mentally ill former camp inmates encounter on a daily basis". Among them also the man central in *Do you understand now why I cry...* This is hardly surprising because Milikowski was the one who sent him to Bastiaans. A few years later he revealed that, although he did not suffer from any kind of syndrome, it was him whom Van Gasteren initially asked to be the man talking about his camp experiences under the influence of LSD.[35] He declined but declared himself willing to look for another candidate. He then discussed it with a former prisoner friend and both he and his wife expressed their willingness to cooperate in the experiment. According to Milikowski, the LSD treatment had brought his friend a lot of good. "He looks younger, he is capable of doing so much more, he can *live again.*"[36]

Although in his own review Milikowski called the film "a human tragedy well captured by both psychiatrist and filmmaker", that he contradicted Bertina's criticisms didn't mean he fully approved of it. After all, the social context in which trauma can arise was absent. In his view this context was that a lot of camp survivors still were told not to whine and/or that they just wanted to be a hero or a martyr; see Bertina's comments. He baptised this way of looking at the war and its victims "a kind of *reversed* KZ syndrome". Doctors, politicians, citizens: they all said they sympathised, but at the same time they did not want to be reminded of the horrors. In other words, the camp survivors were only allowed to suffer passively. And this although, according to Milikowski, the relationship between camp and suffering was "a scientifically proved fact". He concluded that those who nevertheless denied this simply didn't want to see misery. And not just the misery of the past, but neither the present one. They didn't want to accept "that the reality of the Vietnamese people is the same as that of the former Nazi-camp prisoners". This also was one of the major problems Bastiaans' patient suffered from. He simply could not convince his surroundings that fascism was still out there. He was genuinely afraid of what he saw happening in the world. In other words, resistance fighters were traumatised not so much from all they had been through but because they saw the world learned nothing from their anti-fascist resistance and, therefore, their suffering had been in vain. They were thwarted in their persistent resistance because they were seen, also by the psychiatrists treating them, as pitiful victims of an earlier war and not as the militant anti-fascists they still were. The interview ended with the words: "What I am about to say is illusory. But I believe that if we had come back into a world in which you saw: they've learned from it, we would have found therapies in society itself."[37]

Bertina couldn't let it pass. He came up with an elaborate response, which started and ended with putting on a sackcloth.

> I would like to state that if *anything* in my review of *Van Gasteren's film* has given the impression of being an attempt at lay psychiatry *against* the scientific authority of *Prof. Dr. J. Bastiaans,* I am willing to withdraw my entire review. (…) My necessarily clinical evaluation of a film, which can so easily give rise to emotional misunderstandings, in no way implies that the undersigned is unwilling to show consideration for what psychiatry has come to know as the concentration camp syndrome and all the unimaginable suffering associated with it.[38]

However, the many words between this opening and closing quote make clear that he stood by the crux of his criticism, which was that the film had failed *as a film.* Contrary to what many thought (and condemned), Bertina said he did not want to present a medical opinion but wanted to put forward his opinion as a non-medical viewer. He only had written down what had come to his mind when watching the documentary, assuming these thoughts would roughly coincide with the thoughts popping up in the minds of other non-medical onlookers. In other words, what he wanted to do, and what he would continue to do and defend by virtue of his position, was to give a critical assessment of a medical registration presented by the filmmaker as *cinéma vérité.* Most critics were silent about this. It was always only about the registration itself and not about the way in which it had been registered. In this respect, the film simply wasn't that original. There were countless examples of *cinéma vérité,* for example about "a gay Negro" or "an American voyeur and exhibitionist on his pleasure trips in Las Vegas". Usually, all these films were highly regarded by critics "as a record of human authenticity, which may be critically discussed". And now a former concentration camp inmate joined the line.[39]

Cinéma verité, and certainly in case the subject is the treatment of troubled war victims having lived through the horrors of concentration camp reality, is primarily intended to provide insight into the matter. Those who know much about it or have experienced it themselves, will pay little attention to the cinematic qualities, but mainly look at the registration itself, and identify with the patient who wants to be released from his torment. "They know what he's talking about when fragments of memories come alive, albeit put into words rather vaguely." The critic, however, is not a part of this group and will therefore look upon the movie with different eyes; the eyes of someone wanting to be informed about the subject by means of a film. He looks at how the filmmaker – who is not a physician either – worked; what he did to clarify all he wants to convey. It's not for nothing that Bastiaans stated plainly that it's not his film, but Van Gasteren's.[40]

The proof of the pudding is how to make the medical story cinematically clear to an uninitiated audience. Bertina included himself in this last category and, if the movie ever will by publicly broadcasted, this undoubtedly will include almost everyone watching. But, he went on, this was exactly where things had gone wrong. Even though a lot of suffering was shown, even though regularly you saw a man crying, after everything was said and done the film, and therefore Van Gasteren, had revealed little. Overall, the film was completely medical, devoid of a cinematic-dramatic raison d'être. Therefore, a wider display was pointless. The viewer wouldn't understand the incomprehension the man felt and, Bertina feared, would lose all interest in him. At least that was exactly what had happened to him and which is why he searched for another account that could explain "the motives of the 'leading role'". Sadly this "was conceived as a psychiatric lay judgment".

> Here and there it was suggested that the movie *Do you now understand why I cry...* is a shocking movie. I fear it's quite the opposite, namely that when broadcasting it on tv most spectators will find it a boring picture. Exactly that should not happen to Prof. Bastiaans' patient.[41]

Pleas from opponents of public display, including medics, failed to prevent an attempt to accomplish just that, despite prior agreements and the patient's reticence. Members of the former resistance were sent a pre-printed postcard. The only thing they had to do was sign it and send it to Bastiaans. It gave him a means of pressure in his plea for wider dissemination. The card accidentally miswrote the movie's title, not using the courteous word 'u' but the familiar word 'je' (in English both 'you'). Karel Hofman, who was interviewed by the *Algemeen Dagblad,* didn't have a problem with this. On the contrary. It showed a geniality that reflected the atmosphere of an LSD treatment, or at least the atmosphere of the treatment of that particular patient. Hofman had been imprisoned in Amersfoort and Vught and in the interview he described the horrific torture he had undergone and witnessed. To recover from and escape these haunting images, he had undergone the above-average number of eight LSD sessions.[42]

Of course, readers couldn't know that the horrors dished up by Hofman almost certainly had only happened in his head.[43] To by far the most of them it didn't occur that, if only in the struggle for their own survival, camp victims could partly have been perpetrators – a prominent theme in the work of Andries Kaas.[44] And it certainly didn't occur to them that victims invented horrors to which they were exposed – only to often really believing in them afterwards. As said: victims were taken at their word. Those who doubted were despicable creatures downplaying Nazi-terror.

Hofman had initially been so shocked by the film and so thrown back into his war past that he opposed showing it to a wider and non-medical audience. However, Bastiaans asked him to let the film sink in for a while before making a final judgment. In this pause he indeed changed his mind.

> This film must be on television, albeit with an introduction by Professor Bastiaans. It will become clear that without medical supervision LSD is dangerous. But I now believe that everyone should know what the concentration camp syndrome is, why for no immediate cause ex-prisoners are mentally broken twenty-five years after the war. And I also want a TV broadcast to show all doctors and all housemates of ex-prisoners and resistance members, but also themselves, that the concentration camp syndrome is real. In this way many people can be spared unnecessary suffering.[45]

As mentioned, it only came about a few years later. Until then, the film had been shown to a restricted audience only. It, for example, featured at a scientific conference on drugs and addiction in Zurich in 1970 – where, by the way, the chairman of the United Nations Commission on Narcotics expressed his conviction that marijuana would soon be legalised.[46] Nevertheless, it was the film screening in The Hague in the presence of the

Queen, that Bastiaans himself singled out as the event turning the KZ syndrome into a familiar concept. Due to the enormous media attention the premiere managed to achieve, from that moment on the Dutch people were aware that men and women who had experienced and endured the horrors of war and internment, could still experience problems years and years afterwards.[47]

6. THE WORKING GROUP CAMP SYNDROME

An important player in opinion making on the KZ syndrome was, of course, the Jewish community and thus the *NIW.* It devoted half a page to a lecture Cohen had given on it to the Dutch Society for Jewish Science in September 1970. He also discussed "the startling" film by Van Gasteren, which "in a very penetrating way shed light on the tragedy of the returnees".[1]

Cohen also went into the history of the syndrome and the circumstances leading up to it: abuse, chronic malnutrition, forced labour. He pointed out the possible physical consequences (damage to blood vessels, and to muscle, nerve and brain tissue), and explained its development (from physical illness via apparent recovery to renewed physical problems, also because of overestimation of what one was able to do, and clear mental issues because of this). Due to the absence of physical evidence, the term "pension-neurosis", lingering in illness to ensure and secure pension benefits, was used regularly in the 1950's. According to Cohen, it was precisely the other way around. Often people went back to work too early rather than too late.[2]

This attention to pension-neurosis wasn't in itself conducive to an empathetic relationship with the ones psychologically suffering from war experiences.[3] But it had a flip side. Through discussing it, Cohen advocated a broader application of the reversed burden of proof when applying for benefits; a burden of proof that became increasingly difficult to provide as the time span between war and application grew. According to Cohen, the assessing authorities should prove there was no correlation between symptoms and war history. And preferably a doctor who himself had a concentration camp history should have the final say. Norway and France already had similar arrangements. In Norway, a committee concluded that for 208 of the 227 ex-concentration camp prisoners examined, the problems were wholly (the most) or partly (a few) attributable to the war. On top, their disability percentages were mostly adjusted upwards, and not for a tiny bit. For example, initially there had been six people who had been declared 100 percent disabled. The commission now stated that this percentage had to be allocated to 59 others as well. The implicit conclusion is clear: in the Netherlands many received a disability pension that was too low rather than too high as well. "These were just some of the important topics masterfully brought up by Dr. Cohen. They will occupy the minds as long as the generation of the great catastrophe lives and thinks and relives and commemorates its events."[4]

It was no coincidence that Cohen addressed the benefit issue. First, the reversed burden of proof didn't yet apply to those interned solely because of racial persecution; those who were persecuted not for what they had said or done, but merely for what they (in the eyes of the occupier) were by birth. And secondly, the pension issue once again came into the limelight because Prime Minister De Jong set up a working group in July 1970, perhaps in response to a letter, dated May 1970, from the German Prince Bernhard, the husband of Queen Juliana, and, in spite of a past in the German national socialist party, hero of veterans and former resistance fighters. This working group had to investigate how soldiers who had been in the resistance and/or had ended up in a German camp, could be helped financially and socially. Six months later, however, it was discovered that the working group had still not met, not even once. It consisted of representatives from the Ministries of CRM, Interior and Defence, who referred questions about it to the chairman. After all, he was the one who had to ask the working group to gather. However, this chairman, Noordhoek Hegt, said he wasn't aware of being appointed chairman of anything. Yes, he had someone on the phone once mentioning such a topic, but he never received a written confirmation. He said to be stunned that he was expected to initiate deliberations about "the interests of several hundred Dutch people, who almost had given the best they had for their country – their lives – and who now, 25 years after the war, were still waiting for a thank you from that same country, the Netherlands".[5]

This state of affairs concerning the military men who had been in the resistance and/or concentration camps, particularly agitated Henk Vonhoff, Member of Parliament for the liberal-conservative *Volkspartij voor Vrijheid en Democratie* VVD (People's Party for Freedom and Democracy). In blatant contrast to, for example, POW officers or the ones who had been able to cross the North Sea to England, the so-called *Engelandvaarders* (England sailors), they received nothing, not even proper social-medical support. He therefore applauded that Bastiaans and Cohen started to educate military doctors about the mental and physical mutilation from which many people over fifty, and with them their families, still suffered. Among those mostly young doctors, there was a lot of incomprehension, arising out of ignorance. The last time a military doctor had attended a conference on these issues was in 1961. The *Jan Soldaat* (Tommy Atkins) of May 1940 had been the victim of this negligence. Consequently, Vonhoff took it upon himself to write a letter to the Civil Service Pensions Committee asking them to find out what could be done for them. *De Telegraaf* concluded its coverage with the words: "Since the Netherlands have been liberated, they have bumped their heads against a wall of incomprehension for 25 years now. Cap in hand they beg for some lousy millions. And for preferential treatment. That's all they ask. It this too much?"[6]

Finally, State Secretary Kruisinga set up the Post Concentration Camp Syndrome Working Group shortly after this interview (in short: the Working Group Camp Syndrome). Noordhoek Hegt indeed became chairman. The military medical service was represented by the then highest military medical officer Arnoldus 'Bob' van Overeem, the man who attended the international conference on KZ syndrome nine years earlier. Bastiaans and Cohen were the primary medical advisers.[7] However, the working group was no longer limited to former soldiers, but focused on all concentration camp victims. It was intended to provide advice "on the treatment of the concentration camp syndrome, and on the provisions for the victims that were in order". Its first task was to answer the question of whether the camp syndrome could and should indeed be regarded as a scientific fact. "Assuming this is the case", it was subsequently necessary to determine the approximate number of people suffering from it and how many of them received the diagnosis so far. If there was to be a legal regulation, answering questions like these was necessary. In addition, it also was necessary to consider whether a special institute for research and treatment should be set up.[8]

When the working group was called into being officially, Kruisinga – who warmly thanked Bastiaans, Cohen and Speijer for all the work they had already done in this area –[9] noted that Dutch doctors still had a serious knowledge gap concerning the syndrome, and that its existence was still doubted. He therefore took an affirmative advance on the question about the syndrome's existence. Because many symptoms only gradually manifested, it had taken a long time before the problem was recognised. This had led to insufficient scientific understanding. As a result, the victims weren't always given the financial backing they had deserved in retrospect.[10]

The installation was followed by two days of emotional parliamentary debates about a state pension for Jewish war victims, in which, for example, from the general gallery a 55-year-old war invalid threw a prosthesis into the hall. The first requests for such a pension dated back to 1965, and, pointing at the psychological consequences of the war, poet and Dachau survivor Ed Hoornik had made a strong case for it at the Auschwitz commemoration in 1968, which was repeated on television shortly afterwards.[11]

A motion to this effect was submitted by the Social Democratic Member of Parliament, Joop Voogd. It was passed by the Dutch house of representatives, the Second Chamber, but the government chose to ignore it. This again resulted in a motion of 'no confidence' against State Secretary for CRM, Hein van de Poel – who didn't want a state pension – which only barely escaped acceptance.

According to Van de Poel, the so-called National Group Regulation Prosecution Victims 1940-1945 was completely geared to the psychological needs of the war victims and based on the General Assistance Act. The latter immediately formed a hefty stumbling block, which increased the psychological needs. A pension was seen as the acknowledgement of a right, while this arrangement gave the feeling that people had come under the care reserved for the poor. But, Van de Poel assured, the scheme was really only based on the social assistance act and had nothing to do with the so-called support pulls of old. It gave full security and was paid out as if it were a pension. The only difference was that it was a supplementary benefit and therefore wasn't intended for people with sufficient income of their own to maintain their previous financial level. He had discussed it with De Wind, who agreed with the arrangement.[12]

It was no coincidence that Van de Poel specifically mentioned De Wind's name in the interview. In the magazine *Vrij Nederland,* originally set up by the resistance, he stated that the State Secretary had no insight into the clinical picture of camp victims, something Van de Poel justifiably argued. He had been secretary of the Extraordinary Pensions Council for twelve years and, therefore, looked at thousands of pension reports. Also, because of this, he had been in frequent contact with "the doctors who have studied this matter extensively", including De Wind.[13]

Voogd calculated that around and about 2300 Jewish survivors were eligible for a state pension. This came down to about 22.5 million guilders (€10 million), an amount that, according to many, shouldn't be difficult to obtain. But first of all, the government, read: Van de Poel, questioned the calculation of the number of people, and thus the financial consequences. Van de Poel thought 23,000 would be a better estimate than 2300, partly because he wanted to include those who had been in hiding. If these were left out, it in fact was said that the suffering of one group, the camp survivors, had been more severe than that of another, those who had been in hiding. He rejected this weighing of suffering, this hierarchy of hurt. Van de Poel was willing to acknowledge that the Jewish group was special. But, he said in an interview with *de Volkskrant*, "If you make an arrangement for this group today, you will be confronted with another group striving for the same arrangement tomorrow". Therefore, separation was impossible. A government shouldn't put anyone above another. "The Chamber always says that *this group should have priority.* This in fact means: Only this group should come into this special position. Yet no one dares to say *this group alone*."[14]

When asked whether he wasn't ignoring the medical-psychiatric discovery that camp survivors, people who "lived in the shadow of death", have their own syndrome and therefore form a separate group, Van de Poel replied:

> I have assumed that access to the so-called National Group Regulation, under which these victims fall, should be as flexible as possible. That the disabled do not have to prove that there is a relationship between the disability and the war years. As a rule, we accept this relationship without question. To that extent we do indeed recognise this special psychological disability, but we do not isolate this group. We allow all the disabled who, objectively, have been persecuted to fall under the National Group Regulation.[15]

The reversed burden of proof therefore applied. "Anyone who is a Jewish victim and an invalid, will be helped," Van de Poel said. Those who continued working despite having problems, the invisible invalids, couldn't take advantage of the scheme. Therefore, their doctors should encourage them to stop working when labour in fact was too hard. Then they too could make an appeal.[16]

The discussions about Van Gasteren's film and financial compensation for war victims took place in the midst of a national discussion about whether or not to release war criminals. This discussion (re)started in the mid-1960s. Willy Lages, due to poor health, was released in 1966. He died in 1971. The Minister of Justice, Carel Polak, called for the release of the other three in 1969. However, on the advice of the Supreme Court and after fierce opposition in the Second Chamber, he refrained from doing so. Polak's reasoning was that the government had to accept the view of the majority of the Chamber, for he believed this to be the view of the majority of the population as well: "Life imprisonment isn't a punishment too severe for what some people can do wrong and have done wrong." Thus, they had to remain in detention because of the ongoing suffering of their former victims; because of "the psychological, yes physical impossibility" of these victims "to accept a possible release".[17] It prompted the *NRC Handelsblad* to pay lots of attention to the KZ syndrome; a phenomenon which, according to the author Cohen, had been researched far too little. In the Netherlands it was written about by merely eight doctors.[18]

First, Cohen's article, 'Vechten om ziek te zijn' (Fighting to be sick), contradicted the idea that the syndrome was a mental illness, even though six of those eight physicians were psychiatrists by profession. The physical problems that occurred during camp life should anything but be neglected.

Apart from that, there was the psychological stress of that 'life'. It was precisely because of unfamiliarity with the syndrome and its causes and symptoms that Bastiaans and Van Gasteren came up with the film *Do you now understand why I cry*.... Cohen agreed with Bastiaans that thanks to the extensive newspaper coverage following the first screening of the picture the Netherlands had become familiar with both the syndrome and the LSD treatment used by Bastiaans. "But in my opinion, the most important thing is that the new Dutch generation of doctors has studied the German concentration camps and their consequences – at least, in contrast to other universities, the ones educated in Leiden."[19]

The second important element Cohen brought forward was that the KZ syndrome wasn't riveted to concentration camp survivors. German soldiers who had been in Russian POW camps, at sometimes 40 degrees below zero, often showed similar symptoms, as did American soldiers of the Korean War, 1950-1953. In North Korean POW camps they had been kept from sleeping deliberately. Furthermore, familiar problems could be detected in people who had experienced a peacetime disaster: an explosion, a shipwreck, a plane crash, and so on. He therefore introduced the term disaster syndrome, a kind of PTSD avant-la-lettre.[20]

Finally, the third element Cohen pointed out was the progressiveness of the condition. In a longitudinally survey, 1950-1966, of a Danish group of about 370 people, no one had shown a decrease in disability, only an increase. Why, Cohen wondered, should this not hold true for the Dutch, especially since compensation mechanisms diminish with age? The problem with aging was, it has been said before, that it becomes increasingly difficult to determine what resulted from war-related stress and what from the aging process and/or after-war stress. This didn't imply questions had to be asked when granting a pension. It did imply, however, that, as was the case in Denmark and Norway, only the degree of disability determined the amount of the benefit. A physician shouldn't be asked to determine which part of a disability percentage was attributable to the war and which was not. A past in the resistance and/or in a camp had to suffice, an arrangement which, Cohen knew for certain, surely the ex-resistance members wouldn't take advantage from. "Often the Norwegians and Danes have served as an example in this matter. Perhaps they could be so once more: it would constitute a definitive closing piece of the Extraordinary Pension Act."[21]

Cohen, who extensively reported about his own war past and the camp horrors in general, not failing explicitly mentioning Aus der Fünten, didn't find it strange that young ignorant doctors at the Extraordinary Pension Councils were sober and reserved and showed minimum understanding for former camp inmates. But it was strange that older doctors, who had lived through the war themselves, not seldom behaved in the same manner. Here the system took its revenge that, when deciding on a pension, only current complaints were considered and not the circumstances in which the applicant lived during the war; circumstances, moreover, which weren't easy to talk about for applicants. Therefore, he pointed at the need to keep on asking questions continuously; to ask consciously what happened to them during the war. For example, women had to be asked explicitly whether they had been raped. Only then this would be admitted and could trauma be explained. And, especially as regards former Dutch prisoners, the failure of the Dutch Red Cross should never be forgotten. Unlike other national Red Cross Societies, it hadn't managed to get food parcels into the camps. "Many ex-inmates have made no secret of their bitterness towards me about this. It's impossible to estimate how many Dutch human lives were lost because of this lack of daring, courage, and initiative of the Dutch Red Cross."[22]

Cohen pointed out that the quoted Danish study also had a look at 52 ex-camp residents claiming to be healthy. After the survey, this group had shrunk to 12. Of the other 40, 17 immediately filed a claim. Although the other 23 admitted they also suffered from the syndrome, they decided to continue working. This, however, came at the expense of their private lives and of the few physical and mental reserves they still had. It was only a matter of time before they would visit a pension board too.[23] Cohen apparently failed to notice the discrepancy between his generalisation of the syndrome and his desire to focus less on the current symptoms and more on the past cause. He also didn't question whether it had been the investigation itself that had caused the problems to surface. All it had done, he said, was to make the camp survivors become aware of their victimhood and the problems it had caused. And he said that it was good.

7. THE ADVENT OF THE POST CONCENTRATION CAMP SYNDROME CLINIC

A month after Cohen's extensive article in the *NRC Handelsblad* and a few weeks after the debates about the National Group Regulation, a new chapter in the KZ syndrome story was opened. Noordhoek Hegt's Working Group Camp Syndrome presented its interim report to Kruisinga. It referred to the difficulties war victims encountered on their return due to, for example, a lack of societal understanding and difficulties in obtaining work. In the case of many Jewish victims, they moreover had to discover they were (almost) alone in the world. Furthermore, again symptoms were mentioned such as early aging, high disease rates, and an increased risk of premature death. This report too estimated the number of people still suffering from the great mental and physical strain caused by the war at 'several thousand'. It also endorsed the view that KZ syndrome or (post) concentration camp syndrome were incorrect names because they didn't cover the full package. The cause, it said, should be considered of lesser importance than the symptomatic effects, which could also be witnessed in people who had been in the resistance without being captured; in people who had gone into hiding in difficult circumstances; who had completed their military service under extreme conditions, as well as among those "who had been victims of other forms of man-made catastrophe". In addition, the report mentioned the generation transgressing effects of the syndrome.

> These effects have not only been observed in the victims' peers, but in particular in the victims' children. They have grown up in a family situation in which the sufferer of the syndrome was unable to lead the upbringing in an appropriate and healthy manner. According to the report, it may be expected that these consequences will have their disease-inducing effect into future generations.[1]

It was a description of the (possible) victims, which made it clear that releasing the cause as defining characteristic would result in many more than a few thousand receiving the diagnoses, and that the syndrome wouldn't disappear once the war generation deceased.

The State Secretary thereupon decided to follow the advice to set up a special clinic and to enable its establishment financially. Moreover, it would be examined whether in due course more special clinics should be built. The first one would have twenty beds and provide space for about 200 outpatient treatments per annum. On top, scientific research had to be done in the field of the post concentration camp syndrome; the term that, despite the simultaneous criticism of its exclusive instead of inclusive nature, was increasingly used for the delayed psychological problems of war victims. A suitable location was discussed with the municipality of Leiden – the territory around the Jelgersma clinic coming to mind. If all went well, it could be opened within six months. To arrange this a separate foundation was set up, the Foundation Post Concentration Camp Syndrome Centre, chaired by the former Director-General of Public Health, social physician Piet Muntendam. Prince Bernhard was asked to take on the role of honorary chairman, which probably must be seen in the light of the fact that one of the initiators of the foundation was a close friend of his: former resistance fighter Hans Teengs Gerritsen, chairman of the Natzweiler committee, and its representative in the COVVS Confidence Committee. Teengs Gerritsen himself became vice-chairman. According to him, Bernhard had continuously said to Kruisinga: "Just tell me what I can do and whom else I should contact." Teengs Gerritsen also involved his good friend Piet Maliepaard, a communist, former Spanish Civil War volunteer and survivor of Dachau. He was admitted to the Jelgersma clinic, also referred to by people like him as 'the Jel', in 1970. Teengs Gerritsen had visited him there on a regular basis.[2]

A few years later, Teengs Gerritsen declared it a major shortcoming that he hadn't come up with the idea of a special clinic earlier. After all, the problems of camp survivors had been known for much longer. He found treatment in the Jelgersma clinic itself undesirable because of its unpersonal, cold atmosphere. He even considered it "a kind of KZ". Nevertheless, it was of the utmost importance that the new clinic was placed in the vicinity of the psychiatric centre. "We have to be close to Professor Bastiaans, because this psychiatrist in particular feels the wavelength of the bruised former concentration camp prisoners so well."[3]

De Tijd sent an editor to Oegstgeest to interview Bastiaans about the developments. It led to the article 'After 26 years a clinic for victims of concentration camps. People who have remained psychologically wrecked after the war'. In the interview, Bastiaans said that there are 15 to 20,000 Dutch people, so indeed a lot more than 'a few thousand', for whom the war continues to "root in their memory" so severely that it makes them ill, age quickly, and die prematurely. Together with Speijer, for years he campaigned for such a clinic, but, although almost no one had left the camps mentally unscathed, hadn't found an audience for it until recently. However, the group of medics who after the war recognised that a problem had arisen, was small. The medical profession focussed more on biological phenomena and therefore did not know how to deal with psychological complaints. “Forget and don’t complain” was the motto presented to war victims in the 1950s, the decade characterized by silence about the past and the eyes firmly on the future. This of course was impossible because emotionally the war, the memory of the war, dictated their lives. Because, Bastiaans explained, their past had been blocked, so to speak, their treatment had to be aimed at guiding them through the hell called concentration camp once more. Only then their problems could be solved. Only then the restlessness in their heads would disappear, an effect his patients had confirmed. Various techniques were available to achieve this, including psychotherapy, hypnosis, meditation, and psychogenic medication such as LSD. In particular these latter means enabled to have the experiences “come back in full force” in a medically controlled setting; a necessary step in the direction of processing and healing, of true liberation.[4]

According to Bastiaans, most victims now were in the third phase of the syndrome. The first phase, the immediate post-war era, was typified by nervousness, fatigue, and nightmares, mostly suppressed by means of repression. The second phase was typified by physical complaints resulting from the mental problems and the initial repression. Now, after having been able to adjust twice, the mind had lost its power to adapt once more. The clinic therefore was built late, but certainly not too late because it indeed was not only intended for camp survivors. According to Bastiaans, it, in any case, would prove its use to the children of the survivors. But for the survivors themselves as well the clinic had anything but been built in vain. It would be beneficial for them that they could now be treated in an environment in which they could feel at home. At the clinic they could expose themselves freely because the doctors working there understood their past and problems. It was logical that this was a small medical group, Bastiaans said, hinting at his own past in the resistance. “In fact, you have to have experienced it yourself to be able to help these people.”[5] That his own resistance days had soon be over because of the leg injury he received, wasn’t mentioned.[6]

In the families of the camp victims Bastiaans saw as well how important shared experience was.

> They sit and watch television. Suddenly images of Vietnam war misery or wherever appear on the screen. The own experiences come back in full force and family members who saw those TV images also, but have no difficulty processing them, say: “Why are you so upset about this?” As a result, they feel misunderstood, even in their own home, their own intimate environment.[7]

8. THE BREDA THREE

> It seems that only recently doctors discovered how serious long-term effects of war suffering can be. In addition, until now blocking problems has been fairly successful. But for some reason, when you're not expecting it, the syndrome pops up like an abscess.[1]

When, mid 1971, newspapers reported on the importance of the new clinic, possible lacerations due to the release of the Breda Three, Kotalla, Aus der Fünten and Fischer, didn't yet play a role. However, this was exactly what Minister of Justice Van Agt argued at the time, after having been advised in this sense by several judicial courts. Ultimately his efforts proved as fruitless as those of his predecessor Polak. Aus der Fünten died in captivity in 1979 and the other two shortly after their eventual release in 1989. The emotional discussion that ensued from the intention to pardon placed the spotlight once again on the fate of Dutch Jews, both the victims during the war as the survivors thereafter. Some described it as a nice side effect.[2] To others it was sickening. Apparently, a discussion about perpetrators was necessary to do justice to victims; apparently, pity for the persistent imprisonment of the perpetrators was necessary to realise the lifelong suffering of their victims.[3]

That the discussion became so heated was partly because Van Agt – who was opposed by some of his colleagues in government as well – gave in less quickly than Polak had done. What followed was a genuine media storm, including mostly furious letters to the editor in which regularly the political, international situation was just around the corner. For example, according to a letter writer in the communist *De Waarheid* Van Agt had to worry more about the thousands of, mostly communist, innocents who groaned in Indonesian prisons than about three guilty criminals in a Dutch cell.[4] This media storm turned the discussion about the release of the three into a key moment in the acceptance of psychological trauma by Dutch society.[5] And, it made clear how much newspapers and television could shape and change public and political opinion.

A few weeks after the debate ended, the massive media attention tempted sociologist Jan Godschalk to analyse the role played by the relatively new medium of television. The title of his piece in the *NRC Handelsblad*: 'The blow-up effect of television information' speaks volumes.

The effect was twofold. On television, an event seemed more comprehensive and impressive than it actually was. Because of television coverage an event became known to a far larger audience than just those who were on the spot. The role of opinion makers from politics, science or interest groups was crucial in interpreting this information, which made him mention Bastiaans.[6] Precisely in a case like the Breda Three, "in which it was impossible to determine objectively the rightness of a decision, non-political, or even scientific figures" rose on "the ladder of credibility". Consequently, of a politically rather colourless former resistance fighter was said that he was a friend of Prince Bernhard – probably Godschalk referred to Teengs Gerritsen. And consequently, the role psychiatrists, and especially Bastiaans, played in the debate was huge. "As a modern dowser standing above the parties" he was entrusted with the task of pointing out "where the source of the truth was to be found".[7]

Indeed, Bastiaans could not be kept away from newspaper columns or TV screen in those weeks. This media storm thus led to his definitive breakthrough as an authoritative participant in discussions about the consequences of war (and all kinds of other issues at play in the Netherlands). He was mentioned, spoken about, or interviewed in hundreds of articles in 1972, especially from February to April. One sign of this breakthrough was, for example, that the then-known Rabbi Avraham Soetendorp successfully summoned the Second Chamber to watch *Do you now understand why I cry...* before making a final decision, in the hope and expectation it would make them rejecting release.[8] And so they all gathered in the evening of February 23, in the presence of Van Agt and State Secretary for Justice Hans Grosheide.[9] It didn't stop there. Following the screening for MPs, on 26 February the social-democratic *Verenigde Arbeiders Radio Amateurs* VARA (United Workers Radio Amateurs) broadcasted the film in its entirety on television, preceded by an introduction by Bastiaans. It was much watched, although some viewers probably regretted that to make room for the film the first episode of an almost certainly somewhat more light-hearted British series about depraved women had to be cancelled.[10]

On 19 February, Bastiaans informed *De Tijd* that the discussions about the release of the Breda Three led to renewed anxiety attacks among camp survivors. Many of his patients, he said, were quite annoyed about Van Agt's plans. Still, they were filled with feelings of revenge. However, medically speaking, whether the three were or weren't released was of little consequence. Neither decision affected treatment and healing process, positively nor negatively. What did have an influence, however, and a negative one at that, were the regularly recurring discussions about release, for they time and again confronted former inmates and resistance fighters with their painful past. Therefore, it might be better to release them, although it probably would be smart not to set all three of them free at the same time. “Then we’re done with it. Otherwise, in two years’ time we will have the same unrest again.”[11] It was a position based on medical considerations, but a week later the lawyer Van Agt pointed at them as well when uncovering his intention to release the three one by one instead of simultaneously. After all, Bastiaans had “demonstrated”, as *De Telegraaf* wrote, that simultaneous release would seriously shock his patients.[12]

Bastiaans thus took a position contrary, firstly, to the 1959 appeal of the War Criminals Release Committee of which he had been a member; secondly, to that of the Vice-President of the Foundation Post Concentration Camp Syndrome Centre, Teengs Gerritsen, and thirdly, to that of the board of the Dutch Association for Psychoanalysis.[13] It’s unclear whether it was partly due to this resistance in his own circles, but a few days later it turned out that his opinion wasn’t carved in granite.

Opinions against release were medically substantiated as well. The chairman of the Auschwitz Committee, Jos Slagter, repeatedly referred to the KZ syndrome when arguing that the three should remain where they were.

> I will feel so broken if they are released. I am sick, but not even very sick. I feel abandoned. I’m voicing the thoughts of thousands. The KZ syndrome. The after-effects. That is the nowadays’ reality. The KZ syndrome culminates after a quarter of a century. The older you get, the less distracted you are by your career. There are those who just sit at home waiting to die. If you’ve ever been in the city of death, something inside you changed for good. The old wounds don’t ever heal.[14]

He rejected Bastiaans’ position that the discussion should end and that therefore letting go wasn’t such a bad idea. Instead, an arrangement had to be made making clear once and for all that imprisonment for life was their fate. This too would bring peace of mind.[15]

On 22 February, a few days after the article in *De Tijd*, Bastiaans, according to some TV critics, stated in a television programme that release could cause aggravation of the illness of several of his patients.[16] But, according to other TV critics, he was silent about the consequences of release. He only said his patients needed psychological and material security. The continuous discussions revived old fears, such as feeling of betrayal.[17]

Like *Trouw* by means of an interview, *Het Vrije Volk* went into more detail regarding Bastiaans’ point of view in an article headlined ‘Prof. Bastiaans warns against acute worsening of disease’.[18] Bastiaans had seen that Van Agt's intention almost immediately led to an exacerbation of his patients' complaints. Incidentally, in the interview he seemed to indicate this had more to do with the fact that they didn't agree with Bastiaans' opinion than with the political discussion. High blood pressure became even higher, heart and rheumatic ailments increased. On the other hand, those on the mend became much calmer. If it was up to them, the three could leave. War victims who were able to look past their emotions again and regained their senses – in other words: who were successfully treated by him –, shared his point of view.[19] But whatever the decision would be, he would definitely advise the committee to improve facilities and treatment options for war victims quickly and strongly.[20] However, this doesn't change that the observed increase in complaints was at odds with his statement of a few days earlier that neither pardon or permanent detention effected the healing process.

Bastiaans' position in favour of release didn't change despite the increase in complaints witnessed in some of his patients, something he explained in a letter to Soetendorp, and what he would tell the parliamentary committee one day later. In *Het Vrije Volk* he expressed his understanding for the view shared by many that there never should be a pardon. "But who guarantees this Never?" It was a view the newspaper expressed by stating:

> Bastiaans says that his patients first and foremost want rest. And because he has no guarantee that if the three remain in prison their release will never be discussed again, he is inclined to say: set them free.[21]

After the Second Chamber screening of *Do you now understand why I cry...*, on the eve of the big debate about the three, it became clear Bastiaans started to doubt his initial views. Indeed, a number of war victims as well felt that it would be best if the three just disappeared out of the Netherlands, but it had also became clear that a large majority thought that releasing them would be catastrophic. As a physician, he, therefore, faced a dilemma. Release was a one-time shock, permanent detention meant chronic torture because the three were allowed to submit pardon request after pardon request. Consequently, they would be all over the news again and again.[22] He himself still leaned towards release but underlined that scientifically sound information about the effects of pardoning the three were absent.[23]

And, as said, there was a great numbers of war victims. Earlier Bastiaans said that hardly anyone left the camp undamaged. After *Do you understand now why I cry...* was seen by the MPs, he not only said he hoped the politicians would now understand a little more about the KZ syndrome. Above all, he emphasised that only about eighty people could be helped each year, while there were "thirty to forty thousand people" suffering from it.[24] These were numbers repeated in an interview with *Trouw* and simplified to "just under 40,000" in the *Limburgsch Dagblad* (Limburg Daily).[25] This meant a sudden increase of 100 percent from the numbers mentioned by Bastiaans a little over a year earlier and even a tenfold increase of the numbers mentioned by Van Emde Boas in 1969. This also meant that the vast majority of them never had been in a concentration camp and thus in a literal sense couldn't suffer from KZ syndrome.[26]

The increase was explained by references to Jews and resistance members who hadn't been deported, people in hiding, people set to work in Germany, Sinti and Roma ("Gypsies") and "Dutch people who had been interned in the Japanese camps"; a group of which a few years earlier was said that mentally speaking they had suffered little from their hardships.[27] All kinds of different groups were thus swept together into one psychotraumatic safety net simply because they all were defined as war victims. The *NRC Handelsblad* wrote (and endorsed): "All these people still suffer the consequences. One can say they have a life sentence, because, according to Prof. Bastiaans, the last phase of the concentration camp syndrome ends with death."[28] The camp syndrome had become endemic as well as epidemic. The latter not in the sense that it was contagious – although it was said to pass on from parents to children – but in the sense that continuously new groups suffering from it were added to the original one. The syndrome was here to stay.

Coincidentally, on that same day, 24 February, these large and ever-increasing numbers were implicitly questioned by the then well-known Jewish publicist Henriette Boas, who lived in London during the war and afterwards emigrated to Israel for several years. According to Boas, it wasn't the war-experience itself that made victims sick. It had more to do with the way they were treated and dealt with by the surrounding society. Like Cohen, she pointed to Israel as the land providing the answer.

> All Jews who survived and even their children for most part, are said to be traumatised for life. However, the population of the State of Israel consists largely of survivors of concentration camps and other persecutions, and of their children. Nevertheless, although the living conditions are much more difficult, and, on top, there is a relentless threat of war violence, they are much less war traumatised because one is much less fixated on one's personal past than on the collective present and the collective future.[29]

Like, for example, Abel J. Herzberg, prominent member of the Jewish community, Bergen-Belsen survivor and author of the *Kroniek van de Jodenvervolging* (Jewish Persecution Chronicle),[30] Boas spoke out in favour of releasing the Breda Three, "despite the statements of renowned psychiatrists like Prof. Bastiaans" (whereby she must have meant emphasising the aggravation of the disease, not, of course, the pro-release stance he took at the time). She was convinced that releasing the three wouldn't increase the suffering of war survivors, as the release of other war criminals hadn't done before. She wondered whether anyone would really think at night, before going to sleep: "Thank God, the Breda Three are still imprisoned. It makes me sleep more peacefully." And if there was such a person, "wouldn't it be better to try to get him or her over this dead centre instead of fixating him on it?"[31]

Boas will have found it problematic that, a few days later, Israel joined the opponents of release. Shortly before the decisive debate, Israeli Foreign Minister Abba Eban stated that in the eyes of Israel in the case of genocide leniency is out of the question. He reminded the Dutch government that, when their death penalty was commuted to life in the early 1950s, the three had already been pardoned (by the way forgetting that, according to the then government, this almost certainly meant that they would be released after about twenty years).[32]

Although on 23 February Bastiaans was still in favour of release, together with his opponent Soetendorp he organised the screening of Van Gasteren's film for politicians. Keeping in mind the numbers of psychologically troubled mentioned by him, Bastiaans' intention will have been that showing the movie could contribute indirectly to fulfilling his wish that the Dutch government would invest more in victim support. But he seems to have underestimated the direct effect of the screening on political decision-making about the Breda Three. That effect was severe but contrary to his wish to release them. The display played no small part in turning the initial political majority in favour of release into a minority.[33] The parliament acknowledged that its decision was largely motivated by the estimated psychological consequences for the war victims. [34] The film also affected Van Agt himself, although in his case this did not lead to a change of opinion. It's said he was deeply impressed and moved by the psychological effects that (the discussion about) release had on the war survivors. He took Bastiaans aside during the session of the parliamentary committee. The psychiatrist remarked about this conversation: "I believe that the minister initially based himself mainly on the human application of the legal principles towards the Breda Three, but that now he much more wants to take the consequences of release for the victims of war into account."[35]

In an interview Bastiaans said that in his two-hour meeting with Van Agt he suggested the idea of a survey among the war victims and that the minister was seriously considering this. Admittedly it would not be easy to trace those tens of thousands of victims, but the various war organisations should be able to ensure this. The problem with this proposal was that it ran counter to Bastiaans' own idea of preferring a hefty blow above recurring torture. It prompted the interviewer to ask what his position would have been if there had been the possibility of keeping the three locked up without any prospects of pardon; the position of Auschwitz Committee chairman Slagter. Then, Bastiaans said, "this is what I would have preferred".[36]

Bastiaans' opinion, which gradually became less and less firm in favour of release, was the most important medical thermometer for the MPs.[37] However, he was anything but the only psychiatrist who had something to say about the matter. A large demonstration against release had taken place in Amersfoort on 23 February. The Amsterdam Jewish psychiatrist, resistance fighter and Auschwitz and Buchenwald survivor, Max Hamburger, was one of the speakers. He in particular resisted release because the three never showed any remorse. They probably hadn't. But this wasn't the only thing bothering him. Their victims, he said, had been "neglected and neglected by successive governments and large groups of the Dutch people". Time and again, Dutch post war society had shown it didn't want to be confronted with the years of war and occupation.[38]

Armand Sunier got involved in the discussion as well. He was the director of Jewish Mental Health Care and of the Sinai Centre in Amersfoort. Four to five thousand Jewish camp victims had been nursed there from 1960 onwards (to later switch to a more general target group later). He stated that if the Breda Three indeed were released the former inmates' emotions will again become topical without even carrying "a germ of a solution". They then will feel "placed back in the danger zone".[39] In other words, don't do this to the victims.

On 24 February 1972, the day after the parliamentary screening of *Do you now understand why I cry...*, the hearing by the Permanent Committee for Justice took place in the Second Chamber's meeting room. It completed Bastiaans' transformation from proponent of release to its opponent. Nearly forty organisations applied to be heard. Ten minutes each, which meant the meeting would last approximately seven hours. Bastiaans spoke on behalf of the Jelgersma clinic, Teengs Gerritsen on behalf of the Camp Syndrome Clinic Foundation.[40]

It was, to put it very mildly, a rather tumultuous gathering. Proponents of a pardon, such as the Catholic peace movement Pax Christi and the Coornhert League for criminal law reform, described in *De Tijd* as an association of alternative lawyers, were regularly stopped from speaking. With similar regularity it was argued that pardoning would strike an unbearable blow to all who survived the Nazi-horrors.[41] No fewer than 35 organisations said that the effect release would have on the victims was their most compelling argument.[42]

Remarkably, the representative of the Coornhert League, professor of law Louk Hulsman, also referred to the medical side of the story, but in his case to support his position; a position mainly based on the fact that further detention contradicted the principle of effectiveness, which should be always kept in mind when sentencing. However, Hulsman – who, like his fellow lawyer and former Professor Van Agt, in a letter to the *NRC Handelsblad* was accused of sailing "under the false flag of science" –[43] added to his legal reasoning that if he understood Bastiaans and *Do you now understand why I cry...* correctly, it was clear that continued detention did anything but help the victims, whilst rekindling the discussion with every request for pardon worked negatively on the minds of those suffering from concentration camp syndrome for sure.[44] It was exactly the view that Bastiaans held. At least, that's what Hulsman thought.

As said, when, shortly after Hulsman, Bastiaans held his speech he did so in a room cluttered with emotions. The atmosphere was set by hostility to those advocating a pardon and by emphasising the enormous and terrible psychological consequences release would have for camp survivors and former resistance fighters. Hostility towards proponents also set the stage outside the Chamber, including threatening letters and "unsavoury telephone calls", especially addressed at Van Agt. Several times this led to temporary relocations of family members of proponents, in a single case even to police surveillance, and, in the afternoon prior to the public broadcast of *Do you now understand why I cry...,* to a bomb threat in the VARA studio.[45]

After it already was threatened a few days earlier, the VARA again was called by a woman who announced that at half past four a bomb would detonate. According to the *Leeuwarder Courant* (Leeuwarden's Paper), it was placed because of the broadcast of the film, according to other newspapers, however, because according to her the VARA advocated the release of the three. To be on the safe side, the broadcast of a live concert including audience was cancelled.[46]

It soon became clear that Bastiaans no longer was on Hulsman's side. Although Bastiaans denied having changed his mind,[47] little was left of his earlier plea in favour of a hefty blow, or as the *Limburgsch Dagblad* and *Tubantia* stated: "Even Prof. Dr. Bastiaans of the Jelgersma clinic was more dismissive of the government's position than the day before" when he introduced Van Gasteren's film to the MPs.[48] It was a twist of which, with a sense of understatement, Prime Minister Barend Biesheuvel said: "In recent days Prof. Bastiaans' position was quite subjected to change."[49] He left it at that. He assured he would consider all arguments but didn't want to go into those of the professor any further, nor of those of other psychiatrists at that.[50]

During the hearing, Bastiaans stated that the "so-called legal limitations" of the sentences of the three didn't outweigh the medical consequences of continued mental and physical suffering of tens of thousands. Previously he limited his remarks to what he observed within his own patient group of a several dozen people, but now he spoke about the entire population of camp survivors and former resistance fighters. Moving the three back to Germany would bring certainty to a small group, but uncertainty to a vast majority.

> For many of them, the period 1940-1945 lives as if it was yesterday or even today. For them, the suffering is not time-barred. And the potential release of the Breda Three has sparked fear and anxiety all over and has already in many exacerbated the symptoms of post concentration camp syndrome.[51]

So according to Bastiaans, the rights of perpetrators were outweighed by the suffering and insecurity of the victims. Although 27 years in prison was worse than the death penalty, and as a human being he opposed this, as a doctor he was obliged to look first and foremost to what is best for his patients, what is, in other words, best for the victims – according to *De Tijd* mentioning the number 30,000 and according to *Trouw* 40,000. For some of them release was acceptable, but to the majority pardon was "the deepest insult to their own existence and to their beloved deceased. They accept the risk that new requests for clemency will periodically lead to the same discussions and therefore to a temporary or permanent aggravation of their illness".[52] He had to exchange his initial preference for a blow for regular torture because the majority of the victims themselves wanted it. It was a twist with consequences. The movie of him treating a KZ syndrome patient made many change their ideas already, or at least made them doubt, and now Bastiaans' "impressive scientific account" did the rest. It, *De Telegraaf* wrote, was "of great significance for the turnaround" from proponent of release to opponent many MPs and ministers went through.[53]

Tubantia kept it more general, saying that the testimonies of some psychiatrists, in addition to Bastiaans, Musaph and Sunier, about the KZ syndrome many war victims suffered from, impressed the most.[54] Sunier said that release "would destroy all the recovery work of years" and that he feared he would then have to welcome "a multiple of three" at the Sinai Centre.[55] And Musaph stated that the government had no moral right to consider release until all necessary financial, social and medical assistance measures were taken that the victims needed.[56] According to *De Tijd,* in the days of the film screening and the hearing, the group of supporters shrunk from 80 to 37 (in the end it turned out to be 61). Certainly, the paper wrote, as Bastiaans said as well, a small group of war survivors would be at peace with their release, but the bulk of them would get sick or even sicker than they already were, an effect that most likely would not be temporary.[57]

One of the MPs changing from proponent to opponent was lawyer Aart Geurtsen. He was not just any MP. He was the Justice Department spokesperson for the VVD, one of the parties taking part in the Biesheuvel cabinet, which had taken office in 1971. At the time of the pardon discussions, he also was chairman of the Parliamentary Judiciary Committee. His empathetic demeanour during the hearing earned him the respect of many. In an article published in various newspapers, he explained his turn. It's striking that it kept pace with Bastiaans' change of view and that the screening of *Do you now understand why I cry...* played a major role in it. Initially, he was in favour of release. Like Bastiaans, he feared "that the repeated discussion about whether or not the three should be released again and again would revive the victim's past and confront them with the loss of so many loved ones once again". In retrospect, he thought this was too rational an approach. It had begun to waver while watching the movie. In it, the patient suddenly exclaimed: "Please, understand what I'm saying!" It had been that cry of despair which had made him think a pardon could be wrong.[58]

The hearing perpetuated the doubt. In it only generally known facts about the reality behind words like Amersfoort, Natzweiler, Auschwitz were presented. However, in this setting, they very much came to life again and once more became "a terrible reality". Geurtsen could only immensely admire those who had the courage to tell their stories. For them, the hearing must have been torturous. Moreover, the psychiatrists' stories presented their "moving, yet almost clinical diagnosis". They too made clear that for many release would at least have temporary, but more probably long-lasting consequences. The decisive factor was a conversation during a short recess, which was called because emotions ran wild. Geurtsen spoke a man who was totally upset. He suddenly crumpled up and said the worst thing Geurtsen heard the entire day: "How I would have loved my children to have been spared it."

> It was then that I realised that whatever ethical or other considerations there are, they can never justify people having to go through again so painfully what has been done to their children. From that moment on I am convinced that if this issue is concerned with humanity in criminal law and its application, then it's about humanity and solidarity towards and with the victims first and foremost and not towards the perpetrators. As long as such deep sorrow can be

> evoked in people who have been told that their executioners and those of their children may be released, releasing them is the most inhumane thing we can do.[59]

Of course, Geurtsen added, the Netherlands is a parliamentary democracy, and in such a system free speech is guaranteed. This didn't alter that in the discussion that necessarily ensued, the victims were entitled to the support from all the Dutch, and that they would not be abandoned by them once more. For then they knew "that all has not been in vain, and that their sorrows will not be neglected".[60]

Geurtsen wasn't alone. Many initial proponents followed in his footsteps. Releasing the three would be an abomination to the victims of the Nazi regime. As a result, also releasing them one by one received no support.[61] In this the victims' wishes, partly expressed by the psychiatrists, were decisive. Even though proponents of release weren't blind or deaf to the interests and pain of the victims either, in their eyes the "fight against injustice and inhumanity", exactly the fight that was fought during the war, had to carry more weight. However, the argument that detention went against the norms of the criminal justice system, was dismissed as cold and heartless. For example, left-liberal MP Anneke Goudsmit, initiator of the hearing, said that the rules of criminal law weren't written for the extreme crimes committed from May 1940 to May 1945.[62]

Goudsmit expressed an opinion shared by psychiatrist Jacques Weijel, professor of social insurance and survivor of Theresienstadt. People need to be sure that real evil will not go unpunished. This hadn't been the case during the war, resulting in mental injuries. The idea that maybe this once again wouldn't happen certainly played into the turmoil over the three. No, Weijel confirmed, taking revenge didn't help, but mercy was no solution either.[63]

The government, although not bound by a parliamentary decision as regards pardoning convicts, decided not to proceed with Van Agt's plan. A lengthy newspaper article by Hulsman on February 28 – 'Pardoning the Three: the lesser of two evils' – could do little to change this.[64] It will not have helped that on the same page as his plea the reasoning of Van Agt's predecessor Polak was brought back to memory: there can be no question of release if the Second Chamber and therefore the Dutch people oppose it.[65]

Even a large article in *De Telegraaf* by the then eminent professor of law at the Catholic University in Nijmegen, Frans Duynstee, no longer had any influence on the outcome. Duynstee focused on the emotional atmosphere and the subsequent threats because they were a hindrance to a balanced judgement. He was astonished that due to these emotions some

MPs preferred not to show themselves to stay out of harm's way. And he found it worrying that in just a few days Bastiaans had changed his mind. Pressured by the reactions, he had come to a position that was the complete reversal of his earlier one. This new position, that medically spoken detention was preferable to release, subsequently dominated the hearing.[66] Implicitly diametrically opposed to Geurtsen, he wrote:

> Everyone will understand that people who are sick as a result of what they suffered during the occupation have feelings of revenge and express them. But who can maintain that government policy should orient itself on this and that it should step aside for it? We would be treading a path which in the long run would make the humanisation of criminal justice impossible. Victims of offenses could start to influence the nature and severity of the punishment. Starting with war criminals, it's very doubtful whether one will have sufficient strength to resist the penal system from being dominated by the human urge for revenge any further. Why, in principle, should revenge be legitimate in the case of war crimes but not in the case of other serious crimes against fellow human beings?[67]

Not only from a legal, but also from a psychiatric point of view Bastiaans was criticised. According to psychiatrist Jan Lumeij Bastiaans' argumentation was unsound, as, by the way, was Musaph's. Based on mental health arguments Lumeij argued in favour of release and therefore spoke about Bastiaans' latter plea against a pardon. However, his remarks can also be related to Bastiaans' earlier point of view. According to Lumeij, in his reasoning the honourable professor put aside his psychiatric expertise. Instead, he based his opinion on his involvement with war victims, who continuously told him release would have a disastrous effect on their state of mind. This, however, should not play no role at all in a psychiatric opinion. After all, one also couldn't advise a woman to marry a man because he threatened to commit suicide if she didn't. It was precisely this threat that was detrimental to mental health.[68]

The motion arguing against release was discussed in the night of 29 February to 1 March 1972. A large majority of MPs backed it, both from opposition and government parties. The debate, followed by millions of Dutch people on radio and television, again led to emotional scenes in as well the MPs' benches as in the public gallery.[69] An attempt by Van Agt to have a group of experts decide on further decision-making failed as well. It concerned doctors, lawyers, war victims, and members of the former resistance. They not only had to look at social reactions and consequences but to consider the physical and mental condition of the Breda Three as well. Various newspapers reported that it was an idea Bastiaans was anything but happy with. He would have liked to have previously an opportunity to investigate the consequences for the victims of the resulting postponement of the decision to release the Breda Three one by one or detain them permanently.[70] It's a comment suggesting he felt that he should be consulted prior to any cabinet decision related to war syndromes.

It doesn't alter that all in all Bastiaans could be satisfied. In addition to his speech during the hearing, the outcome of the parliamentary debate on 29 February was heavily influenced by the decision of the VARA to broadcast *Do you now understand why I cry...* with him giving the accompanying commentary, a few days before the parliamentary debate. This again turned proponents into opponents, both in parliament and society. The version was the most recent one, shown at the Fifth World Congress of Psychiatry in Mexico in November 1971, including images of the patient shot some years after the original film had been made.[71]

9. THE TV BROADCAST OF *DO YOU NOW UNDERSTAND WHY I CRY...*

> These days television helped to 'rediscover' the victims of the German concentration camps. Rediscovered in quotes, because they have been with us for 27 years, but now, in the discussion about the Breda Three, their need penetrated the public mind and can be used as a strong argument against pardoning them.[1]

These are the opening lines of an article called 'KZ victims "rediscovered" on TV' published on 26 February 1972. It was written by Jan Bank, then television critic for *de Volkskrant* but from 1988 to 2005 professor of Dutch history at Leiden University. Bank wrote this on the eve of the broadcast of *Do you now understand why I cry...*, but nevertheless already felt that the familiarity of terms such as KZ syndrome and the general compassion for those who suffer from it couldn't be explained without pointing at this fairly new medium. He used the words "the reality of" which means that Bank himself had no doubts about the existence of the syndrome. The government recognised and acknowledged this reality as well, but too late and, moreover, even then highly insufficiently. Most importantly, though, his article dealt with the wave of emotions triggered by the proposed release. For this too he blamed the government. It had come to this only because it had allowed it to come to this. It was an emotionality which came to the fore perfectly in a television report made of a gathering of former prisoners and resistance members. First, they were addressed by Cohen and Goudsmit, subsequently by Bastiaans. The last one addressed the issue of victims' needs "in a committed and at the same time distant manner".[2]

But the historian in Bank could not just point at the emotions. He wanted to analyse as well. In his view, the emotions could only in part be explained by the suffering inflicted. The same was true for the feelings of guilt the Netherlands had after it became clear how large the percentage of its Jewish population was that had been deported to the extermination camps, or rather: after it had become clear it had them deported. Among other things, this was nourished by a two-thousand-year-old "Christian tradition" of anti-Semitism. It also had to do with the Zeitgeist. Firstly, there was the end of pillarisation, the system in which groups like Catholics, Protestants and socialists lived, although fairly peacefully, next to each other instead of together. As a result, the choice "for or against releasing the three" changed from a collective decision driven by a party or a newspaper to an individual one. More important, however, was the humanisation of criminal law, not to be separated from this same individualisation. Part of the humanisation was that criminals were increasingly seen as individuals and therefore no longer symbolised, in the case of the Breda Three, a racist and destructive ideology and organisation. The other side of the coin was that arguments from proponents, such as that continuous punishment was meaningless, no longer convinced but only provoked aggression. "Judging by the statements of a number of former resistance members, one gets the impression that humanisation arouses their anger, because it robs them of a possibility of revenge."[3]

The possible broadcasting of Van Gasteren's movie by the VARA was the reason for Bank to write his article, but the VARA came close to cancelling the plan altogether. The idea to show it to the entire population was based on the wish to make the Dutch "widely acquainted with the current problems of war victims, in particular the consequences of staying in German concentration camps called KZ syndrome".[4] Because the broadcaster was convinced the ministry owed the screening rights, the Minister of CRM, Piet Engels, was asked for permission. Based on the agreements made with Bastiaans and Expogé in 1969, the association of all except communist ex-political prisoners, he said he didn't think this to be a good idea. At the time it was argued that there was a good chance broadcasting it would have adverse consequences for concentration camp victims. There was no reason to believe this would have changed in the meantime. However, the TV critic of *Trouw* suspected that Engels was rather afraid to stir up emotions even higher than already was the case.[5]

According to the *Leeuwarder Courant* the most striking aspect of the film was the relentless demand for understanding, something that also echoed in the protests against the release of the Breda Three. Release was imagined as an official end of a past which, according to the opponents, hadn't finished at all and probably never would. This incomprehension had typified the refusal of Engels and had only deepened the perceived powerlessness and insecurity of the camp victims.[6]

However, a spokesmen of Engels' department assured that the minister hadn't given his advice – so: not 'protest', let alone 'ban', the word used on the TV news shortly before the broadcast on Saturday evening – in his capacity as Minister responsible for broadcasting affairs, but because he was responsible for overseeing the interests of the war victims as well. He had carefully listened to the views of Dordrecht lawyer Gerhard Charles (Charlie) Aalders, chairman of Expogé. Contrary to Bastiaans, who was consulted too, Aalders still considered broadcasting the movie to be irresponsible. Therefore, there was no question of an attempt to censor or ban. However, he added, should the VARA decide to go ahead with its intentions, any negative consequences for the victims were entirely "the personal responsibility of Professor Bastiaans".[7]

Shortly after the broadcast of *Do you now understand why I cry...* Aalders died of a heart attack at the age of 59. Although both his family and his physician denied there was any relationship between his death and the broadcasting of the film – Aalders had been suffering from ill health for some time – Bastiaans, after having stated that he was not implying that they were wrong, couldn't restrain from pointing out that heart failure was a hallmark of the concentration camp syndrome.[8]

Engels was anything but the only politician questioning the VARA's plans. Early April, the lawyer Isaäc Diepenhorst, MP for the Christian *Anti-Revolutionaire Partij* ARP (Anti-Revolutionary Party), wanted to know whether Bastiaans hadn't acted in violation of medical professional secrecy by agreeing to the broadcast. Physician Louis Stuyt, Minister of Health on behalf of the *Katholieke Volkspartij* KVP (Catholic People's Party), replied is was certainly possible that medical-ethical boundaries were overstepped.[9] Stuyt's answer bewildered Bastiaans. He thought it was incomprehensible because actually it was the exact opposite. Broadcasting the picture "had been a matter of the highest ethical considerations". Apart from the fact that some sort of first aid had been arranged for troubled viewers and that as far as known the broadcast hadn't claimed any casualties, the patient who was questioned in the film consented to the broadcast. And moreover: "We had to do something for the war victims."[10]

Bastiaans opposed full public display in 1969 and initially took this same view three years later. However, he assured late February this was before he knew that, because of first rate medical supervision, there were no risks involved. Around and about twenty psychiatrists reported to him to be willing to render aid to viewers who, as a result of the broadcast, had gotten mentally disturbed.[11]

The pressure of the moment made medical-ethical objections against broadcasting to an audience larger than physicians and medical students, put forward in 1969, fluid. But that the couple who starred in the movie had given up any hesitations regarding a public screening, silenced critical opinions in 1972. Still, every day they were grateful to Bastiaans for the LSD treatment the husband had received, and they had come to believe that broadcasting could help other war victims. This was confirmed in the media. In an article in *Het Parool,* the patient and his wife announced that the day after the television broadcast they received a phone call from some acquaintances. “Only now, after all these years, had they come to peace with the death of their daughter (in Sachsenhausen), because only now had they understood what her fate would have been had she survived the war.”[12] Or, as it was said a few years later in *Het Parool*: “Surviving camps is worse than dying.”[13]

On the advice of Bastiaans and after the board of the VARA had seen the film, the decision to indeed broadcast the movie was finally taken. Expert guidance had to be provided, but as mentioned, that had already been taken care of. Before and after the broadcast, the film was commented on by psychiatrists Hugenholtz, Van Tol, Weijel and, of course, Bastiaans himself. Nevertheless, his cooperation had been less obvious than one might think. On Saturday morning he announced not to cooperate. According to him, the film had nothing to do with the discussion on the Breda Three and therefore didn’t point in any direction, neither in favour of nor opposed to release, which would have been surprising indeed because it outdated the discussion several years. However, he decided to change his decision because in his eyes the film could contribute to “a calmer judgment about the future prospects for victims and about the options for assistance and treatment”.[14]

Weijel, personally in favour of gradually releasing the three, commented right from the heart and left nothing to guess about his feelings towards the Dutch government. Until recently it might indeed have been better not to throw the film out in the open. However, after everything this “short-sighted and stupid government unleashed”, it could only bear witness to an ostrich mentality “to be against it out of fear everything will be stirred up again”.[15] Judging by *de Volkskrant* and *Het Parool,* he added that the authoritarian way in which Biesheuvel and his followers reacted to the emotions they themselves evoked, displaying a “tough governmental attitude”, could only be characterised as “polarising between revenge and mercy”. Governing in a democratic way, Weijel said, “means being careful with the feelings of all the people in the country”. 40,000 men and women protested at the Dockworker, commemorating the February strike and testifying against release. This pointed at “a multitude of people who have been hurt” proving that “a large group of ordinary people feel unhappy with the blunt policy of their own government”.[16] Often, Weijel went on, expressions of revenge, as heard by the Dockworker, were “expressions of a powerlessness to really grieve, to really vent”. The same was true of mercy. This too was often an expression of impotence because the government didn’t come up with adequate solutions.[17]

It was a view endorsed by Hugenholtz, professor of anthropological psychopathology and long-standing medical advisor to the Foundation

1940-1945. The man who two years earlier published an article titled 'Unfinished Past' in which he analysed what it really meant to be in the resistance, said that the government could have started the discussion about the three in many ways. Almost all would have been more satisfying than the actual path chosen, and almost all would have required a lot less of the resilience of those involved.[18]

After the film was broadcasted the VARA had six telephones available, manned by people who in the afternoon were prepared by Musaph. They had to process so many phone calls that not all could be answered. The numbers mentioned vary from 600 to over 800. Later on, about 2000 letters were added: 1500 to the Ministry of Justice, 175 to Bastiaans personally and the others to the VARA. Those who did have their say generally reported that it was good the film finally had been shown to a large audience. According to Bastiaans, these telephone calls proved they had succeeded in "casting oil on the highly stored waves of emotions".[19]

According to *Het Vrije Volk,* there had been no negative reactions whatsoever, citing, it said, the VARA and Bastiaans.[20] But that's a bit on the optimistic side. According to Bastiaans, Van Tol and Weijel, two-thirds of the callers expressed their agreement. However, according to them, the VARA itself and to the *NIW,* there also had been about ten, often economically and/or politically motivated, cases of anti-Semitic verbal abuse. Also, about fifty people indicated that television was meant to entertain; an opinion for which the *Nederlands Dagblad* had just one word in store: eerie.[21] Striking had been the large number of reactions from people who had been in a Japanese internment camp, who, for example, said that what they had been through had been "just as bad, if not worse", or: "of course not as bad, but we feel as if the Netherlands have abandoned, have forgotten us." Twenty to thirty disturbed people were forwarded to the expert team.[22] If they lived in the vicinity of Amsterdam, maybe, the somewhat cynical poet and journalist Nico Scheepmaker wrote, they could be forwarded to the *Binnengasthuis* (Central Hospital) where a number of medics was present, "ready to personally receive overly shocked viewers". He even heard that, just to be on the safe side, in the Wilhelmina Hospital some beds had been left empty.[23] In many cases, according to Bastiaans, those referrals led to an appointment with a psychiatrist, which easily could be the first step towards recovery.[24]

In spite of his mild cynicism, Scheepmaker, who a short time later became known to the general public because of his book *Cruijff, Hendrik Johannes, phenomenon,* was very enthusiastic about the film and the decision to broadcast it. In his TV column 'Kastje Kijken' (Watching telly) he described it as "a statue for the tortured twentieth century man". It, for the first time, made very clear that despair is "an integral part of your personality". The Dutch population should therefore be grateful to the VARA that it had not backed away from its intentions "despite the enormous pressure the government" had exerted on it.[25]

Like Bank, Scheepmaker looked at the broadcast in a broader sense. Showing the picture hadn't been a cinematographic and psycho-hygienic act alone, but a political one as well. Although in itself, as Bastiaans stated, the film had nothing to do with the ongoing heated discussion, Scheepmaker judged that showing it was indispensable for obtaining the correct information about the matter and thus for a well-considered opinion about whether or not the Breda Three should be released. The VARA therefore rightly thought that a film considered indispensable for the decision-making of members of parliament, was indispensable as well "for all other fully-fledged, articulate Dutch inhabitants".[26]

The reviewer of *Trouw* was equally enthusiastic and advocated repetition. After all, the film "proved" that with the assistance of LSD "many of the approximately 40,000 psycho-traumatic war victims" could be cured. For this the only thing the government had to do, was to dig a little deeper into its pockets making an extension of medical and social facilities possible. "This too is a very positive tenor of the film."[27]

Herman Hofhuizen of *De Tijd* and Wim Jungman of *Het Parool* were among the few reviewers putting question marks. They were in the respectable company of Duynstee, according to whom the broadcasting, although clarifying, was very indiscrete. Again, Bastiaans was his main target. Although in *De Tijd* the psychiatrist said that many of his patients still bore feelings of revenge, Duynstee hadn't seen any evidence of this in the film. The man at the centre of it was "rightly against the Nazi system, but precisely not against the individual criminals".[28]

Hofhuizen agreed. The VARA had broadcasted the film to help the Dutch population form an opinion about the three, although Bastiaans himself said it was neither in favour of nor against release. This raised the question how it could help that population to reach such an opinion. In addition, Bastiaans spoke of "a professional film, like one on a kidney transplant". He put the emotional side of it into perspective by saying that any emotional movie could upset a person. He thus created the impression that television viewers "in a clinical manner had to look at something completely clinically". He therefore doubted whether Bastiaans correctly assessed the situation that had arisen. According to Hofhuizen, a lot of people watched the film "with an anything but clinical eye". He used Weijel's words about the government's blunt policy as evidence for this.[29]

The decision to proceed to public broadcast was therefore not approved by Hofhuizen. This had nothing to do with the movie itself. It was of an "unassailable integrity and also a poignant document". It was the political context on which his doubts were based.

> That it was shown on the screen at this moment, in these eventful days when honourable people, who on completely honourable grounds plead for releasing the three, must be placed under police guard, seems to me a highly debatable matter. That the VARA confronted us insistently with a horrifying problem for more than two hours on Saturday evening may perhaps be called an act of bravery. But an act of bravery is not always and under all circumstances also an act of wisdom.[30]

This was the approach of Jungman too, the TV critic of *Het Parool* who already had written pieces for, among others, this former resistance paper during the war. He as well said the film was a "gripping document about helping a man to be able to say farewell to the past". But it was decided for a good reason to only show the film before a limited audience in 1969. Yes, he wrote, there had been discussion among the VARA staff. And yes, their intention hardened by the pressure the government exerted on Bastiaans not to broadcast or to cooperate with broadcasting. It was unclear whether this pressure was the result of public health concerns or more opportunistic reasons. And yes, when Bastiaans decided to resist government pressure, the VARA had done everything possible to minimise the risks. But all this failed to change Jungman's view that it would have been better had the decision to screen the picture been cancelled "as a final argument against a questionable and pitifully presented government decision".[31]

It was, Jungman continued, illustrative of "the polarisation of points of view, the flare-up of passions, that, at a time which was the least suited to confront a broad and uneducated public with it" since 1969, it nevertheless was decided to broadcast the picture on TV. Such a lack of knowledge also characterised the average MP. Yet, as they themselves informed him, the film impressed them so much that it had turned many from favouring to opposing pardon.[32] In other words, the broadcaster that received a bomb threat, perhaps because of an alleged pro-release stance, broadcasted a picture that, although it was neither pro or con, played a major role in the Second Chamber's decision to oppose release. This, Jungman's point was, went far beyond the journalistic task of informing an audience. This was, intentionally or unintentionally, nothing but influencing in favour of continued detention.

In the week after the broadcast, Bastiaans, Van Tol and Weijel presented a "quickly made booklet", entitled *Leven na een Oorlog* (Living after a War). Although the issue of the Breda Three was not explicitly addressed, the date of publication was no coincidence, which is clear from the fact that it contained an article by an editor of the VARA about the public reactions after the television broadcast of *Do you now know why I cry*... In the booklet, the treatment with psychotropic drugs was positively discussed. The numbers 30 to 40,000 were repeated, to which was added that there were also "several millions of Dutch people with distressing memories from the war". Although they probably didn't have a real syndrome, their experiences were and remained a burden all the same. In addition, it was reiterated that the syndrome wasn't linked to the Second World War. According to Van Tol, it could arise anytime and anywhere "where the free expression of opinions and feelings is suppressed, and people are left behind powerless".[33] It isn't without reason that in the meantime also the term 'after-pain syndrome' was proposed to emphasise the general character of the KZ syndrome.[34]

The collection of articles was intended "to provide a large public with insight into the psychological consequences of war experiences and into the forms and possibilities of the treatment thereof". According to the publisher, the *Nationaal Centrum voor Geestelijke Gezondheid* (National Centre for Mental Health), the need for information about it suddenly increased rapidly. It was hoped that the booklet could help victims to recognise the symptoms of the KZ syndrome more quickly, to discover they were not alone, and that they could seek medical attention. In addition, it was hoped that the collection would help people without damaging war experiences to better understand the victims and thus improve assisting them in their distress.[35]

The extensive attention the collection received in the newspapers must be explained entirely from the context of the trial against the Breda Three and the broadcasting of Van Gasteren's film. The booklet itself, in fact, mirrored the speed with which it had been put on the market. In appearance it resembled a student's term paper more than a professorial publication. It was little more than thirty pages printed one sided, with a green front on which the title was typed, held together by a ring binder. It's also striking that on the front it states: "with the cooperation of, among others, prof. dr. J.A. Bastiaans, D. van Tol, neurologist and prof. dr. J.A. Weijel", while only two others contributed to the collection. But they were journalists, not scientists, or, more specifically, not psychiatrists.[36]

Living after a War was critically discussed only by the Protestant-Christian newspaper *Nederlands Dagblad*, although the basic attitude and conclusion were as positive as with other papers. This already is clear in the opening sentence by psychiatrist Pieter Leendert Los: "This collection was created in a week and bears the traces in the form of *otherwise unimportant carelessness*." (Ital.: LvB) What followed was a summary of the various articles. The criticism focused mainly on Van Tol's article and especially on the passages about LSD, a drug the reviewer called "this dangerous poison". On the one hand, Los was pleased that Van Tol warned against non-medical use. On the other hand, he contradicted his comment, which had also come up in Van Gasteren's film, that LSD had the advantage over hypnosis or pentothal – a short-acting, hypnotic, sedating barbiturate that has been used earlier and more often than LSD – that nothing discussed during the course, faded from memory. Certainly, in the case of hypnosis, Los hadn't noticed a disappearance of the memory of what had been said and happened during the treatment either. All in all, however, the collection was a warning to be welcomed "that we must give our bruised fellow man the opportunity to speak out" and that we should never prevent war victims from "expressing their emotions".

> The one who is so harassed that he no longer finds or thinks he can't find understanding even in church or his family, he for whom doors are truly shut because people find it boring to listen to his stories because they think entertainment is more important, shouldn't be ashamed to enlist the help of professionals. He shouldn't reach for a cigarette, a drink or LSD: After 27 years there really are a number of people who finally understand why he cries.[37]

Bastiaans didn't want to stick to this thin collection of a few short, hardly original articles. He, firstly, advocated a central treatment institute for war victims that should set up discussion groups throughout the country as well, delivering outpatient care, for example in the form of creative, expressive and occupational therapy.[38] He, secondly, also announced that he was taking part in a working group consisting of three psychiatrists, a sociologist and two VARA-journalists, aiming to publish a real book in the autumn of 1972, about the reactions to the discussion about the Breda Three and the broadcast of the film of Van Gasteren, who became the secretary of this working group. The victims of German and Japanese camps would take centre stage. Only this announcement of a possible release in about halve a year of a book on the KZ syndrome, received wide press coverage already.[39] It was never published.

10. THE INFLUENCE OF THE BREDA THREE DISCUSSION

Meanwhile, during all the almost literal clatter of arms, the plans for the construction of a KZ syndrome clinic progressed. Naturally, this was profoundly influenced by the Breda Three discussion. Although the general public had become aware of the reality of the camps in the 1960s already, according to *de Volkskrant* the actual victims remained invisible until the debate about the three and the TV broadcast of *Do you now understand why I cry…* Suddenly, what for a long time seemed impossible, became reality: the implementation of the long-standing plan to create a special clinic for them.[1] One of the readers of *Trouw* suggested that the three should only be released on the condition that Germany would pay for the construction of the clinic and the subsequent treatment of the thousands of traumatised Nazi-victims so they would be cared for well and free of charge, and perhaps even be cured.[2]

Therefore, the Foundation Post Concentration Camp Syndrome Centre was obliged to comment when, at the height of the Breda Three debate, mid to late February 1972, the news was spread that the construction could start at the beginning of April. Teengs Gerritsen, who declared use of force was to be expected if the three were to be released,[3] said:

> In these days of understandable emotions about three war criminals, once again the visible and audible tragedy of all the thousands who can't possibly break free from the horrors of war has become apparent. I do agree with the socialist MP Voogd, who seriously fears several war victims will die if the Breda Three are released. It for certain will accelerate the death of many former resistance fighters and Jewish people.[4]

He would rather have waited with his announcement that indeed a centre for people suffering from KZ syndrome would be opened in Oegstgeest, until all necessary permits from the hospital committee and the Ministry of Finance had been received. However, all the commotion about the Breda Three made him decide to make it public prematurely in the hope that, not in the least because of the support of the Queen and Prince, "soon something substantial will be done about the suffering of the victims of war criminals".[5]

Teengs Gerritsen was certain. The pavilion or rest home, words he preferred above clinic, became "a devilishly nice thing" with a medical exterior completely separated from the living area in the middle. Bastiaans would be the clinic's consultant. International interest was immense because no such institution had ever been built before. He didn't know exactly how many potential patients were involved but suspected the number ran into the thousands. Therefore, the intended twenty beds certainly wouldn't be enough, even though the first intention wasn't so much treatment on the spot as familiarising doctors throughout the country with the syndrome and its treatment methods. However, if need be, naturally deliberations about how to expand the capacity would start. Although some of the victims had already been treated in the Jelgersma clinic, this wasn't deemed satisfactory because of the, as it was called, frustrating presence of other patients suffering from other psychological problems. Contrary, in the clinic "they can talk to like-minded people about the same topic. The phrase 'You don't understand what I'm talking about' will no longer have to be uttered."[6]

That almost immediately substantial aid could be delivered, was directly related to the Breda Three discussion as well. Besides that the discussion had led to cancelling their intended release, another outcome was that the government had informed the *Bond van Nederlandse Militaire Oorlogsslachtoffers* BNMO (Association of Dutch Military War Victims) that it was prepared to assist it with the aftercare it rendered. Concretely, this meant that it soon would send proposals "for aid to the neglected groups of war victims". This could include pension rights, financial assistance for medical treatment, and social support. *De Volkskrant* didn't beat around the bush. "This sudden government interest is the direct result of the overwhelming response to the revoked decision to release the three German war criminals."[7]

Bastiaans, "the great expert on the concentration camp syndrome", the paper added probably unnecessarily, was asked to set up a catch-up programme for "war victims suffering from unhealed psychological and social wounds". He wanted to start with a cautious inventory of those affected, also to determine priority in treatment. In addition, the therapy they received had to be well organised. Referring to the common belief that the appointment of a group of experts was just an attempt by the government to put the issue of the Breda Three on hold, at least temporarily, he observed: "I am convinced that by providing more security for the affected groups, making treatment and counselling financially possible, a calmer assessment of what should be done with the three Germans will soon develop."[8]

The discussion impacted pension schemes also. At first, Minister Engels had no intention of changing financial regulations because he believed they had been improved considerably already. Moreover, the number of applications had increased considerably already as well. However, after his attempt failed in the previous Cabinet De Jong, Voogd again tried to arrange a separate scheme for Jewish war victims. Another motion was put forward by the Portuguese-Jewish doctor Jacques Baruch, MP for the party *Democratisch-Socialisten '70* DS'70 (Democratic Socialists 1970), a recent conservative split from the social-democratic *Partij van de Arbeid* PvdA (Labour Party). Although, like Voogd's did, this motion decoupled the payment from the Social Assistance Act as well, it didn't involve a separate arrangement for Jewish survivors. It was intended for all war victims, including those of Japanese internment camps.[9] Therefore, Baruch's motion appealed to both a larger and a younger group of victims. Many of the internees in the Japanese camps had been children, while the number of children who survived a German concentration camp was virtually nil. Together with the second-generation problem, still to be discussed, it was another reason that there was no question of "the war victims eligible for medical and social assistance becoming scarce".[10]

It was Baruch's motion that was accepted eventually. The National Group Regulation Prosecution Victims 1940-1945 was thus converted into the Prosecution Victims Benefit Act. At long last Voogd too voted in favour of this arrangement. Although it didn't go as far as he would have liked, it was an improvement over the previous regulation, in particular because of the decoupling of assistance.[11] However, due to the consternation about the possible release of the Breda Three, soon this arrangement came to be discussed. The Biesheuvel cabinet began to work on a law explicitly regulating benefits for those who were "persecuted by the enemy occupying powers for their race, religion or world view, or for their participation in the resistance", as well as for those who "became disabled or whose pre-existing disability was aggravated as a result of persecution or persecution circumstances". Once again, when reporting on these pension debates the papers took a step in heightening the numbers. When mentioning the usual numbers 30 to 40,000 the *NRC Handelsblad* added: "only those affected directly".[12]

In addition, both the *NRC* and the *NIW* stated there were "people in their daily environment (woman and children)" who suffered from the consequences as well. In the newspapers not only resistance fighters, but war victims in general usually were male. And then there were the tens of thousands of Dutch people who were weighed down by "extremely frightening memories of, for example, the *Arbeitseinzatz* (compulsory work placement. LvB) or going into hiding''. The *NRC Handelsblad* wrote this in the first of three full-page articles in which Bastiaans got ample opportunity to speak and in which, respectively, the clinical picture of the KZ syndrome, material support and social guidance were put in the spotlight. It stated that now it was scientifically proved that with the passage of time the syndrome's symptoms did not weaken but strengthen.[13]

The new law, regulating financial compensation for medical and social assistance in addition to pension rights, had to come into being around May 1972. Before that, talks would take place with all kinds of social organisations, such as the *Stichting Joods Maatschappelijk Werk* JMW (Jewish Social Work Foundation). According to *Trouw,* this foundation had some more groups to add to the list such as married female victims of persecution, who up to that point hadn't received any benefits.[14]

Shortly after the discussion about the three had ended, Voogd didn't spare himself in an interview with *Trouw*.

> I couldn't explain to myself that I was an MP for five years already and ignored the issue all the time. After all, we could all have recognised the problem long ago from Prof. Bastiaans' dissertation, which was published in 1956 (1957. LvB).
>
> When trying to explain this, three points seem important. The inability to imagine what those people have been through. Then there are the so-called '*Spätfolgen'* (the consequences that have only emerged in recent years). And the third important point is that, if you try to realise what those people have been through, you actually stop thinking about it because you can't possibly figure it out. You're going to transpose it onto your own family and then you say: stop right there.[15]

The soldiers who took part in the resistance and who hadn't been made POW were heard by the preparatory committee too. They weren't awarded a pension for their war activities – which had partly brought them into hiding, prison, or camp – although soldiers who had been in the German *Arbeitseinsatz* received one; a situation called insane in the Second Chamber already in 1970. Some of them suffered from the concentration camp syndrome as well, but, according to MP Vonhoff, they didn't dare to make this public out of fear it would be detrimental to promotion opportunities. Moreover, according to their champion and Natzweiler survivor Major Godert Willem Baron van Dedem, many of them dreaded the re-examination, possible disapproval, and because of this early and therefore lower pension, which only resulted in further aggravation of the complaints. Although in fact they already had collapsed, they dragged themselves through the rest of their service. It was frustrating that for years, with very little result, Van Dedem tried to get the Ministry of Defence to take responsibility. In any case, two interdepartmental commissions, set up with the help of Bastiaans in 1970, didn't bring the problem any closer to a solution. And:

> On my initiative, Professor Bastiaans gave a lecture on the post concentration camp syndrome last year – in front of all military doctors. That is hardly enough and, moreover, a bit late if one assumes that the Military Medical Council must have been aware that this professor already had obtained his doctorate in 1956 (1957. LvB) on this subject.[16]

Dedem also pointed at the international conference on belated effects of war experiences that was held in 1961 already and where the mentioned and then Lieutenant Colonel Van Overeem was present. Had he not, Van Dedem asked, already at the time could have taken charge of the medical and social supervision of military resistance fighters? Furthermore, the remark of another military doctor had always been in his mind. "I don't understand what you're so concerned about. If those people have died, isn't this problem solved automatically?" "Such a comment devastates me. I can only hope that it's not typical of those wanting to continue to discriminate against military resistance fighters."[17]

As a result of the discussion on the Breda Three the world changed for Van Dedem as well. Suddenly, he became a frequent guest at various ministries invited to submit his demands. Not that the doors had been hermetically closed in the past. He had his say before the Parliamentary Defence Committee in the autumn of 1970. This led to one of the two interdepartmental committees mentioned, to publish its first report in April 1971, a year after it had been founded. However, it contained little more than the recommendation to open a clinic for KZ syndrome patients and to recognise the disease. On top, three days later the De Jong cabinet fell. He again was able to address the Parliamentary Committee halve a year later, during the discussion of the Defence budget of 1972 in the autumn of 1971; a meeting characterised by several fierce interruptions because State Secretary Adri van Es "once again tried to hold back on the case of the post concentration camp syndrome". For example, the general in KVP service, Joop van Elsen, demanded proposals in this direction within two months, otherwise he himself would draw up a text; an interruption widely acclaimed. Nevertheless, the discussion about the Breda Three that started shortly afterwards revolutionised the entire playing field. When, one day after the decision to not release the three had been made, the Parliamentary Committee again debated with the State Secretary, "the issue was settled quickly".[18]

Van Dedem seized the opportunity and presented his demands: double-counting pension years for soldiers in the resistance and the camps, like those who had been able to travel to England were entitled to; free medical care for them and their families after being granted redundancy pay or pension; social counselling also after retirement; a benefit of 100 percent of the last salary received. *Het Vrije Volk* was confident that all four of them would be granted.

> It doesn't look as if the MPs will once again allow themselves to be confused by the remark that a separate regulation for military personnel is not the right way to go. On the contrary, it seems that the government will still be ordered to prepare the military arrangement for all other former resistance fighters as soon as possible, so that at last, 27 years after the war's end, also for them liberation can start.[19]

And this is what happened.

11. The construction of the Post Concentration Camp Syndrome Clinic

The very day Van Dedem formulated his demands, the news came that at least one necessary condition would be met soon: Prince Bernhard would drive into the earth the first pile of the KZ syndrome clinic on 17 April 1972.[1] The construction costs, for which the government issued a guarantee, were estimated at approximately 3.5 million guilders. For the time being, it indeed would have twenty beds, enough to treat an estimated eighty patients annually. In addition, an outpatient clinic was established for approximately two hundred patients every year.[2]

It was not surprising it was Bernhard who was granted the honour to perform the construction's beginning. The considerable problems the national foundation responsible for building the clinic encountered when acquiring the territory, were solved through mediation of State Secretary Kruisinga on the one hand, in spite of his LSD aversion, and Queen Juliana and her husband on the other. Bernhard even was so enthusiastic about Kruisinga's role that he "spontaneously, but also a bit naïve" proposed to name the pavilion after him. This, however, met with resistance from medical experts. They thought "that the patients with their specific disturbances would not be able to detect anything of a particular wavelength necessary in the proposed name". Moreover, Kruisinga himself, who was still convinced in 1971 that it was impossible to take appropriate measures for a separate group of war victims, said that to attach his name to the centre went a bit too far.[3]

W.L. Meijering, the Medical Inspector for Mental Health in the provinces North-Holland and Utrecht, was considered the perfect candidate for the position of medical director because he had been director of the Military Neurosis Hospital in Austerlitz, until it was closed down in 1963. However, his appointment proved to be a lot more difficult than at first sight. In his new position he had to regularly meet with Speijer. Speijer investigated abuses at the Dennendal department of the Willem Arntsz psychiatric clinic in Den Dolder. There, many thought, the anti-authoritarianism of the late 1960s and early 1970s had gotten somewhat out of hand. One of Speijer's conclusions was that Meijering, the Health Inspector responsible for Den Dolder, intervened too late. As a result, he was suspended. Mediation had to ensure the two wouldn't be at each other's throat every time they met at the clinic or at 'the Jel'. However, this problem resolved itself by the early retirement of Speijer, announced a few months later. He then emphasised that this had nothing to do with the animosity between Meijering and himself.[4]

Another problem was that, although usually Speijer and Bastiaans saw eye to eye, in this case – for a short time – Bastiaans agreed with the decision to make Meijering director. According to *de Volkskrant*, this was because Meijering had been in Sachsenhausen for six months and therefore could connect with the patients not just professionally, but historically and emotionally as well. He had, so to speak, that special wavelength that according to Bastiaans was so enormously important. On top, Bastiaans thought, Meijering's ideas about the problem were in line with his own. Furthermore, Bastiaans said that one could hardly blame Meijering for the absence of a more direct connection between the centre and the Jelgersma clinic, no matter how much Bastiaans had wanted the pavilion to become an organisational part of it. Meijering had no part in this whatsoever.[5]

The director had to receive a medical staff of three psychiatrists, three psychologists, two social workers, a neurologist, and an internist. The total workforce came to be between 25 and 35 people. One of the three psychiatrists was, of course, Bastiaans. He applauded a separate building, even if he was director of the Jelgersma clinic. Many of his patients felt uncomfortable in a genuine psychiatric clinic. In the KZ clinic they had the opportunity to withdraw undisturbed for a part of the day if they wished.[6]

Indeed, April 17 became the day whereupon it happened. In the presence of, among many others, Bastiaans and Kruisinga, Prince Bernhard covered himself in a white plastic coat, said that the arrival of the clinic was an honorary obligation "towards the particularly brave Dutch in the war years", called on the people to donate generously to the Friends of the Post Concentration Camp Syndrome Centre Foundation, donated *f*35,000 (€15,910) himself,[7] climbed into a pile driver and pressed a button, after which the machine started doing its job with characteristic hellish noise. Shortly before, Muntendam, in his capacity as chairman of the Camp Syndrome Centre, gave the linguistic kick-off of the construction by saying that the Second World War was by no means a thing of the past. "The horrors still are active, which has recently become apparent again", of course referring to the debate about the Breda Three. It had to be the first pile of a building resembling a hospital as little as possible. It had to be cosy, inviting for making contact. The reason was that no effort should be spared to avoid camp associations. That's why it had real carpet on the floor in order to prevent the sound of footsteps resembling the sound of camp guards' boots. For the same reason the rooms looked like hotel rooms instead of hospital ones. "Memories of prisons and claustrophobic experiences had to avoided". On top, the building would not be rectangular, "but as open as possible".[8]

The long history of the building was recalled, a history that, according to *Trouw,* showed how slowly the insights necessary to take care of camp victims penetrated the minds of doctors, politicians, and ecclesiastical authorities alike. This history started when Bastiaans asked the Foundation 1940-1945 to set up a consultation bureau for ex-resistance fighters in 1951. This foundation, which surprisingly enough only played a minor role in the development and dissemination of the knowledge of psychological war effects, was established at the end of the war to support disabled resistance members and the families of killed resistance fighters. However, it rejected Bastiaans' proposal, because, it said, ordinary institutions were sufficiently equipped to meet all necessary research and treatment needs. In addition, at the time the number of psychiatrists interested was limited.[9] Muntendam commented: "It only recently became general knowledge that the supreme oppression of the human soul is the key point of the KZ syndrome."[10] He added that the fact that the pavilion was built on the site of the Jelgersma clinic had to be seen as a tribute to Bastiaans. Or, as *de Volkskrant* wrote: the choice was of a personal nature. He was the pioneer who treated dozens of psychologically war damaged already.[11]

As had been the case when *Life after a War* was published, striking the clinic's first pile into the earth was extensively covered by the media. This was attributed to the Breda Three discussion. It had ensured that the Dutch people were aware of the existence and meaning of the KZ syndrome. It now was of the utmost importance that this focus wouldn't fade again because then the victims would be pushed back "into the isolation in which they thrive so badly". There still were between 30 and 40,000 victims, a number of which previously the *NRC Handelsblad* already indicated it could well rise. It did so again, now taking time as reason: "As years go by more cases can 'come loose'".[12]

In his speech Muntendam referred to suchlike matters as well. The Breda Three discussion revived the horrors of thousands: concentration camp victims, resistance members, and also those who were in an internment camp in the Netherlands East Indies or forced to work in Burma. It was another sign that the Indo-Dutch population was increasingly drawn into the syndrome discussion and seen as one of the groups in psychological need.[13]

Of course, Bastiaans was interviewed in *Trouw.* Unavoidable question: how many patients are we talking about? The answer: at least 10,000 need immediate care. Of them about 3,000 were Jewish. And then there were about 30,000 people living in the danger zone: all those who had been in German or Japanese camps but hadn't yet reported problems as well as their children. They too would likely become psychologically or psychosomatically ill "due to the pressure of the parents' suffering",[14] or, of course, their early passing.[15] The concept of "the second generation", a term originally used for children who had been in camps or in hiding,[16] was born, and the first generation embraced it. One of Bastiaans' patients said to *Het Vrije Volk* in June 1972:

> A few months ago, Meijering said that this clinic will only exist for about 15 to 20 years, because by that time the war generation would no longer be around. But this will anything but put an end to the suffering, because all those tensions in the families of war victims are transferred to their children. Having been brought up in such an environment they too will be traumatised. I'm allowed to say this. We have three girls in their early twenties, and a 17-year-old son. The latter one should not have been born. I should have known that by this time the youngest would develop mental problems. He already has.[17]

Meijering, however, had already retracted his words, which probably were meant to be a joke. He too didn't expect a quick disappearance of the syndrome. Indeed, it became increasingly clear that children of actual victims developed problems also. A whole new generation arrived, and then yet another one. It was a view Eva Tas of the Auschwitz Committee endorsed: "A grandchild, a girl of six, was meant to stay over at one of ours. But at night she suddenly wanted to return home. She didn't want to stay the night because she was afraid the police would come and pick up Grandma and Grandpa during the darkness."[18]

The news coverage of the event – an event that, *Trouw* was eager to emphasise, hadn't been influenced by the Breda Three discussion –[19] was generally factual and positive in tone. The communist daily newspaper *De Waarheid* was the exception to the rule. In an article entitled 'When driving a first pile. Authorities discover a new syndrome' it stated that, factually, there was no reason at all to pay any attention to the event. A pile was driven into the ground, there were some unavoidable solemn acts, and there were some equally unavoidable speeches. However, it was precisely these speeches that called for attention, and, once more, acknowledgement played a major role in this. Like Van Agt and Biesheuvel had done during the discussion on the Breda Three, both Prince Bernhard and Muntendam called acknowledgement of war victims of the utmost importance. The lack of it played a major role in the victims' problems.[20] Muntendam, for example, recalled how severe the consequences of their hardships were, or rather, how great the consequences could be if they *felt* that victimisation wasn't recognised and acknowledged. "The feeling of not being recognised or not fully recognised as a war victim, that is: as a former combatant, often contributed to aggravation of the diseases and to premature aging and death."[21]

"One could", *De Waarheid* scorned, "almost believe that instead of a post concentration camp syndrome there is a 'not being recognised' syndrome." For certain a physician like Muntendam, who rightly stated the war wasn't over yet, should know there was no such thing. He too, like some politicians, only adopted a tune like this because of the resulting political and financial advantages.[22]

In his speech Muntendam described the syndrome as a complicated interplay as well as the outcome of psychological and physical developments, directly resulting from the mental and physical stress of war. In other words, he described "an *illness*" caused by the concentration camps. This disease was known shortly after the war already. And now, "27 years later (!)" the first pile was driven into the ground for the construction of an institution to assist those who had become ill. So, the only thing that was acknowledged was a lack of attention, and that, until now, the minuscule group of medics who looked after the sick were denied the means to do this properly. Bastiaans already raised the problem in the 1950s but hadn't been able to start his treatments at the Jelgersma clinic until 1964, a clinic of which Muntendam now said it was completely unsuitable for this category of patients. And even so. Eighty patients per year could be helped, while according to Bastiaans' statement, at least 30,000 people in the Netherlands were suffering from the syndrome.[23]

Sure, it was about time the clinic was established and having it meant a huge improvement in comparison to the recent situation. Not long ago concentration camp victims were told that it couldn't be proved their heart condition had anything to do with their wartime past, or even that "probably the austere camp life had had a beneficial effect on the heart". According to *De Waarheid,* it was medical views like these that, together with the Dutch government's policy, caused the ailment to aggravate. After the war, it had made many resistance fighters and concentration camp survivors wonder why they had taken up arms against Nazism.

> Collaborators again were clothed with economic and political power. Germany was rearmed. Efforts were made to oppress the Indonesian struggle for freedom violently. The Catholic Party KVP preached mercy to Nazis and all their accomplices. And the effort many ministers, especially from that same KVP, made over the past ten years to get convicted war criminals out of prison

> has been far greater than the effort to alleviate the plight of the victims. It speaks for itself many people were sickened by this.[24]

The war experiences laid the foundation for the syndrome, the post war experiences made it manifest, exacerbated or even caused it. Especially the last two cabinets, De Jong and Biesheuvel, had done everything "to sprinkle hands full of brine into wounds that never healed. If there is to be an 'acknowledgement', this is it. And from now on the government should pursue a policy aimed at preventing the release of the three and any further discussion on it."[25]

The construction process was expected to take seven months. But, *de Volkskrant* reported, a first problem had already arisen. Minister Mauk de Brauw of Science Policy and Higher Education refused to make the pavilion part of the Leiden University Clinic and thus of the Jelgersmakliniek, its psychiatric department. According to De Brauw, this would harm the general, national character of the clinic. Firstly, this meant it had to be given an autonomous structure. Moreover, although naturally some cooperation with the Jelgersma clinic would be possible, this meant that more staff had to be recruited than initially planned. In addition, it would also become more expensive to get it up and running.[26]

A month before the opening of the clinic, Maliepaard, who, as said, was closely involved in its foundation, gave a lecture on it in London, at the annual gathering of former resistance members. He said only the Netherlands struggled with a KZ syndrome problem, because of years of neglecting the war victims' post war problems. In comparison, communist Maliepaard pointed at the Eastern bloc countries. There, he claimed, the victims were given status and had been taken care of immediately after the war ended. In the Netherlands, the syndrome developed precisely because of the lack of such governmental intervention. He didn't spare the Foundation 1940-1945 either. It too, for a long time, avoided the problem of psychological care for concentration camp survivors. Fortunately, in the shape of the clinic, change was imminent. However, it was a change in fits and starts, referring to the question whether Bastiaans was or was not going to take on a prominent medical role in it. Leiden University announced that in case this question was answered affirmatively, Bastiaans had to give up his professorship from Leiden University, and thus his position at the Jelgersma Clinic. With some right, it very much doubted whether a combination of professorship, directorship of the Jelgersma clinic, and directorship of the centre was humanly possible.[27]

Because of this conflict between Bastiaans and the Leiden University, quickly followed by the probably not entirely unrelated departure of Speijer, the entire department of psychiatry was in danger of "being beheaded", as

De Telegraaf wrote. The staff turnover was enormous. Van Tol left as well. That this conflict was called irreconcilable was also due to a simultaneous disagreement about a structure report accepted by the faculty, which, in spite of being co-author and signatory, Bastiaans ultimately didn't agree with. As a result, the future of the Jelgersma clinic, of the adjacent municipal psychiatric institution called Endegeest, and of the university's psychiatry department itself was up in the air. The Jelgersma clinic, the report stated, had to be disconnected from the university hospital. It was too far away, about four kilometres. The psychiatry beds had to be moved to the academic centre, an action with which Bastiaans on second view wholeheartedly disagreed. On top, although many employees held him in high regards as a clinical specialist, they also felt that, in accordance with the psychiatric Zeitgeist, psychiatry should develop in a more biological direction. Therefore, they considered a psychoanalyst and psychosomaticus like Bastiaans less suited to continue to act as head of the department.

Furthermore, all this was followed by a dispute between Meijering and Bastiaans. The first one was appointed medical director and Bastiaans professor director; titles already containing all the ingredients for a competency conflict.[28] Not for nothing, Bastiaans' professor directorship was soon converted into an advisory position. This, however, many believed to be an insult for the man who more than anyone else knew what the KZ syndrome entailed and what its sufferers needed. It's unclear how far all this impacted the construction process, but the completion date was postponed. 1 March 1973, became the date the building was supposed to be ready, a date that indeed was met, after which it was widely said that the construction process had gone smoothly and swiftly.[29]

As if to give him some support in the various conflicts, Bastiaans was awarded the so-called Forester Prize early in February 1973. It was presented to him a few days before the clinic's opening. He received it for his contribution to "a better understanding of victims of war and resistance – and especially the ones suffering from the so-called concentration camp syndrome". He was praised by the Foresters' chairman, Joseph Kleerekoper, a man who had lost much of his family in the Shoah. Through his work Bastiaans "served humankind and restored the victims' humanity". Besides money, the prize consisted of an image of a deer, that "symbol of meekness". To Bastiaans the award served as an encouragement to continue with his work despite all obstacles. Certainly, since *Do you now understand why I cry...* some progress was made in the Netherlands in the treatment of war victims with psychological problems. Nevertheless, in his opinion aid still only scored a meagre 2 on a scale from zero to 10.[30]

Shortly thereafter, the day finally came. Centre '45, the name the clinic was given, was ready to welcome patients. Although the official opening by Queen Juliana would not take place until 16 May, Muntendam spoke some words. "Here work will be done that we never before experienced in the Netherlands. This is a monument built by the Dutch people, and it's meant to assist the best part of them."[31]

People in need of the assistance the clinic was meant to provide, could immediately report to the desk for specialist aid without the intervention of a general practitioner; usually the road patients have to take in the Netherlands. An estimated half of them could do with home treatment, the others stayed in the clinic. In accordance with the architect's commission, it indeed more resembled an "atmospheric winter sports hotel than a hospital", as the *Algemeen Dagblad* wrote. According to *de Volkskrant,* this "distinctly contrasted the run-down clinic" where Bastiaans worked; an old villa that was part of the Jelgersma clinic. And *De Waarheid* too pointed out that the word 'clinic' in fact was incorrect because the building was furnished "very comfortable, cosy, and modern".[32]

One of the first allowed to view the pavilion was the man who had been central to the film *Do you now understand why I cry...* and whose name was finally revealed: Joop Telling. He took the opportunity to call the clinic's capacity a drop in the ocean. The WUV pension act had come into effect just one week before and already 6000 people had registered to claim damages. (Ultimately, about 100,000 people would do so. About 30,000 applications were granted.)[33] Therefore, Meijering expected that it would be necessary to train psychiatrists throughout the entire country to meet the demand.[34]

Despite all the struggles between Bastiaans and the Jelgersmakliniek on the one hand and the Leiden Medical Centre on the other, the *Algemeen Dagblad* said that, nevertheless, there was a close contact between the clinic and the university hospital, also regarding psychiatric treatment. Remarkably, the newspaper wrote that in the case of a KZ syndrome LSD sometimes was the only means providing a solution. However, at the time only two permits were issued for a medical use of the drug. One had been granted to Wil Arendsen Hein, the director of a psychiatric clinic at the town of Amersfoort, the other was for Bastiaans in his Jelgersma clinic. But, as said, he was merely an adviser to Centre '45.[35] In other words: LSD was not allowed to be used at the centre and there was nothing to indicate this would change in the future. Typically, the clinic's LSD treatment room, planned by Bastiaans, was only partly finished at the time the centre was declared open.[36]

De Waarheid had sent a journalist to cover the happy day of the clinic's opening too. Remarkably, and tellingly, the headline of the article only spoke of a centre for victims having fought in the resistance. It was a curtailment that also characterised the article in the social-democratic *Het Vrije Volk,* although its headline limited itself more generally to victims of war.[37] *De Waarheid* also pointed at the amazement about all the publicity in circles of concentration camp survivors and resistance. After all, the capacity of twenty beds stood in stark contrast to the chronic mental and physical suffering of tens of thousands. The newspaper also wrote that Muntendam's answer when asked why it had taken so long, was incorrect. The problem, he said, was unknown until the mid-1950s. Like Maliepaard, *De Waarheid* pointed out that immediately after the war in Eastern European countries attention had been paid to the problem of concentration camp victims and resistance members in word, writing, and treatment, something that in the West only characterised France.[38]

The communist daily also discussed the problems surrounding Centre '45 itself, which apparently had arisen "given the argument between some resistance members and the board during the press meeting". The complications were discussed that led to fierce debates between supporters and opponents of Bastiaans. The paper concluded that Bastiaans had in fact been side-lined by dismissing him with an advisory role and depriving him of the directorship. He hadn't been invited to the viewing either.[39]

To celebrate the happy occasion, *Het Vrije Volk,* which by that time had shrunk from the largest Dutch daily in the mid-1950s to a Rotterdam city newspaper (only to cease to exist in 1991), decided to interview Meijering. However, it did note that Bastiaans was attached to the centre only in an advisory's role, although he, and no one else, had been the man who, in recent years, ensured that the voices of the victims, who mostly kept silent about their past, were increasingly heard. On the one hand, this provided more financial security through the WUV and, on the other hand, resulted in this special clinic. And still, as director of the adjacent Jelgersma clinic, he was confronted with "the psychological aftermath of the war years" on a daily basis; with people who "decades later still are haunted by the most horrible nightmares".[40]

In addition to focusing on the clinic, the interview with Meijering was characterised by reflection on a related issue. At the time there was a lot of controversy in the Netherlands about the role the Jewish writer and economist Friedrich Weinreb played during the war. Was he a charlatan who had only tried to save and enrich himself during the war, as Abel Herzberg said? Or was he a hero without whom many more Jews would have lost their lives, as, for example, Jacques Presser believed?[41] *Het Vrije*

Volk was one of Weinreb's defenders. Meijering had heard that Weinreb had said that the KZ syndrome should actually be called a society syndrome. In part Meijering agreed. Society hadn't exactly responded well to former resistance fighters and camp survivors struggling with mental problems. But the arrival of the clinic proved that the turning point was there.[42]

The interview made clear that twenty beds could indeed be a bit on the tight side. When asked who was eligible for treatment, Meijering said that in addition to groups mentioned more often, like resistance fighters, Jews, gypsies or Jehovah's witnesses, people belonging to neither of these groups but nonetheless suffering from psychological or physical consequences caused by their war experiences, for example because of severe malnutrition, would be welcomed as well. In addition to talking about "people" with, for example, irritable relationships with "women and children", he now also explicitly referred to the survivors of the Japanese internment camps, as well as the second generation, turning the centre into a place of "a kind of family treatment".[43]

As mentioned, Meijering expected about eighty to ninety inpatient and two hundred outpatient treatments. Whether this was enough remained to be seen, but doubts were warranted because already 13,000 people had registered. They received group therapy as much as possible in day treatment. Only the severely physically affected patients, who required permanent assistance, remained in the clinic day and night.[44]

Meijering's concerns weren't limited to the demand side. The supply side was reason for concern too. In other words, there was not nearly enough staff. "Actually", he told the *NRC Handelsblad* that very day, "there are only two psychologists and one and a half social workers." He did expect, however, to have sufficient nurses available by the time of the actual opening. But getting an extra psychiatrist remained problematic,[45] even though the whole adventure had started with a psychiatrist, Bastiaans. But he was and remained only an advisor.

Mentioning Bastiaans touched on another important point: the ban of LSD. Meijering didn't regret this. After all, it was a highly controversial drug. However, should someone urgently feel the need for an LSD treatment, Bastiaans could be called in at the nearby Jelgersma clinic. It was a comment criticised by Telling, despite all his appreciation for the clinic itself. The LSD cure had been of great significance to him. The centre should offer this possibility as well.[46]

The most remarkable aspect in the *NRC* interview was that Meijering, who in *Het Vrije Volk* still had drawn all kinds of groups into the target group, tried to reduce the number of people who could seriously get into trouble. A rare event in the history of the KZ syndrome. "Not all ex-prisoners suffer from it," he said. And there were many who could be helped by their GP or a local psychiatrist. However, he didn't add the words 'if they feel the need to do so'. The word 'ex-prisoner' may not directly mean that a syndrome was present, it did automatically mean that there were psychological problems. As a result, the centre also began to provide psychological counselling for these people and their families; a time-consuming activity because, for that, social workers had to visit those families. He hoped a solution would be found for the hefty costs involved; a solution that could come closer if the public made substantial donations to the Friends of Centre '45 Foundation.[47] According to the *Limburgsch Dagblad,* at least the first team of Ajax, the world's best football team at the time, would play a short match against the builders of the clinic on Wednesday 23 May. The proceeds would come to the benefit of the centre.[48]

That Meijering also looked at social circumstances as the cause of the problems of war victims is indicative of the different approach he and Bastiaans had. Was it indeed all about individual troubles, based on personal youth problems and personal experiences during the war, as Bastiaans thought, or was there some truth in Meijering's view that at least an underlying social problem is present as well? If so, a solution had to be sought and found at that level too.

It was an aspect of Meijering's views that came to the fore in an interview conducted a few months later. Globally speaking, he said, there was no reason to put things into perspective. There were still many countries in which torture and war crimes are daily business. Thus, it was an illusion to think that once the Second World War generation had perished, the syndrome too became a thing of the past. For this to happen, much more should be done to prevent war, torture, and other human rights abuses. Healing should always come second.[49]

Not only the man who became director was sought out by the newspapers. Of course, this applied to the one who hadn't been given the position as well: Bastiaans. The report of the interview *De Tijd* had with him opened with the story of British aviator Henry McAnelly. He regained his memories of the events of Market Garden, September 1944, after Bastiaans took him from the Jelgersma clinic to the former battlefields of Arnhem and its surroundings. He still was very grateful to Bastiaans for this, and for everything else the latter had done for him. The emotional and medical-ethical discussion surrounding the broadcast of the film *Do you now understand why I cry...* was called into remembrance as well. Meanwhile, the film was also broadcasted on Belgian television and by an American TV station. The latter unfortunately and coincidentally did so precisely at the time the first Vietnam POWs returned. It was the reason why Bastiaans regretted this broadcast. As a result, the transfer of knowledge the film intended threatened to become political propaganda.[50]

The opening was typical of the admiring, uncritical tone of the rest of the interview. Bastiaans was one of the first and few to care about the fate of war dead, and two decades later little changed. And that, he said, despite the fact the Netherlands harboured "about ten to twenty thousand people for whom the war misery they have endured continues to root in their minds". Although they as well were physically liberated in 1945, psychological liberation hadn't occurred. To accomplish the latter, a psychotherapeutic return to the hell called concentration camp was necessary. It was typical of the attitude of most newspapers that, unlike many doctors, the Catholic *De Tijd,* although extremely critical of the use of LSD for personal pleasure, had few problems with using such psychotropic drugs for treating the KZ syndrome.[51] The question raised in the medical literature as to whether the efficacy of the therapy, if any, was due not so much to the drug itself, but also, or even above all, to the calming environment and/or the patients' trust in the psychiatrist was nowhere reflected upon in the newspapers.

This is not to say the criticism LSD use received and the ensuing political-social pressure to stop using it, wasn't discussed at all. It was, including its medical therapeutic use. This was done by asking Bastiaans, as said one of the two psychiatrists still allowed to use the drug, what he thought of the critique. He answered that criticism on medical usages had more to do with fear than with science. This answer was subsequently adopted uncritically.

> People think too magically about it. It is feared that if psychiatrists continue to use it, it could easily find its way into another market. I must of course account for each amount carefully. The accidents that happened during medical use were due to failing guidance. A patient who has been given LSD should not be left alone for one minute.[52]

It gave Bastiaans the opportunity to express his own criticism of colleagues who, despite all evidence to the contrary, still had problems with psychosomatics, with psychological backgrounds of physical manifestations, despite the fact that it provided conclusive explanations for many cases of, for example, breathing difficulties or stomach ulcers.

> I believe that a certain predisposition may lead to certain sensitivities, but the outbreak or worsening of a disease is usually determined by conflicts impossible to process. It's amazing, but, for example, I have given people with asthma the same kind of LSD treatment as sufferers from post concentration camp syndrome and doing so have cured their ailments.[53]

This only was strange on the face of it. According to Bastiaans, all psychosomatic disorders were "based on a kind of private KZ syndrome" usually resulting "from an uncomprehending, too dominating or psychologically neglectful environment".[54] Unfortunately, the interviewer didn't elaborate on the possible consequence of this: an almost unlimited increase in the number and type of people who could suffer from KZ syndrome. Its definition would, therefore, drift away so enormously from the one given by Musaph and certainly from the one in the *NIW*, that it lost all meaning.

12. THE OPENING OF CENTRE '45

Although already partially in use, in May 1973 the official opening was due at last. To mark the occasion the *Maandblad Geestelijke Volksgezondheid* was entirely devoted to the KZ syndrome. It was the issue in which Hustinx argued a preference for the term EESS, explained in more detail in the introduction. Meijering wrote an article about and entitled 'Concentration Camps'. The issue was sent to all general practitioners and psychiatrists in the Netherlands to inform them about the symptoms and possible treatment of the syndrome. In general, the journal wrote, it was to be cheered that the centre had been established. Meeting others who suffered from the syndrome could have a liberating and stimulating effect and thus promote healing, although for this to really happen it also had to be ensured that the patients wouldn't get isolated from society.[1]

In the previous weeks, obviously starting on 5 May, Liberation Day, some newspapers looked ahead. For example, Emmy van Overeem, the religious exception of the generally secular *NRC Handelsblad* and married to a man on war benefits, wrote that despite all the festive sounds surrounding the opening of Centre '45, there was nothing to be happy about. In view of the gigantic demand for help, the number of people who actually could be helped was too small for festivities. And the demand didn't get any smaller. According to her "an enormous wave of post concentration camp victims" could be seen coming at the horizon. Nevertheless, it was a good thing and high time that the centre was opened. The concentration camp survivors' resilience was exhausted; a process that had gained momentum because of the Breda Three discussion. They no longer could bring themselves to suppress their fears and depressions. At least, now some of them no longer had to be helped "in the cold Jelgersma clinic".[2] Nevertheless, it implied a clear critique of the time span between the war's end and the centre's arrival. It was a criticism *De Waarheid* had spewed already, and Van Overeem wasn't the only one endorsing that newspaper in this respect.

According to *De Tijd,* many interpreted the name, Centre '45, "as a permanent reproach". The figure served as a continuous reminder that the liberation happened decades ago and that not until now a clinic was opened for those still struggling with their war experiences mentally and physically. Meijering responded to such comments by saying that there was no reason to blame anyone because at the time no one could have foreseen that many problems would manifest themselves only years later. In addition, it was thought that the already existing problems could be solved through usual medical routes. Unfortunately, this turned out not to be the case. However, the interviewer recalled that Bastiaans proposed to the Foundation 1940-1945 to set up a social-medical consultation bureau for former resistance fighters already in 1951.[3] In other words: the name could be pictured as a reproach indeed, something *de Volkskrant* thought as well. "The Centre '45 was anything but established too early and for many it came too late. No one knows how many former camp residents, who could have been helped, have since died because of their bitter experiences."[4] But all in all, the paper continued, one could also say the centre had been built rather quickly, given that the first pleas for it were made in 1970 and how desperately slow the Dutch government usually acts.[5]

The many years that had passed since the war had ended weren't the only point of criticism. *De Tijd* interviewed R. van Dam, one of Bastiaans' patients.[6] Bastiaans, he said, had been the one who stood by him, who understood him, who understood "us". But because of certain intrigues, invisible to him, this very man was set aside. "I received an invitation to attend the opening of the centre in Oegstgeest. I'll go, but I'm afraid that a whole bunch of dignitaries will crowd around the queen again. And where will Bastiaans be?"[7] This, however, didn't take away that he was positive about the centre in itself and that he didn't want to blame anyone for it being too little, too late. "In the first years after the liberation we too didn't realise that things were that bad with us. It's late indeed, but as long as our boys are treated optimally now, it isn't too late completely."[8]

Van Dam also broached a problem that was, he thought, purely hypothetical; hypothetical because the centre was assigned its patients by the Foundation 1940-1945. It only did so if a resistance past was proved or if the patients were granted a war pension – again showing that admission was seen as acknowledgement and non-admission as denial of it.[9] What, he wondered, if someone had the same kind of problems, joined the patients, after which it turned out he had fought on the enemies' side? If such a person would receive help in the centre, he nor the others would accept it. Meijering couldn't ascertain this would never happen, ranging from people who voluntarily had gone to work in Germany and therefore had to endure bombing raids, to soldiers and medics who had been part of the Dutch SS Eastern Front Legion. He saw a solution to this ethical problem, which arose because doctors are obliged to provide help without regard to a person's beliefs or past, or the cause of the problem. They would receive help, but not in the Centre. There the 'without regard' didn't apply. The beds were intended for people who had been active in the resistance and/or had been imprisoned in one of the camps only. This wasn't just better for the peace of mind of the patients, consequently it was better from a medical point of view, including the former Germany friendly patients. Because former resistance fighters or camp survivors wouldn't accept them, splitting the two groups could only speed up the healing process of both.[10]

It couldn't be much more obvious that by now terms like KZ syndrome or (post) concentration camp syndrome started to feel wrong. With the increasing focus on symptoms as a decisive diagnostic factor at the expense of war-rooted causes like dehumanisation, deprivation of liberty and the resulting fear of death, those responsible for sending people to the camp could now get the diagnosis as well, even if they weren't welcome in the centre especially set up for treating those suffering from the syndrome. Thus, it isn't surprising that around this time alternative terms such as EESS and disaster syndrome emerged; terms that had a much more general timbre and content.

The suspicion raised against the clinic because of the minor role Bastiaans had gotten was unfounded, Meijering told *De Tijd.* Bastiaans already had enough on his plate with his professorship and his directorship of the Jelgersma clinic. "Should he now also be charged with the management of Centre '45?", he agreed with the university rhetorically. In addition, Bastiaans was chairman of the Advisory Board of the Centre '45 Foundation, the name the Post Concentration Camp Syndrome Centre Foundation adapted after the opening. This ensured contact and cooperation. Other than some, he thought it not at all strange that people with the syndrome could now be treated in the Jelgersma clinic by Bastiaans as well as in the centre not by him. There were psychiatrists all over the country treating people with war-induced problems. They probably stayed with them. So why couldn't the others go to the Jelgersma clinic anymore?[11]

It was an answer that couldn't convince *De Tijd,* which took a much more critical stance in the interview with Meijering than when interviewing Bastiaans two months earlier. After all, in the Jelgersma clinic Bastiaans could use LSD. Because he wasn't affiliated with the centre, the patients there were deprived of that treatment even though they might need it. It gave Meijering the opportunity to criticise the government's "weird" LSD policy. Why did it fear this drug that much? Certain measures seemed to be the result of panic rather than ratio.[12]

Meijering assured that, if in need of an LSD treatment, patients will be referred to the Jelgersma clinic.[13] A miraculous situation, *de Volkskrant* wrote. Wasn't one of the reasons for the construction of the centre that the patients in the Jelgersma clinic didn't feel comfortable because of its appearance and because there they were surrounded by real psychiatric patients, which negatively influenced their treatment?[14] One of the centre's patients expressed this some months after the opening as follows:

> Last year, when I was in the Jelgersma clinic, I noticed it clearly: group formation. There were also drug and alcohol patients, and somehow, they never become one community with the war victims. Here in the centre, we are one group. Every Tuesday when I come here, I see old friends, my own Natzweilers. We can bring our wives along, while at Bastiaans' clinic we couldn't, because of a lack of space.[15]

The articles that appeared around the official opening paid ample attention to the holiday resort-like appearance and design of the centre as well, referring to it as a small Hilton hotel. Although Bastiaans wondered whether the patients would feel at home, Eva Tas was pleased[16] and so was the patient referred to above.

> The new centre in Oegstgeest is a relief, an oasis. In the 14 weeks that I've been going there now: it's great, the way the staff familiarised itself there in such a short time, the way you're received. We are sorry for the prof, but here on the other side, in 'the Jel', he never had enough space for this.[17]

It doesn't alter that Meijering had some reservations too. Of course, it was a positive thing that the attractive design prevented unnecessary stress situations and that existing stress was reduced or even removed. However, it also entailed the danger that a patient really felt on vacation, so that after returning to his normal environment, his problems would return just as hard. Moreover, the danger was that precisely because of the contact between the various patients admitted, all the pain and misery endured would be rekindled. But, Meijering said, this was one of the tasks the staff had set itself. It had to ensure that a good helping and healing therapy emerged from the conversations resulting from the patients' encounters.[18]

During the official opening by Queen Juliana, with five of the twenty beds occupied, Muntendam pointed out that the treatment in the centre deviated from the usual hospital interpretation of that word. The pillars on which this treatment was based were understanding and tranquillity: "the tranquillity of the house, of the living room, of the terrace and the garden, where one can linger to listen and speak." After she as well pointed out that for many the opening of the centre had come too late, Eva Furth-Halverstad, the representative of the resistance organisations, pointed at the importance of 'understanding'; understanding the victims of war, particularly psychologically. It was Bastiaans who was to be thanked for the considerable increase in understanding among government and medical professionals in recent years.[19] Incidentally, one of those present told her that she was "just a victim" and not someone from the "active resistance". Apparently, *Het Parool* wrote, people from the resistance feel superior to those who "merely" had been in a concentration camp.[20]

It was not the only time that day Bastiaans was mentioned – who had come to the opening with a wooden sculpture of a pointy head intended for Teengs Gerritsen because, the latter had remarked during one of the regular conflicts in the foundation board the psychiatrist gave him one.[21] The controversy between Bastiaans on the one hand and the boards of the university and the foundation on the other casted a shadow over what should have been a festive event. It was a controversy made public by his patients. Bastiaans, they said, was the only one who really understood their problems, so he should have been the centre's director.[22]

The day after the opening, the conflict led to headlines such as 'Quarrel at opening of new war victims clinic', 'Syndrome specialist Bastiaans side-lined', or 'Relentless power struggle eliminates Prof. Bastiaans. Clinic for victims of KZ syndrome failure?'. These articles made clear that not only *De Tijd* was completely in favour of Bastiaans. *Tubantia,* for example, concluded that what should have been a glorious day for the psychiatrist had turned out to be a major disappointment.[23] *Het Nieuwsblad van het Noorden* wholeheartedly agreed. In addition to a minuscule article about the opening of the centre, it published a hefty article entitled 'Professor Bastiaans victim of university power struggle'. As a result, the opening of the centre turned into a sad personal drama for the one who had championed its creation like no other.

> The man, who for years fought to give adequate treatment to KZ syndrome patients, has been side-lined by a relentless power struggle within Leiden University. The spokesmen of ex-prisoners were dragged into this. Their feelings and emotions, already so lightly touched after everything they experienced in the war years, are affected. Wild outbursts are the result.[24]

Bastiaans wasn't allowed to speak during the opening, according to *De Telegraaf* in order to guard the royal family from a riot.[25] In protest against this Maliepaard, a great admirer of Bastiaans and his method, didn't use his right to speak; he was replaced by Furth-Halverstad. Even the presence of Juliana and Bernhard, *Het Nieuwsblad van het Noorden* and *Tubantia* wrote, couldn't dissuade him from his decision. According to Bastiaans, Maliepaard would otherwise have had to reveal everything that disturbed him during the entire process, and he didn't want to do so in the presence of the queen. A year ago, Bastiaans had been promised he could speech at the opening, two months ago he noticed he had suddenly disappeared from the list.[26]

It was the apotheosis of a fight that started early 1972. At that time, as mentioned, some members of staff of the Jelgersma clinic, his old companion Speijer among them, criticised Bastiaans' psychiatric insights that, they claimed, were outdated. This obviously had consequences for the centre he wanted to lead, which was seen as his hobbyhorse. In this endeavour he was supported by a large number of former camp inmates. After their treatment in the Jelgersma clinic he was nothing short of their medical hero. But most members of the foundation board, as well as national leaders in the field of mental health, didn't want Bastiaans to be the centre's director. They chose Meijering "when Prof. Bastiaans was in the US".[27]

This was a misrepresentation. Apart from the fact that Bastiaans visited the World Psychiatric Congress in Mexico, not in the United States, the decision on the directorship was made at a meeting early in 1972 that Bastiaans attended. Given the choice to remain a full professor or to become a professor by special appointment and director of the centre, which he regarded as "an institution closely linked to my clinic", he decidedly opted for the full professorship. An extraordinary professorship meant that he had to stop training upcoming psychiatrists, which he had, in his own words, done with one in four of all Dutch psychiatrists at the time. It was impossible for him to end this.[28]

But, several newspapers continued, whether he had agreed to withdraw from the directorship or not, and whether the decision was taken in his presence and with his consent or not, it certainly was a painful decision for Bastiaans' patients, who, moreover, announced not to trust Meijering's treatment method. Like the foundation board, Meijering saw the new accommodation more as a kind of reception centre, while Bastiaans and his colleagues believed that KZ patients should have their own, real hospital.[29] In other words: actual, individual treatment instead of rest, understanding, group discussions and a listening ear.

De Telegraaf extensively discussed the affair too. That Bastiaans wasn't allowed to speak at all and that Maliepaard no longer wanted to, were "just a few examples of a conflict already on the brink of erupting". Emotions ran high, with Bastiaans "trying to persuade employees and sympathisers not to launch public actions". It was highly regrettable that the conflict between Bastiaans and the foundation board wasn't resolved prior to the centre's opening. As a result, it had become completely separated from Bastiaans' vision in design as well as purpose. He envisioned the centre as a university clinic, closely associated with the Jelgersma clinic, because in his eyes treating war victims was an essential part of modern psychiatry. However, the university board supported the decision that it should become a rural centre without university ties. This changed

Bastiaans' role in the centre. Instead of being a therapist and co-determiner of the policy to be pursued, his position became that of "well-known but not very influential" chairman of the Advisory Council, and even this for merely a one-year period only.[30]

The advisory role was uncertain for a long time too because the board of the foundation believed he, in case Meijering and his colleagues turned to him for medical advice, could not be both chairman and consultant. To the great dismay of his sympathisers, he still had to make do with the beautifully situated but completely outdated Jelgersma clinic. There he had tried to transform Leiden psychiatry in line with his insights for years, but until then hadn't seen a fifth of the promises made to him when he was appointed turn into reality.[31]

De Telegraaf linked the conflict of the foundation and faculty boards with Bastiaans to the latter's use of LSD. Although the very film in which someone was treated with LSD had significantly contributed to the arrival of the centre, the drug itself had to stay outside of it. That film also sharpened already existing contradictions and created new resistance. Although war victims had some questions regarding the clinic as well, because of their aversion to being seen as 'patients', this new resistance mainly manifested itself "in the medical-psychiatric sphere and the Leiden medical faculty, which already was in conflict with Bastiaans about the future structure of psychiatry". Consequently, the Jelgersma clinic remained Bastiaans' domain. In the centre, outpatient care and day care through psychological and social assistance were paramount at the expense of "direct psychiatric aid to people in need". The mere twenty beds had to remain empty as much as possible.[32]

That's how it came about, *De Telegraaf* continued, that Meijering instead of Bastiaans became the director of Centre '45, while, according to the newspaper, in no way he had earned any spurs in the field of clinical psychiatry. He had been a Mental Health Inspector for eleven years and made only one, far from glorious public appearance during that period. He played "an astonishingly passive role" when in Den Dolder "the sharpest staff conflict about abuses that ever hit a Dutch institution erupted". Moreover, he was the man who said that in ten, fifteen years' time, "when the last of the survivors has deceased", the "all memory of concentration camps banishing, but according to many rather sterile" centre could still serve as a nice motel, close to the main highway. Such a comment – which continued to haunt Meijering – wasn't seen as funny. On the contrary. It gave testimony to an enormous lack of understanding "for the much broader scope of the generations who tried to survive psychic dynamite".[33] In other words: whatever one might think of Bastiaans, Meijering in any case wasn't the right man to lead the centre. According to *Tubantia,* even his camp past began to turn against him. Some of his former companions felt he should not treat but be treated.[34]

Thus, the opening of the clinic hadn't become an undivided festive pleasure which tempted the *Algemeen Dagblad* into an interview with "its maligned spiritual father" as well. He too made no secret of the fact that, he claimed, the underlying reason for his subordinate role was that influential figures in the ministry felt that medical LSD use was considered not supportive in the fight against drugs, even though this non-addictive substance was initially created for psychiatric use. Of course, like any drug, LSD could be misused for purposes it wasn't intended for. This didn't make it any less valuable as medication. The chance that he might be able to apply his treatment method in the centre at some point in the future did, however, not increase. "It has already come that far that the board is warning against my methods." This could very well turn against the board and its centre. Some representatives of camp victims' associations, including E. van Hemert of the Pelita (oil lamp) Foundation, representing the interests of survivors of the Japanese internment camps, already said it would advise its members to visit Bastiaans only.[35]

Several newspapers reported on Bastiaans' disappointment and resentment and not only because the centre didn't have a university affiliation. The foundation board had "treated him in a rude and anything but tactical manner". At first it asked him for his opinion about what should and what shouldn't be done, but this increasingly lessened over time. As a result, he said, albeit certainly unintentionally, some apparently small, but in fact very important measures were taken that could have an inhibitory effect on the patients' treatment. He was given far too little say in the appointment of the centre's staff, that as a result, including director Meijering, lacked the specific expertise required for treating war victims. In doing so, he contradicted his opinion, written down in *de Volkskrant* earlier on, that he and Meijering were on the same page medically.[36]

Bastiaans called his position as chairman of the Advisory Council a sham. That council was a cumbersome body that hadn't engaged in any activity yet. He also accused the well-known Dutch physician Pieter Baan of inciting the staff of the centre against him. Baan, who a year earlier had been a mediator in the dispute between Speijer and Bastiaans and who discussed Bastiaans' thesis very positively in the *NTvG* in 1959,[37] was famous for his treatments of criminals, but at the time he was Chief Inspector for Mental Health and administrative advisor to the centre as well.

Baan was in favour of a national, non-university institution. According to him, many patients had to be helped which was impossible with Bastiaans' method, which, according to Bastiaans, he thought to be too traditionalistic. Furthermore, Baan would blame him for having given permission to broadcast Van Gasteren's movie on television. Baan was and remained in favour of releasing the Breda Three, while, Bastiaans stated, "I knew from my experiences with ex-resistance fighters and camp victims how serious the consequences of the discussion about the intention to release were for their psychological condition and declared myself an opponent". Bastiaans forgot (?) to mention that he too for a long time was in favour of release, precisely because of the effect of a recurring discussion if the three weren't released. Anyway, "this profound difference of opinion became the main source of the difficulties".[38]

Maliepaard and most of the other patients endorsed Bastiaans' criticism. They thought non-experts had gotten their hands on the centre. With their emphasis on psychology and a listening ear, they had strayed far from the original goals: medical care for people with KZ syndrome. Bastiaans did support these goals. Therefore, although Teengs Gerritsen had begged Maliepaard to continue to advise Meijering about social problems, Maliepaard refused. He, *Tubantia* wrote, had taken sides. "As a rock in the surf he stands behind Professor Bastiaans."[39]

Het Parool as well gave Bastiaans plenty of scope to air his grievances. However, it ended its article with the positive remark that the centre really wasn't as bad as Bastiaans would make believe. The day-to-day cooperation between the Jelgersma clinic and the centre didn't appear to be bad, which wasn't surprising because some of the centre staff had indeed been hired after a recommendation by Bastiaans. At that time there were 35 people, including three psychiatrists. According to the *NIW*, they made use of the findings of the ex-camp inmates and psychiatrists De Wind and Cohen. Referrals back and forth were made without any problem, even if a patient from the centre felt he needed LSD to really make the therapy profitable.[40] The chance on that happening was not inconceivable, according to *Tubantia,* because Bastiaans' LSD cure had "quite a lot of success". It was now up to Meijering to achieve the same result with methods considered incorrect by Bastiaans. Given the history, the newspaper had its doubts.

> What could have become a crown on all the (relatively few) activities the Netherlands employed for its former resistance members (it is known that Queen Wilhelmina was deeply disappointed about this) has become a pool of human misery. The pioneer is side-lined. When the first pile was driven last year, he asked the board of the foundation to have a word. He was advised not to. You can have your say at the official opening, he was told. Bastiaans, however, had to keep his mouth shut today. Muntendam, the man who had to

> be made enthusiastic by Maliepaard and Teengs Gerritsen and who was finally prepared to take on the presidency, would then take charge of the speech. Piet Maliepaard, a roaring lion, if necessary, threw his head back.[41]

In response to the problems with the centre, in an interview with the *NIW* Bastiaans discussed his LSD treatment in detail. He explained why this method couldn't be applied by just anybody, including, should it ever be allowed, the staff of the centre. Moreover, by no means all psychiatrists wanted to use the hallucinogen, even if they had no problems with the drug itself. The sessions were intense and time consuming. The doctor had to stay with "him" throughout the entire session and maintain psychological contact. Those sessions were aimed at reliving the camp hell, "but now in an atmosphere of intense humanity and together with the therapist". The psychiatrist held his hand, listened closely, cried with the patient. Bastiaans ensured that complete identification, and with it a complete blurring of the doctor-patient relationship, was not forthcoming, but they were quite familiar with each other. Doctor and patient were "friends or like father and son".[42] His nickname 'daddy Bas' didn't come out of the blue.[43]

Although the sessions were time consuming, the *NIW* continued by stating the duration of the treatment was much shorter and more successful than the often years-long psychoanalytical sessions without additional psychogenic drugs. After several LSD trips and even more conversations, the patient often was able to calm down and come to terms with his memories. However, despite the presence of three psychiatrists in the centre, individual psychiatric treatment focusing on mental problems was replaced by group sessions, and attention to physical ailments and social (dys)functioning. However, according to Bastiaans, the individual aspect was necessary. That had to be the start. Only then "the rest could have its turn".

> I hope the Centre's colleagues will see this. I can only render advice because I'm not involved in the treatment at the Centre '45. Nevertheless, I am very happy the Centre has finally been established, because patients can now be treated in a much more suitable environment than in our old-fashioned and on the upper floors barred clinic.[44]

Two days after the opening, when Prince Bernhard, among others, began to make efforts to reach a compromise,[45] an analysis in the *NRC Handelsblad* by the later science editor E.J. Boer tried to throw water on the fire. Boer also referred to the role LSD played in the conflict. According to him this was at the heart of every other problem, that easily could have been solved if not because of the hallucinogenic therapy. The problem, however, was that after the broadcast of the film *Do you now understand why I cry...*

successful treatment of war victims was identified with LSD by the general public as well as war victims themselves. According to Boer, even a film crew from America arrived to interview Telling. This interview became part of the American screening of the film. As previously described, this long-planned broadcast took place just as the first POWs returned from Vietnam, which gave the film an unintentionally topical political accent leading to misinterpretation in the USA as well as in the Netherlands.[46] And as said, also by Bastiaans himself.

Bastiaans, Boer continued, undeniably did ground-breaking work with his patients who walk through fire for him. But according to Meijering the belief they had in his method, which for several reasons he thought incorrect, was misplaced. Boer therefore rejected the suggestion that Meijering disapproved a good methodology merely to maintain his prestige vis-à-vis Bastiaans, but this didn't alter that also in the current construction Bastiaans could continue to use his knowledge to the benefit of war victims. The interests of the patients were thus safeguarded. In short, it was time to bury the hatchet.

> Meijering is director now. And he certainly and conscientiously will discharge his duties as director and doctor. He is skilled and one may wish that he is given full cooperation to bring his unique and difficult work to a successful conclusion. As long as emotional spectators (patients or non-patients) don't add fuel to the fire, the work can be done.[47]

Boer will have regretted that, at the same time as he typed his piece, three things nullified the possible positive effect of his soothing words. Firstly, former resistance fighter, lawyer, mental health expert, former MP for the PvdA and prominent member of the centre's board, Jaap le Poole, indicated that he was not sure whether a compromise between the fighting parties was possible. Le Poole was also the one who conducted the investigation resulting in discouraging a public display of Van Gasteren's movie in 1969.[48] Secondly, Bastiaans gave an interview in which he fully expressed his grievances. Thirdly, someone in governmental circles in The Hague was busy stoking the fire again.

Le Poole, the one who had come up with the name Centre '45, was interviewed by *Het Parool,* which in an article of 19 May still spoke about the new clinic "of Prof. Bastiaans".[49] He started by saying that he would try to keep his emotions out, although this would be difficult after all that was said and written about him by Bastiaans and his friends. He reduced the crux of the matter to two points. Firstly, Bastiaans wanted a firm bond between the clinic and the centre. This was impossible. The entire board of the medical faculty was against it, and as far as Le Poole could see, rightly so.

Furthermore, Bastiaans' wish to provide the patients with individual psychiatric care was completely unrealistic given the enormous size of the group.[50] In effect, this means that, by putting the number at tens of thousands, which underlined the urgency of the problem and the need for treatment, Bastiaans himself dug the grave for his method based on individual sessions.

Le Poole added that according to many experts, including psychiatrists whom Bastiaans had trained himself, the analytically oriented method he had in mind had at most a minor effect on the fifty- or sixty-year-olds concerned. The title of *Het Parool* article was therefore 'Experts doubting the Bastiaans method', a rare exception to the rule of praise that usually set the tone.[51]

The interview with Le Poole was reproduced as an insert in a larger piece, an interview with Bastiaans himself, entitled: 'In this matter bad things happened'. He said he had been too trustful. In the article, the day of the opening, the day he hadn't been allowed to speak, was described as one of the most difficult days of his life. In short, it was the kind of interview that didn't exactly increase the chance to compromise. It's conceivable that Le Poole – who foresaw that in the future judgments about Bastiaans, at the time almost a saint to many, might be harsh –[52] was asked for a response. In the interview Bastiaans called him the great catalyst of the conflict. Despite this, some letter writers didn't get it. One of them was Trix Terwindt. She was one of the victims of the so-called *Englandspiel* (more on this later) and a passionate adept of Bastiaans. She thought he should have taken control of the centre. Le Poole was not a psychiatrist. Therefore, he had no clue. Therefore, his views on the matter were null and void.[53]

According to Bastiaans, that Le Poole joined the board at Muntendam's request considerably exacerbated existing problems. For example, the meetings were suddenly moved to the so-called neutral The Hague. A secretary who, for a whole year, had put in a lot of effort to make the arrival of the centre possible, was suddenly fired for talking to the press, which, according to Bastiaans, she hadn't done. From that moment on, Le Poole and Meijering discussed everything outside of him. It had also been Le Poole who turned against his wish to be both adviser and consultant to the centre and who bluffed the board with shrewd legal arguments. If the Foundation 1940-1945 hadn't insisted, he even wouldn't have become chairman of the Advisory Council.[54]

Bastiaans didn't think that the expertise and experience of him and his staff would be neglected. "After all, you don't offer a piece of your property only to be told later: we have nothing to do with you." He assured that even in the situation that had arisen he and his people remained ready to give all their strength to the salvation and healing of war victims and their loved ones, but for this, certain conditions had to be met. In short, they came down to the fact that, firstly, he had to have a say in the admission policy because Meijering lacked the experience and knowledge to do so. Secondly, it had to be possible to give LSD in the centre as well because, once ready, the room in the centre especially designed for this, was much better suited than the room in the clinic now used. And thirdly, the centre had to become a 24/7-clinic instead of the Monday-to-Friday day care clinic it was now.[55] It's highly questionable whether Bastiaans didn't know in advance that these conditions would never be met.

Bastiaans looked back on the past few months, for instance on the broadcast of Van Gasteren's film. It had given many people the impression that he was administering LSD to everyone. This wasn't the case. Of the hundreds of resistance and camp victims he treated over the past ten years, he administered LSD to no more than 20. It wasn't true, he said, perhaps in an attempt to take the edge somewhat off the interview, that LSD was at the centre of the controversy. There were differences in treatment methods between him and the practitioners at the centre, but these weren't as great as often suggested and on top only partly concerned the use of psychotropic drugs.[56]

Maybe Bastiaans was right in denying that LSD played a major, let alone central role in the conflict, but the drug certainly was part of it, and probably to a greater extent than he would have the readers believe. Meijering swore to him that the Ministry of Health, and in particular the department of pharmaceutical inspection, was adamantly against the use of LSD. If this was true, it was incomprehensible to Bastiaans. He simply couldn't believe that someone would object LSD treatment in the centre when given under his supervision.[57]

Bastiaans admitted that initially he opposed Meijering's appointment. This was solely due to the fact that at the time Speijer had still been his colleague. Speijer and Meijering hadn't been on speaking terms since the Dennendal affair. After Speijer's early retirement, this objection disappeared. That was not the case, however, with the conflict concerning the place of psychiatry in the new university hospital to be built, leading up to Speijer's goodbye. In Bastiaans' view, this was the real background to the controversy over the centre. Bastiaans wanted a large clinic, with at least ninety beds, combined with a manifold of outpatient options. Only then could he fulfill his task teaching new generations of psychiatrists. However, the faculty didn't agree and opted for a much smaller clinic.[58]

All these "extremely unsavoury" things made Bastiaans bitter about the past and (thus) little hopeful for the future, although he kept hoping the compromise attempts of Bernhard and others would be successful. "Because it's rather unpleasant if you have spent twenty years of your professional life dealing with the mental problems of resistance and war victims, and once the clinic, for which you have made the plans yourself, is finally there, you are set aside."[59]

After the resentment between Bastiaans and Meijering and Bastiaans' interview in *Het Parool,* complication number three remained: the oil thrown on the fire in The Hague (which eventually would bring some tranquillity as well). Naturally, questions about the conflict were also asked at the Binnenhof, the centre of Dutch government. This even happened the day after the opening, and it was Eibert Meester who did so. He was a member of the Senate for the PvdA and a long-standing authoritative member of that party, who, however, drifted somewhat towards its margins in the years before. It was no surprise that exactly he was the one asking questions. He had been in the news a few weeks earlier because he was given a royal award. He received it at the Jelgersma clinic where he was treated by Bastiaans because of the psychological problems resulting from his past in the resistance and the time he had spent in camp Amersfoort.[60]

Meester, who, like Boer, attributed the conflict above all to disagreements about whether LSD should be used, asked Harry van Doorn and Irene Vorrink to conduct an independent investigation into the course of events at Centre '45. They were the ministers of CRM and Public Health respectively in the centre-left cabinet of Joop den Uyl, also PvdA, which had just taken office one week earlier. According to Meester Bastiaans should be put in charge and it also should be made possible for him to take his own employees. Moreover, the patients now being treated by Bastiaans in the Jelgersma clinic had to be granted access to the centre too. Meester wanted to know whether indeed decisions were made, like the appointment of Meijering, which went against the intentions of Bastiaans and former State Secretary Kruisinga. He also wanted to know whether the economic and medical aspects of the centre's treatment were sufficiently monitored. By this he was referring to the rumour that a bed in the centre cost *f*400 (€182) a day, while in the Jelgersma clinic it was only *f*200 (€91). Bastiaans hoped that he would have been able to continue his treatments with new resolve in the centre, LSD and otherwise. Financial barriers like this could frustrate these intentions. Furthermore, Meester wondered whether Meijering was the right man to lead the centre, given his role in the Dennendal affair and because he had admitted not to have any experience in the field of assisting war victims. Had sufficient account been taken of Bastiaans' objections to Meijering? And finally, Meester wanted to know whether the ministers as well believed "that the activity of some officials to undermine the authority of Prof. Bastiaans and the publicity about it are particularly damaging to the peace of mind of KZ syndrome sufferers".[61] These questions turned out to be the prelude to his own political downfall and to the first real dent in Bastiaans' image. But nobody could have guessed that at the time.

Following questions asked by the staff and the board of the centre, Bastiaans stated, a week after the centre's opening, that a number of comments he made, especially in the article in *Het Parool,* had come across incorrectly. The cooperation between him and the employees of the centre was good. He hadn't wanted to give the impression that the centre's staff in general was incompetent and inexperienced. This it was only so far as LSD treatment was concerned. However, he kept all reservations he had about the policy of the centre's administration, which should ask Vorrink to allow LSD treatments in the centre as well. The former concentration camp inmates insisted on this as well, because of the lack of space Bastiaans had in the clinic.[62] One of them, who deeply regretted the conflict that had arisen, said: "It's a shame Bastiaans can't be here for an LSD treatment. This is necessary to bring people who are afraid to talk into a dream state in order to give voice to their emotions. No, I didn't need it. But 50 percent of us do, I guess."[63]

In a letter to Muntendam, Bastiaans wrote that, in his opinion, it was a matter of consultation between the university and the centre board about what the collaboration between him and Centre '45 in practice should look like, between, more strictly formulated, the university Jelgersma clinic and the national centre. In principle, this had nothing to do with him. In *Het Parool* interview he also only wanted to indicate some general terms and conditions. A week later it could be read in both *Trouw* and in once again *Het Parool* (in an article in which perhaps for the first time the title simply read 'Bastiaans' instead of 'Prof. Bastiaans') that the centre's board thought differently about this. It too quickly had come up with a sharper, more legally valid description of the conditions under which he and his associates were willing to work with the centre. Otherwise, there would be little point in consultation between the university and the centre about this cooperation.[64] This is the state of affairs in which Vorrink decided to accede to Meester's request.

A week after Meester asked his questions, Vorrink asked psychiatrist Jacob Dorsman, Regional Medical Inspector for Mental Health in the provinces South Holland and Seeland, to start an investigation and issue advice on the future of Centre '45. Because of the personal animosity between him and Bastiaans that surfaced a week earlier, she passed Baan, who, from his position as Chief Inspector of Mental Health, in fact was the first person designated to carry out such an investigation.[65]

It is to be hoped, the *NIW* wrote, that success would be achieved quickly and the conflict would end. It harmed the treatment and well-being of anyone in need of medical and psychiatric help. This was not in line with the intent of neither the clinic nor the centre, nor was it in the best interests of those treated in those institutions. For this they had to be centres of rest. Incidentally, it was clear to the *NIW* that it was in the interest of the war victims that Bastiaans was involved in the centre because of his status and experience.[66]

The *NIW* seemed to be getting its way. Early in June, in a meeting of the Advisory Council of the Centre '45 Foundation, of which Bastiaans was the chairman and Meijering the secretary, it was decided that psychiatrist Hugenholtz, also a member of the council, would explore the possibilities for practical cooperation between the clinic and the centre. The meeting reportedly was characterised by a positive and collegial atmosphere. Furthermore, Bastiaans and Meijering would also gather a number of times to try to reach an agreement. Firstly, they had to clearly map out the conflict and then formulate the conditions for cooperation. Ultimately, the final word would be pronounced by the centre's and the university's medical faculty boards. These developments brought *de Volkskrant* to the headline: 'Problems around Centre '45 appear to be solved'.[67]

Whether this was indeed the case is another matter. However, nothing more was heard about it in the newspapers, so calm certainly returned to some extent. It took two years before the centre regained some interest. Then the journalist Ischa Meijer, who survived Bergen Belsen as a child, was allowed to spend a few weeks there for the magazine *De Haagse Post* (The Post of The Hague). He wrote that therapy was greatly complicated "because the patient himself is so intensely focused on the war past".[68] It was at the same time that Meijer published his *Brief aan mijn Moeder* (Letter to my Mother), a book written by a first-generation victim, but seen as a book about second-generation problems. In it he broke the tacit agreement that victims of the Shoah, in this case his parents, should always be spared criticism.[69]

13. THE WAR SYNDROME AND LSD'S MEDICAL USE BOTH CRITICISED AND PRAISED

Taken aside some articles of Bastiaans' involvement in a report on the psychological impact of British internment camps in troubled Northern Ireland, mentioning problems identical to those experienced by Second World War victims,[1] attention for him and traumas arising from war and violence not resurfaced until late 1973. Then the Protestant *Nederlands Christelijke Radio Vereniging* NCRV (Dutch-Christian Radio Association) broadcasted the documentary *En wij, wij leven voort in een doolhof* (And we, we live on in a maze) about what was called the war syndrome. Remarkable about this documentary was that it didn't focus on the problems of the victims of violence, but on what the violence did to the perpetrators: the military. It was made by Henk Mochel, who was already known for *De Milde Dood* (The Merciful Death) an award-winning documentary about euthanasia.

Specifically, the documentary was about a soldier who, to the dismay of many of his former colleagues, talked about executing Indonesians during the decolonisation war 1946-1949. Four years after the VARA reported on war crimes for the first time,[2] this soldier – Gert van Emst, not his real name – admitted having murdered ten Indonesians and that he had become aware that he violated the laws of warfare. Therefore, the word 'guilt', almost absent in the KZ syndrome unless as part of the words 'survival guilt', played a major role in the war syndrome. It didn't alter that the war syndrome was lumped together with the concentration camp syndrome, although the *Leeuwarder Courant* talked about "a kind of branch".[3] This, at least, can be concluded from the fact that, according to *Het Parool,* the documentary brought back to mind the discussion about the Breda Three,[4] or from the phrase in *De Telegraaf* that Bastiaans, who provided some comments afterwards, estimated the number of Dutch sufferers from a war syndrome at 30 to 40,000; exactly the numbers he used for the KZ syndrome at the time. "More than enough", *De Telegraaf* continued, "to show interest in the subject."[5]

Mochel received dozens of responses to his broadcast, mostly from people saying they too suffered from problems resembling the ones he and Van Emst talked about. It was reason for him and the NCRV to invite some of them a month later. They could pour their hearts out in the programme *And we, we live on in a maze...* (same title but now with dots for reflection time). Again, Bastiaans was asked to comment. According to the TV critic of *Het Vrije Volk,* he said some "sensible things". However, he was very surprised to hear him say that people who had fought on the German side during the war and were now struggling with a war syndrome should be helped, but not before all the others had their chance of psychological or psychiatric assistance. "A curious point of view that probably won't contribute to the peace of mind of those doomed to come second place."[6]

It wasn't the only criticism. TV critic Scheepmaker noted that only writers of letters were invited whose complaints weren't specifically addressed to Van Emst. "Some problems" had arisen around him because of the things he said. Then he took aim at emotion TV – in vain. Why were all these people put around some kind of cafe table? And why were their stories interrupted by songs of the Greek composer Mikis Theodorakis?

> Why? To create a moment of rest in between the emotions? For whom, for what? For us, viewers? For the people at the tables themselves? In case I was emotional already, I wouldn't want to hear another Theodorakis song (probably the 'Ballad of Mauthausen'. LvB). Besides, I would have found it anything but pleasant to have to make my confessions 'en plein public', that is to say in a company of people also highly emotional, to have to display my nightmares, marital problems, etc., and to have my tears run free. It now resembled something like group therapy, which couldn't possibly have been the intention.[7]

Scheepmaker also wondered whether it was wise for people of such different backgrounds to be grouped together: from a man who, despite the prison sentence he had to endure for it, refused to fight in Indonesia and was still experiencing the disadvantages of having done so, to a man who said he hadn't taken any prisoners. Did the reason behind their problems no longer matter? Was everything KZ syndrome regardless of background? Had the symptoms been declared sacred? This must have been the reason that, according to Scheepmaker, Bastiaans had been a bit uncomfortable and argued that KZ syndrome should not simply be lumped together with war syndrome (a confusion to which he himself had contributed). The psychiatrist made clear there was a hierarchy between the two. Perpetrators suffered from a war syndrome. Victims suffered from KZ syndrome. Victims had priority. A KZ syndrome had precedence over a war syndrome.[8]

The war syndrome made the news again quickly because of reports about (assistance to) traumatised Israeli soldiers who participated in the Yom Kippur War (October 1973). In addition to the fact that many died at an age when their parents, who were traumatised for the second time now, had been in a camp, reference was made to similarities with the KZ syndrome again.[9] If journalists missed the obvious differences, it can be assumed that readers (and viewers) did too.

The attention for the psychological victims of the Yom Kippur War coincided with the run-up to the commemoration of the February Strike. This gained momentum because it had become known early in February 1974 that 22,000 war victims had applied for a persecution benefit. It was a sign for the Committee to Commemorate the February Strike to let it be known that it was high time that, according to the communist *De Waarheid,* "speedily and generously without any form of political discrimination and bureaucracy" the government would provide in "the financial and social security of former resistance fighters and victims of the German fascist persecution". Also, their number was higher than the 30 to 40,000 Bastiaans mentioned, "because in many cases the symptoms of KZ syndrome only appear after years".[10] In other words, one of the reasons Bastiaans had given when asked why there could be so many, was now put forward to show that this number couldn't be right. The numbers he mentioned were changed from an extrapolation into a minimum.

Only recently, that same *De Waarheid* stated, attention was paid to the fact that the victims of fascism experienced a lot of misery not only during the war, but afterwards as well, and that they had been exposed to a wide range of stress situations. As an example, the paper cited the repeated attempts by various governments to release the four and later three war criminals staying in Breda. Also, attempts to obtain support often ended in severe trials. The newspaper pointed at the bureaucracy, the long waiting times, the many forms, the lack of understanding. They all had done nothing but exacerbate the KZ syndrome, in spite of all the complaints about these complications and numerous warnings against their consequences. It was partly for this reason that Milikowski, meanwhile lecturer at the General Practitioners Institute of the University of Amsterdam, published a book entitled *Sociologie als Verzet. Over KZ-syndroom, gezinsproblemen, sociale en seksuele relaties en agressie* (Sociology as a Form of Resistance. On the KZ syndrome, family problems, social and sexual relationships, and aggression). With the exception of *De Waarheid,* it received little attention from the press. It was too steeped in communist ideology. Nevertheless, *de Volkskrant* praised Milikowski for being one of the first Dutch sociologists who dared to dig into the medical hornet's nest and had gone to war against authoritarian doctors.[11] The paper did not, however, mention that Bastiaans was one of the authoritarian doctors targeted by Milikowski.

Although, five years before, he reviewed *Do you now understand why I cry...* fairly positive, in the chapter on the KZ syndrome Milikowski turned out to be a fierce critic of Bastiaans as well as the Van Gasteren film and the syndrome itself, which, in his eyes, was a mere product of bourgeois psychiatry. He had, he told *De Waarheid,* strong objections to both the way in which the film was made and the final result. The main stumbling block was the focus on individual misery, making the social causes of KZ syndrome disappear behind the horizon. As a result, it wasn't a film in which a position was taken against war and/or fascism. In fact, Bastiaans led the patient's story. As a result, any attempt to extend his story beyond personal suffering was nipped in the bud. The problem had to continue to fit into the psychiatrist-psychiatric patient framework. The KZ syndrome was turned into a family problem and simultaneously "the identity of the resistance member as a resistance member" was lost.[12]

The events of the preceding years made it clear that the government should be counted among those suffering from the reverse KZ syndrome he coined. It wanted to release war criminals and was anything but generous when benefits had to be granted. But the psychiatrists didn't escape his judgment either. By limiting themselves to attempts to combat the psychological symptoms and by ignoring the cause, to wit still existing fascism, the sufferers were turned into dependent and powerless patients. "The former prisoners and many others suffer from oppression and fascism *because they're still present.*" As far as the Netherlands is concerned, he referred, for example, to alliances with "fascist-ruled countries" like Greece, Portugal, or Spain, and to the decolonisation war, which in the Netherlands was referred to as 'police actions', with their "war crimes against the national struggle for freedom in Indonesia".[13]

The crux was that if the assumed background of the syndrome was wrong, the usually applied treatment couldn't be right either. The war experiences were not decisive as regards whether a syndrome would develop or not, the reactions of post-war society and government were. The problem was not family relationships, but the relationship of the whole of society to the KZ syndrome sufferers. How could they be liberated, how could they regain their certainties and their trust in society, when the world threatened to repeat the hell they had lived in and fought against? Their struggle, Milikowski said, hadn't ended when the Nazi armies capitulated in 1945, but continued as long as oppression existed.[14]

Leaving warnings against contemporary fascism out of the medical narrative further exacerbated the powerlessness, Milikowski continued. As a result, the psychiatrists played a major role in creating and perpetuating the myth that the war had created an unbridgeable gulf between former prisoners and former resistance fighters on the one hand, and their post-war environment on the other. They weren't allowed to "become accusers of our society" because "in essence it was a continuation of pre-war times". Moreover, it wasn't coincidental that shortly after the war the government abolished the annual liberation's commemoration. In effect, it meant that "resistance in itself should be regarded as some kind of disease".[15]

Aversion to and struggle against post-war society will certainly have played a role in the problems of some of the former resistance fighters, like the communists among them, but by no means all of them. That is why *Sociology as a Form of Resistance* hardly received any attention from the newspapers as well. This was anything but the case with the book *Allemaal rottigheid allemaal ellende* (All wretchedness all misery) published a year later. It was written by the journalist Wim Wennekes, who knew Bastiaans because he interviewed him two years earlier, shortly before the opening of Centre '45, for *De Gelderlander* (The Gelderland Provincial Paper).[16] It was a book that, according to Prince Bernhard in the one-line preface, should be read by anyone with even the slightest interest in "what happened here during the war and how many suffered from it – and often still suffer from it".[17]

The book was presented in the Van Gogh Museum in Amsterdam in the midst of a small exhibition of work "by victims of KZ syndrome" (not 'by sufferers from'!). They had "found or tried to maintain their psychological balance" through painting or other art techniques.[18] *Vrij Nederland* published an entire chapter of Wennekes' book. *Trouw* wrote that it made more sense "than many war documentaries regularly appearing on the television screen". According to *De Telegraaf,* it belied the question that probably occurred to many whether a book about such a treatment was really necessary. Everyone had already seen Van Gasteren's film, isn't it? However, "precisely because it lacks the surprise and emotional span of the visual report", the book came across better than the film. It could be "processed more objectively". As a result, it most likely produced "less emotional reactions of adhesion and disapproval". *Het Parool* saw the publication as a good reason to give a full-page explanation of matters related to the subject. To mention but a few: the long history of the syndrome, beginning in 1946; the (unknown) numbers of people who were in the camps or in the resistance; the (im)possibility of a benefit; the broadcast of *Do you now understand why I cry …*, as well as the problem of the persecuted homosexuals (sufferers from a Bolshevik disease, according to Arthur Seyss-Inquart, the Austrian, National Socialist Reich Commissioner of the occupied Netherlands). And, of course, this article discussed the still deficient provision of assistance and guidance.[19]

Like Van Bueren six years earlier, Wennekes, as a member of the post-war generation, never quite understood why those former resistance fighters and camp prisoners couldn't stop talking about the war. Their stories meant nothing to him and hearing them over and over was a bit like watching acquaintances' vacation slides. They probably had meaning for the makers, but the viewer had no idea which one. The psychotherapeutic and LSD supported treatments of "a well-known but anonymous Dutchman", conducted and attended by Bastiaans in 1973 and 1974, changed his mind completely. The patient had been a member of a resistance group of which fourteen out of sixteen members hadn't made it to the end of the war. The man, named Willem van Salland, already collapsed for the first time in 1949. In 1960, when the discussions about whether to release the then still Breda Four started, he developed all kinds of physical complaints again. He was sent to the Jelgersma clinic in 1973. *All wretchedness all misery* was the record of the subsequent sessions. In a diary he kept at the time, the patient in question wrote about them: "It's as if you have finally emptied a garbage can with rotting remains." Incidentally, that garbage can had not begun to fill after 10 May 1940, but during childhood already. The treatment had revealed that his youth had "much, if not everything" to do with the situation he found himself in decades after the war.[20]

At the presentation, Bastiaans said to be very pleased that now in book form too a good picture was given "of what is actually so difficult to grasp for those who didn't experience it themselves". First of all, he took the opportunity to refute the doubt about the number of 30 to 40,000 sufferers mentioned by him a few years earlier, which according to some was too high, although, as said, according to *De Waarheid* it actually was too low. Its correctness was demonstrated by the large number of cases that came forward via assistance organisations that since seen the light of day. Probably unknowingly aligning himself with Milikowski in part, Bastiaans said that many who previously lived in silence and misery now stepped into the light because they no longer had the strength to keep up appearances and adapt, also "as a result of the daily confrontation with new war violence".[21]

Secondly, he made a fervent plea for the use of LSD. The good results achieved with the drug, "if applied selectively", were mistakenly surrounded by "fear, mistrust and myth-making".[22] Besides showing that even after thirty years the war still left its psychological mark, the book was also intended to dispel the myths and (consequently) take away the fear. According to Bastiaans, many people with KZ syndrome were afraid to go to his clinic. They thought they were immediately put in an LSD box, both literally and figuratively. But LSD was only administered after extensive, thorough preparation and, moreover, didn't suit everyone. It was especially used on those who repressed their emotions and impressions to such an extent that it had become impossible to process the events they endured.

LSD lifted that brake, allowing previously inaccessible areas in the human brain to break free.[23]

But as much as Wennekes' book was appreciated by the newspapers, and as much as Bastiaans explained and defended the use of LSD and downplayed its consequences and risks, it couldn't allay criticism of its use; criticism that grew fiercer after it became known that, in exchange for a few days' leave, the American armed forces experimented with LSD on Vietnam soldiers. Rightly, Bastiaans argued that experiments like these had nothing to do with his therapeutic use of the drug and that he strongly condemned them too. But it was no coincidence, *De Waarheid* argued, that the number of psychiatrists working with LSD was drastically in decline since the early 1960s. The majority stated that the advantages didn't outweigh the disadvantages. It led to direct criticism from Milikowski on Bastiaans and his treatment of war victims. His method had been a matter of weight once, but not anymore. Not for nothing, Milikowski incorrectly stated, Bastiaans was the only psychiatrist who still used the drug. Therefore, he seriously wondered whether the results were as good as Bastiaans always claimed. To his knowledge, they never were studied or evaluated.[24]

In addition to the question whether LSD actually helped patients, there was another aspect that merited scrutiny and made its medical use questionable. Milikowski's criticism of the use of LSD transcended the treatment of individual mental problems. As described, he kept a sharp eye on its political background and therefore also its political implications. Patients usually trusted their psychiatrist and therefore entrusted him with all kinds of things, especially if he was treating them with LSD, a drug with a disinhibiting effect. This wasn't without danger. Treatment in a university clinic of people, including former resistance fighters with political ideas, clearly referring to communist ideas, could lead to getting into the wrong ears of what had been said during those treatments, after which this information was used against them. This danger magnified in a university clinic like the Jelgersma. There, patient data was available to all kinds of people so that, even if the attending physician himself was faithful to his officially sworn secrecy, someone could get his hands on them. And this was not to mention the possibility that the Homeland Security Service or the CIA would let someone go undercover in a clinic. As an example, he pointed to the break-in of 'plumbers' in the US in the house of psychiatrist Daniël Elsberg, who passed on the Pentagon's reports on the Vietnam War to the press. The danger that could arise from this was obvious, according to Milikowski. After all, many hadn't only been in the resistance during the war. They protested, he repeated, against "fascism, colonial oppression and other forms of oppression in the present" as well. Through LSD use, the views, actions, plans of politically active patients or their friends could reach political opponents and the government.[25]

14. THE FIRST MOLUCCAN HOSTAGE-TAKINGS: WIJSTER AND AMSTERDAM

The criticism by Milikowski and *De Waarheid* only caused a ripple in a pond frequented by just a small part of Dutch society. But even if this hadn't been the case, it would soon have been snowed under by the news that would bring Bastiaans and the camp syndrome back into the news: the hostage-takings by descendants of residents of the Moluccan islands in December 1975, who, after decolonisation, decided to leave for the Netherlands instead of staying in Indonesia. Many of the men among them served in the former *Koninklijk Nederlands-Indische Leger* KNIL (Royal Netherlands East Indies Army). It hadn't been the first Moluccan actions. The residence of the Indonesian ambassador in Wassenaar was occupied on August 31, 1970. The Dutch policeman who patrolled there lost his life. However, this occupation was terminated the very same day. Two more failed actions followed in the spring of 1974 and in the spring of 1975, including an attempt to take Queen Juliana hostage. However, the hostage-takings of December 1975 lasted for several weeks.

On 2 December, train passengers in Wijster, in the North-Eastern province of Drenthe, were taken hostage by Moluccan youths, angry about the conditions under which they had to live in the Netherlands and about the government's broken promise to give their parents and grandparents, who served the Dutch in colonial times, a free Moluccans, independent from Indonesia. The train driver and two passengers were executed. The demands weren't met and after 12 days the youths surrendered. Two days after the start of the train hijacking, a second group occupied the Indonesian consulate in Amsterdam and a school for Indonesian children, located in the same building. One person died, an employee of the consulate. This occupation ended on 19 December.[1] Soon the question was raised what psychological consequences these experiences would have for the hostages.

The medical employee of the *Leeuwarder Courant,* who himself had been in camp Vught, near the city of Den Bosch, pointed out a big difference between the past and present situation; a difference working against the current hostages, so he said. Former inmates like himself were imprisoned for something they did themselves or for something they represented, while the victims of the hostage-takings had simply been in the wrong place at the wrong time. In every other area, agreement was trump. In both cases there was a lack of necessities such as food and water, good sanitation, or room to move. Inmates as well as hostages lacked "a way to get through the day pleasantly enough, a place of their own that is their own, where they can cry or laugh, relax or have sex when they feel like it". And: "At any moment their executioners can drive them from the place where they sit, using rifle butts or shovels. They may be friendly now and then, but they are threatened by a neck shot or a hanging all the time. There is no acknowledgement as a human being whatsoever."[2] However, there was one lucky thing, at least in the case of the embassy's occupation. Unlike the Dutch hostages in Wijster, the Indonesians in Amsterdam had an oriental mentality. As a result, they were able to "withdraw themselves and wait for things to get better".[3]

Once the hostage situation was over, the medical employee said assistance to the hostages should be kept to a minimum, although "of course there always are psychiatrists and psychologists who think it's time to give all sorts of pills and ask the hostages in every detail how they are doing". This "perhaps was useful for those craftsmen, but not for the hostages".[4] Of course, a hospital visit was in order. Of course, there would be crying and comforting. However, other than that, rest was most important, only not through pills. In other words: not providing drugs' assisted rest, but leaving them at peace, in their familiar environment, surrounded by their loved ones, should be the motto. "When all this happens, hopefully there will be no need for LSD to, as Prof. Bastiaans is forced to do, set free the past accompanied by all the yelling, crying, screaming not allowed to be expressed during their time in a concentration-camp or as hostages."[5]

The man must have been disappointed that it was Bastiaans who, during a broadcast in mid-December of the current affairs programme *Brandpunt* (Focus point), of the *Katholieke Radio Omroep* KRO (Catholic Radio Broadcast), insisted on radical psychiatric treatment. Bastiaans said he feared that the hostage-takings would lead to long-lasting, serious psychological and psychosomatic consequences. The hostages would have trouble processing their experiences. Therefore, intensive, professional guidance was more than appropriate. After all, if people are confronted with a situation for which they are not prepared, a physical and/or mental reaction was inevitable. According to Bastiaans, the consequences of a hostage situation were seriously underestimated. To clarify, he cited some of the hostages taken in the French embassy in The Hague and in the Scheveningen penitentiary in 1974. They were observed by a psychiatrist for a couple of weeks only. The obvious suggestion was that a more intensive approach could have prevented the problems, which manifested themselves after several months and which they were facing now. They included anxiety attacks, insomnia, nervousness, depression, and listlessness. Two hostages from the Scheveningen prison confirmed his story. They indeed suffered from psychological problems but had to do without expert guidance.[6]

The day after the broadcast Bastiaans' plea led to the government decision to provide long-term psychological counselling as soon as possible. Prime Minister Den Uyl stated that Bastiaans' words impressed him greatly and that he shared his opinion that good aftercare was necessary. A hostage situation was difficult to process and, therefore, a few days later the State Secretary for Public Health, Jo Hendriks, got in touch with Bastiaans to discuss how best to proceed. Bastiaans thereupon somewhat weakened his alarming *Brandpunt* story. He told the State Secretary that when giving psychological assistance one had to be watchful not to treat the former hostages a priori as patients. He was convinced that many of them were mentally strong enough to process their experiences without extensive aid. If they needed treatment, they had to take the initiative themselves, for example through their GP.[7]

This didn't alter that the emotional neglect at the time of the hostage-taking would certainly break several hostages if they weren't immediately helped. Already the first signs showing this were visible. In *Het Vrije Volk* Bastiaans said that he had urged Hendriks to ensure assistance was available, otherwise it could be too late.

> I told him: the Second World War has taught us a very dearly earned lesson. Now let's not frighten the hostages by talking them into a disease they may not have, but let's do set up a good scientific investigation and ask them to cooperate. On the other hand, their general practitioners should become familiar with distress signals the hostages can send out, consciously or unconsciously. Those distress signals can be like a flu that just won't go away, an imbalance, but also things like stomach ulcers, high blood pressure, muscle aches or rheumatism, coming up months after the fact. These psychosomatic complaints will probably affect the hostages who were among the strongest on the train and in the consulate. People, brought up in a 'don't behave like a child'-atmosphere. The only ones who, in my opinion, will get through these hostages unscathed are the most stable, the real Drenthe-inhabitants, and, strangely enough, also those who were already more or less isolated before it happened. The latter will collapse anyway, simply because every form of isolation will lead up to it eventually.[8]

What had to happen right away was that all hostages were psychologically tested and put under continuous physical control. They all had to be persuaded by a GP or spiritual counsellor to participate in the study. It was certain that problems would come to light such as mortification, anger at both the hostage-takers and the state, inability to put the emotions into words, "Alexithymia this has been called recently", or guilt about the fact that they survived, while some others had not.[9]

The therapy should focus on conversations and involve the entire family. Psychodrama could be applied. This also was used in the Jelgersma clinic, and the results were good. According to Bastiaans, in the case of the hostages, LSD was not necessary for the time being. It was, however, a great pity that the Netherlands still wasn't prepared "to assist people who are caught up in situations like these". By now, there should have been a permanent team. And in any case, such a team should have been formed in the early days of the hostage crisis. Yes, something had been done, but certainly not enough.

> Finally, I do want to say one thing: It's precisely these hostage-taking actions that confront us with an inadequate penal system again. One can wonder if this kind of illness of the Moluccan hijackers, resulting from emotional neglect and manifesting itself in violence, will be cured after 15, 20 years of imprisonment. I believe not…[10]

Het Vrije Volk had these last few sentences followed by the words: "According to Prof. Bastiaans", which suggests a certain distancing from this bouncer.[11] After all, they came down to saying that anyone pursuing a certain ideological goal by force was by definition mentally ill. Thus, this person shouldn't be sent to prison but should receive psychiatric care.

Two days after this interview it became known that a group of experts was going to deal with the reception of the hostages. Th result of Hendriks' consultation with Bastiaans about the best way of rendering aid, was that the GPs remained the first post in the care chain. They would be assisted and informed by a project group: the *Centrale Beleids- en Ondersteuningsgroep (ten behoeve van de Nazorg van Ex-gegijzelden)* (Central Policy and Support Group (for the aftercare of ex-hostages)), more commonly known as the *Commissie Begeleiding en Opvang Gegijzelden* (Committee on Guidance and Reception of Hostages), which resulted in the same abbreviation: CBOG. Of course, Bastiaans joined the committee, together with people from the Dutch Railways, the Medical Inspectorate for Mental Health, the medical psychology committee of the Dutch College of General Practitioners, and representatives from the Ministries of Health, Justice, and CRM.

Probably one of the hostages would be part of the group also. After all, according to Hendriks, outsiders could never fully comprehend hostage experiences. It was not yet clear whether this would be someone from the hostage situation in Wijster or Amsterdam. It was made absolutely clear the CBOG didn't just look at short-term complaints. And, moreover, family members of the hostages could call on the expertise of the group as well. The latter also applied to people who were officially involved in the hostage-takings and to victims of previous hostages, such as those in the Scheveningen penitentiary. On top, the experts had to write down how problems could be identified in time in the event of possible future hostages.[12]

The CBOG started an investigation into the degree of processing, in which all kinds of characteristics were considered. For example, in addition to age, it was taken into consideration what the educational level was or whether the hostage had been part of a group or had travelled alone. If indeed he or she was part of a group, it was also taken into consideration whether it was a group of friends or whether the others were younger relatives for whom they felt responsible. Furthermore, "some social, racial and personality variables were recorded".[13]

After the end of the hostage situation in Amsterdam, Bastiaans elaborated on a point he already discussed with Hendriks: guilt about certain statements made shortly after their release, guilt "about *the fact* that they had been brainwashed".[14] (Ital.: LvB) These statements echoed the understanding and solidarity with the hostage-takers some of the hostages felt. After having made them, some of them were threatened. According to the government they proved that the hostages had gotten into psychological problems; a statement that, as far as *NRC* columnist Van Overeem was concerned, could serve as proof that the government was in need of psychiatric assistance itself.[15]

Bastiaans, however, firmly stood behind the government in this respect. The understanding was explainable. He repeated they had clearly undergone brainwashing – a word, incidentally, that years later was also used by the family of one of the Wijster hostages but pointing at the psychiatrists as perpetrators.[16] Despite that this article mainly dealt with political reactions and further governmental plans, it was Bastiaans' view that graced the front page of *Het Vrije Volk* in huge letters and without quotation marks. This, firstly, shows that not only according to Bastiaans brainwashing should be considered a fact, and, secondly, that it was thought that using his name attracted readers.[17]

In an extensive article printed the same day in that very *Het Vrije Volk*, Bastiaans further stated that showing understanding was a hostages' survival strategy; a strategy not to be shaken off immediately after their liberation. Added to this was "a shared sense of neglect and abandonment". Incidentally, this was not only the key to the behaviour of some of the hostages, but also to that of the hostage-takers. They were emotionally neglected in the past weeks too. In addition, they had been abandoned by both motherland and fatherland. Some became depressed, some apathetic, some aggressive. "Emotional neglect is one of the great roots of violence in our time."[18]

About one of the hostages who had shown understanding for the hostage-takers, Bastiaans said: "When I heard him like that, I thought: Well, father, you are very close to total identification with the views of those Moluccans already. It probably won't be long before he can see things more 'rational' again."[19] In other words, while it was understandable that, given the situation they were in, hostages temporarily connected to the views and actions of the Moluccans, called 'sensory deprivation', it was considered impossible that this understanding was real and long-lasting.[20]

The firmness with which Bastiaans expressed his opinions was not uncontested, although it needed a letter to the editor, written by G.G. van Dam, probably the former member of the Irene Brigade and the English translator of the book *Slag in de Schaduw*, English title: *The Forgotten Battle*, about the fighting in the South-East of the Netherlands 1944-1945 after Market Garden failed. He told *Het Vrije Volk* that he was surprised that from the start so much attention was paid to possible psychosomatic consequences. Among others, he probably pointed at an article that appeared in *de Volkskrant* on 15 December, sub-headed: "KZ syndrome is not to be expected".[21]

There were always situations of emotional neglect, Van Dam wrote. Examples being victims of disasters and the many unemployed in the nineteen-thirties. "They had to get through it themselves, but nowadays everyone seems to have to be guided after only the slightest mischief."[22] Bastiaans, who "may have been an eminent scholar", was one of the causes of this mechanism because of his "great degree of emotionality". Although he said the hostages should not be talked into a disease, he immediately had this followed by a list of all the ailments possibly to occur out of a hostage situation. Continuously emphasising the possibility of psychological problems could only turn them into self-fulfilling prophecies.

> This is precisely the breeding ground for such phenomena. It's quite possible that a few hostages will develop a mild depression. They will rise again. Everyone suffers from emotional neglect now and then. Processing this for yourself is a task that not only the mentally strong can accomplish.[23]

If psychological counselling had to be given, then to the families of those who had lost their lives. They were more likely to suffer emotional neglect "than those who made it out alive".[24] Obviously, this letter had no influence whatsoever on the further decision-making process.

Hendriks officially installed the twelve-strong CBOG on January 14, 1976, now baptised as *Projectgroep Nazorg Slachtoffers Gijzelingen* (Project Group Aftercare Victims Hostage-taking). He declared: "Hostage-takings are acts of violence. That's where threats to life and to security come in, threats that are also executed. People are put under great pressure for a long time."[25] And also:

> Assistance to victims of violence should be studied more, and more systematically than is the case at present. It's possible that from the experiences in aiding victims of hostage situations, lessons can be learned that will improve the aid to victims of violence in general.[26]

In addition to Bastiaans, for example, the psychiatrists Joop van Londen and Dirk Mulder were part of the project group, as well as Frans Huygen, professor of general medicine in Nijmegen. Van Londen was head of the Public Health department of the city of The Hague and later became a top official of the Ministry of Health, chairman of the Assembly of the World Health Organisation and professor of General Health Care in Utrecht. Mulder would play a major mediating role in the next hostage-takings: in the villages of Bovensmilde and De Punt, again in the North-East of the Netherlands, in 1977. One of the hostages as well took part indeed, the physician Benjamin Fanggidaej of the Indonesian consulate, in daily life an insurance expert at the Joint Medical Service in Amsterdam. His experiences were point one of the agenda.

The group had to prepare centrally and support the policy of the already existing two working groups in the north of the country and Amsterdam. To this Hendriks added that for any subsequent hostage-takings, the Ministry of Health would have to prepare an immediate relief plan including guidelines for direct action. After all: "The better the care during the hostage situation and immediately afterwards, the greater the chance after-effects will be prevented." Furthermore, the group had to investigate scientifically what the long-term physical, psychological and social consequences were of the hostage-takings in Amsterdam and Wijster, as well as of previous hostages. Also, it had to advise general practitioners on possible medical consequences of hostage-takings and about the concrete help their patients should receive.[27]

As often happens with such well-intentioned project groups: criticism, justified or not, was inevitable. Moreover, it came from one of the most famous hostages, who on top could easily reveal his resentments: Ger Vaders, editor-in-chief of *Het Nieuwsblad van het Noorden.* The Ministry of Justice and the project group, he said, reacted too officially and unjustly took a wait-and-see attitude. Contrary to the agreements, the project group failed to contact the ex-hostages after a month. (Vaders wrote this on 11 February, so less than a month after its installation.) He, at least, hadn't heard from the group, and with him some of the others he was in contact with. Direct social counselling had taken place, but it was unclear whether this had any effect. Moreover, barring a few exceptions like Bastiaans, the members of the group were insufficiently aware of the tensions hostage-takings could cause. Some of Wijster's ex-hostages still didn't dare to board a train.[28]

One of the examples of carelessness Vaders cited was that of the wife of one of the executed. She wrote a letter to Van Agt. The woman asked whether she could call on the WUV – keep in mind: a pension law for victims of prosecution 1940-1945 – to improve her financial position. She received no response.[29] As with the war syndrome before, it's an example that makes clear that the way in which the problems the hostages, and their families, could face, was shaped by the context of the concentration camp syndrome.

In response, a ministry spokesman said requests for help were still coming in and they would all be dealt with in due course. And Van Londen pointed out that the members of the group didn't visit ex-hostages themselves. This was left to the Dutch Railways, local general practitioners, and social workers. He contested that the members of the group had insufficient knowledge of the subject matter but considered it "inappropriate to specify the specific knowledge of the experts".[30]

Fortunately for the project group, the news thundered on in the form of a renewed attempt by Minister Van Agt, after being asked to do so by the Council of Churches, to set the Breda Three free. In addition to humanitarian and legal arguments, the Council also based this request on medical grounds. After all, with Centre '45, there were better reception facilities for war victims in 1976 than in 1972. Van Agt still held the position that detention was firstly inhumane and secondly a violation of the legal system. Like four years before, this position wasn't shared by the entire cabinet. Minister of Defence Henk Vredeling, for example, threatened that releasing the three would mean the fall of the cabinet.[31]

Vredeling wasn't the only one, not inside and certainly not outside the cabinet. Practically everyone who previously opposed release was still against it four years later, and for the same reasons: the suffering and emotions of thousands outweigh the freedom and rights of a few. Bastiaans also stuck to his (revised) position: releasing the Breda Three would cause too much suffering. He refuted that reception had improved because of the opening of the centre. The number of war casualties simply was too great to be able to do anything substantial there. Treating all the victims still was impossible. Therefore, anyone who advocated humanity towards the three had to assert humanity towards those suffering from a syndrome as well. There were "20 to 40,000" (*Trouw,* March 17, radio/tv page) or "certainly 40,000" (*NRC Handelsblad* and *Trouw,* also 17 March, domestic news page). A good number of them had come into contact with at least one of the three in one way or another. Hence, they had to stay where they were.[32]

And so it happened. However, there were some who used this renewed discussion on the three to point out that psychiatrists, like all physicians, should pay attention not only to existing but to future patients as well. Wim Sprenger, a man who, in those years, regularly appeared in the media as a representative of the Alternative Pedagogical Academy, wondered where the medical protest was against dictators and other politicians who, with their bombs and torture practices took care of countless new victims with psychological problems?

> Has Professor Bastiaans ever heard of preventive medicine? Is psychiatry protesting against politicians who multiply the number of its patients? I would argue in favour of setting the upcoming May commemorations in the context of solidarity with the *current* victims of terror all over the world, precisely to make it clear that we haven't forgotten the Jews.[33]

At the time, this kind of criticism and the problems with the aftercare for the hostages of Wijster and Amsterdam couldn't damage Bastiaans' public stature. However, shortly after questions arose.

15. A FIRST DENT IN THE IMAGE

On 20 April 1975, in his KRO programme *Heel de Mens* (Man in its entirety), television and newspaper journalist Ad Langebent planned to interview Eibert Meester, the PvdA-politician who received a royal award whilst under Bastiaans' treatment for a KZ syndrome. The broadcast was cancelled due to "a mental breakdown". According to *Het Parool,* this confirmed "how gigantically many suffer still from their unprocessed war experiences".[1] In reality, only indirectly war suffering was to blame. Yes, there was a breakdown, but it had more to do with the present than the past. In a small circle, Tini Vogt, the woman with whom Meester had been married during the war, had cast doubts on his war past. This was investigated. The weekly magazine *Panorama* published the story that Vogt was right a year later, in the spring of 1976. Meester had neither a heroic war past, nor had he been in a camp. Consequently, he couldn't have suffered from any psychological damage caused by it. This meant Bastiaans tried to free someone from a non-existent KZ syndrome. It also placed Wennekes' *All wretchedness all misery* in a strange light because the Willem van Salland who played the leading role in the book, was in fact Eibert Meester.[2] The book, intended to educate a lay public about war trauma and the therapy against it considered the most modern, was withdrawn from the market.[3]

Newspapers covered the *Panorama* article early April 1976. This stated that Meester, who spent his wartime days in the city of Zwolle, mistakenly was paid a war pension. He applied for it in 1974 after which it was granted. He was able to convince the Foundation 1940-1945 that he was active during the war, and that these activities caused considerable health damages. This is why he had ended up on Bastiaans' sofa in 1973. Among other things, Meester stated in his application that he attacked a German officer, blew up a ship with aviation fuel, was arrested for carrying explosives and firearms, and was locked up in Arnhem prison. According to *Panorama,* the foundation hadn't been able to confirm the story. It believed him, nonetheless, although objections to Meester's story were submitted by resistance circles from Zwolle. It had been Wennekes' book that gave rise to their suspicions because they noticed similarities between it and the information in the application. Meester, they said, never played the major role in the resistance attributed to Van Salland – a reference to the region around Zwolle – in the book. After having been asked by *Panorama*, Bastiaans confirmed that Van Salland indeed was Meester's pseudonym.[4]

The Extraordinary Pension Council announced that it would quickly decide whether Meester's benefit was too high in relation to his resistance work. Meanwhile, the investigation by the Foundation 1940-1945, commissioned by Wim Meijer, the State Secretary for CRM, after having seen the reports written by the former resistance, was completed and forwarded to the council. After some additional investigation, Meijer would make his decision public. Interestingly, Meester – as mentioned before: a prominent member of the labour party PvdA – received a pension rather high. This was, the *NRC Handelsblad* reported, partly the result of a letter of recommendation from fellow party member and prime-minister Den Uyl. In it, Den Uyl spoke highly of Meester's merits for the party.[5] It gave Bart Lulofs, The Hague editor of the right-wing *De Telegraaf,* a nasty aftertaste, which became even nastier because Van Doorn, the Minister of CRM, had to assess the legitimacy of Meester's pension. He too would, according to *De Telegraaf,* not go down in history as a resistance icon.[6] It was a comment that will certainly have caused quite a bit of sneers in left-wing circles. After all, the same could be said of Lulofs' newspaper, (in)famous for his collaboration with the German occupier.

It would be unique that a war pension inquiry with a positive conclusion, even though Vogt's concerns were known to the researchers, was rerun. The then director of the Foundation 1940-1945, lawyer Huub van de Meerendonk, told the *NRC Handelsblad* that, as far as he knew, it never happened before that a pension was withdrawn because the pension receiver handed over incorrect information. However, because he considered the way in which *Panorama* presented Meester's fantasies to be inhumane, he preferred to wait for the final report to be released before formally responding to Meester's at the time still alleged fraud. Nevertheless, the journalist of the *NRC Handelsblad* who interviewed him wrote he already heard from very reliable sources that the result would be negative for Meester. Not only did he not play a role in the resistance, for some time he even was employed as manager of a company that was essential for the German war effort. Thus, he violated the second rule that was kept in mind for a pension as well, namely that someone had in no way supported the occupier.[7]

Of course, all this raised questions. Was it really "that easy to deceive those having to check whether applicants for an extraordinary pension have told the truth"?[8] Or, on the other hand, given the time that passed since 1945 and the excess of pension applications of which dozens were handed in on a monthly basis: was it even possible to carefully investigate whether an application was rightly or wrongly submitted?[9] Apparently not, because the Van Salland case wouldn't be the last time former resistance fighters protested against war pensions paid out by the foundation because of invented, heroic war deeds.[10]

Besides Wennekes, who himself would suffer from mental break down because of the affair, the people misled included Bastiaans. In addition to, for example, the recommendation of Den Uyl and Meester's Membership of Parliament – MPs don't lie – the *NRC Handelsblad* saw another reason why the first investigation was positive and why it took such a long time to publish the results of the second investigation. Meester was treated for his KZ syndrome by the first and foremost medical authority in the field, professor doctor Jan Bastiaans. How could someone be diagnosed to suffer from mental health issues resulting from certain wartime activities, if those activities never took place? Therefore, the application must have been correct, while in hindsight it could easily have been proved false.[11] As columnist Leo Derksen wrote in *De Telegraaf,* what Meester did during the war years "bordered on the superhuman". Little happened in the world of the resistance or Eibert "had a part in it".[12]

Meester saw the storm coming. Even though the new investigation wasn't officially completed and, therefore, its results were not yet available, he announced on 1 August 1976, that he would leave the Senate because of health reasons.[13] He also said farewell to Expogé.[14] At least that's what *De Telegraaf* wrote. It is more probable that he was disbarred.[15]

Shortly afterwards, the decision of the pension council was released. It indeed confirmed all the suspicions. Meester's pension was revoked. Bastiaans treated and cured someone for a non-existent camp syndrome. Wennekes wrote a book about a treatment that wasn't a treatment. He was interviewed about it by *Vrij Nederland.* His conclusion was that, although Meester couldn't be traumatised as a result of a heroic war past, the man certainly was ill. "And the only question that should be on our minds is, who makes him well?"[16] It was a statement Bastiaans used as well. In the Christmas special of the *Haagse Post* (Post of The Hague) he said that Meester suffered from pseudologica fantastica, which, incidentally and not for the first time, led to the accusation in a letter sent to him of having crossed medical-ethical boundaries, and professional secrecy in particular.[17] Bastiaans said this ailment was fairly common among people who outlived the war years, whereby, aside from Weinreb, he also referred to war criminal Pieter Menten, about whom more later.[18] "What's most fascinating is that Meester is not yet willing or able to admit that he boosted himself on this matter. He's just very outraged… I keep insisting he's even sicker than I thought."[19] With this diagnose Bastiaans exchanged one psychological problem for another. He kept insisting he was right about Meester, but, because of the pathological lying on the part of his patient, he just diagnosed the wrong brain disease. The patient couldn't be blamed for this, nor could he. He was not a police officer looking for the truth, but a doctor helping people. Whether they suffered from one problem or another, was immaterial.[20] He didn't ask why this tendency to lie specifically focused on resistance heroism and war victimhood. Nobody did.

The newspapers agreed with Bastiaans that he wasn't to blame for his *faux pas*. Therefore, the dent the affair could have made in his image was a minor one at best. After all, 'victims' were taken at their word by everyone, and why should the story of a respected Member of Parliament be questioned? Except for a few who had known Meester in the war years, no one had doubted his story, so why should Bastiaans have done so? However, precisely because of the characteristics of a disease of which he knew the existence and of which he even said it wasn't uncommon, he hadn't seen it. That's not a psychiatric job well done. Therefore, there is a much more likely explanation for the mistaken diagnosis. Bastiaans thought that because of deportation and/or resistance participation, sooner or later everyone developed a concentration camp syndrome. He, therefore, had assumed at once that this was the case with Meester also, whose fabled past in the resistance he believed. He hadn't so much diagnosed an individual patient but had thought that what had been the case so often, was the case here as well, and acted accordingly thereafter. In other words, he had traded the truth of the N=1 case study, normally sacred among psychoanalysts, for the truth of the lowest common denominator. This had disastrous consequences. Not so much for him. For his patient.

The only time the role, the expertise, Bastiaans had played in this was mentioned in the newspapers was in early 1978. A good year earlier, two former resistance members had sued Meester because of his deception, but their case was dismissed by the Court of Justice. Meester was in too bad a physical and psychological state to be prosecuted. The former resistance fighters appealed against this. Meester's pension had to be stopped, not just suspended, as had been the case until then. The amount already paid out – approximately *f*100,000 (€45,450) – had to be refunded. At least, they indicated that they would appeal if the answers Van Agt had to give to questions asked by the Senate member for the *Pacifistisch Socialistische Partij* PSP (Pacifist Socialist Party), Joop Vogt, brother of Tini Vogt, weren't satisfactory. One of those questions concerned Bastiaans. Vogt wanted to know which doctor had advised the Court. It would be unpalatable if indeed this had been Bastiaans, which according to Vogt was the case. Because he had been misled by Meester too, and had misdiagnosed him initially, he had an interest in the outcome of case.[21] That no further information was given about this, including whether Bastiaans had indeed been the court's medical adviser, is indicative of the importance the newspapers placed in the further prosecution of Meester. He was both perpetrator and victim, both crook and mental patient, and that's about all there was to say about it.

In any case, the title of the next major interview that Bastiaans gave after Meester's deception had come out into the open, in *Het Parool* of 26 March 1977, will have been interpreted by some readers as self-criticism (which it wasn't): "Problem of war victim not understood". Bastiaans criticised the late establishment, in 1975, of the *Werk- en Adviescollege voor immateriële hulpverlening aan oorlogsgetroffenen* WAC (Work and Advisory Committee for immaterial aid to war harmed), with which the broadening of the number of groups psychologically harmed, had become clear in the naming also. The more inclusive word 'war harmed' increasingly replaced the term 'war victims'.* The WAC had to make an inventory of the entire range of war victims and then advise the government on how best to help them. The reason for the interview was that after more than thirty hearings with all kinds of organisations the WAC had submitted its first report. Such a body should have been set up in the mid-1960s at the latest and not only as a result of the Breda Three discussions and the broadcast of *Do you now understand now why I cry...*[22]

Much of what was said in this interview was a repetition of already well-known information about the KZ syndrome and what to do about it. The most striking, therefore, were the numbers mentioned, picked out of a 1976 WAC-study, and serving as opening of the article: 'For approximately *one hundred and fifty thousand* Dutch people, the Second World War is still not over'. (Ital.: LvB) According to Bastiaans, the WAC-study had shown that in the Netherlands more than 2 million people were experiencing the aftereffects of the war still. The 150,000 *Het Parool* spoke of was the maximum (so not the 'approximate') of, firstly, those who needed short-term social support (100,000 to 130,000) and those who needed longer-term

* Incidentally, the term 'war harmed' would also be considered too exclusive after a while, after which the word *oorlogsbetroffenen* (war affected) became popular. They are terms, cynics would say euphemisms, intended to counteract a hierarchy of suffering. Because the number of actual war victims decreased, they give the impression of a medical profession looking for a new patient file. More importantly, they misjudge the uniqueness of the origin of particular kinds of suffering, especially the Shoah. Mooij commented on this: they formed 'a great disappearing act, with the only advantage that no one had to feel left out'. Mooij, 'De langste schaduw', 280, 286; Withuis, *Erkenning,* 78, 90, 245

guidance by professional workers (10 to 20,000). Bastiaans himself wrote about these numbers in a later article that 130,000 people certainly still needed help, of whom 20,000 were seriously needy.[22] So these 20,000 shouldn't be added to the 130,000 but were integrated in it.

The big question such numbers give rise to, was of course: how does the government intend to assist the aid workers, "especially when considering", Bastiaans said, "that no one is able to do this work all day long"? For that it simply was too hard. "I have seen many young care providers who decompensated (lost their psychological balance. LvB) themselves after having worked for some time." Each year, the group of 20,000 severely affected victims alone – the word 'maximum' was no longer mentioned anywhere – was in need of about 1,000 highly trained psychotherapists, able to work with this particular group. There weren't any. Even from the psychiatrists he trained, only one in five was suited to perform this task. "In many it arouses fears, others often avoid problems by trivialising them." Moreover, it took years to "remain calm in the midst of this problem", and "to take optimal interest in a particular case again and again, and, at the same time, to keep some distance, in order to avoid sleepless nights". Because of this lack of psychiatrists and psychologists there was little choice but to opt for a short-term therapy that at least would make life a bit more bearable for a certain time. For this the non-professional counsellors touted in the report were certainly of some value. "But I do have some question marks – at least with regard to whether the lack of experienced therapists can be made up for in this way. I have my sincerest doubts."[24]

16. 4 MAY 1977: COMMEMORATING THE DEAD

After everything that had happened in the previous year and because of the publication of the WAC report, it was hardly surprising that general practitioner Aart Gisolf, who had a TV show and published in newspapers extensively, devoted his entire page in the *Algemeen Dagblad,* called 'Looking back with the doctor', to the camp syndrome. The immediate cause was the publication of two articles by Dick van Tol about the KZ syndrome, disaster syndrome and traumatic neurosis in the *Medisch Magazine* (Medical Magazine), February and March 1977, psychological diagnoses that had increasingly merged and in time even considered to be more or less equivalent, also by Gisolf.

Gisolf discussed the rapidly changing mental state of marines who, in Rotterdam in May 1940, had defended the bridge over the river Meuse. The four survivors had seen an application rejected for a Military William Order, the highest Dutch military decoration. This was badly processed by three of them.[1] He also discussed the case of a former resistance member who slowly deteriorated mentally, became unemployed and saw his marriage on the rocks.[2] Finally, he addressed the second-generation problem. Because the parents, especially Jewish parents, struggled with problems of their own, they reacted to certain situations as well as to their children's behaviour not in a way considered healthy for the mental development of their offspring. However, the exact consequences of this for the post-war generation hadn't yet been properly researched.

> The 'second-generation problem' is therefore still largely hidden from us. But it's time to take it into account. Few things are as harmful as 'hiding'. That's why it's better to talk about it now. The 4 May commemoration is an annual recurring reason to do this. It would be a tragic misunderstanding to let pass an occasion as such.[3]

But the main part was about the history and symptoms of what "briefly and illogically is called KZ syndrome". It started with the sentences:

> Today we commemorate the dead of the Second World War. But we forget to commemorate the survivors. For many, the war is far from over. Almost every day they have moments in which they experience again and again what happened to them in camp, combat, or resistance.[4]

According to Gisolf, the group suffering from the syndrome seemed to be getting bigger and bigger, for two reasons. More and more doctors became familiar with it, so it was recognised sooner and more often. Even more important was "the fact" that often the syndrome led to complaints after years only. So, according to Gisolf, the complaints didn't form the syndrome. The syndrome was already there, only the symptoms were yet to come. According to him, people didn't so much suffer from it, as fell victim to it. But can a person who is not bothered by anything be said to be ill? Gisolf answered affirmative. "You may ask yourself: Are there also healthy war victims? You could say: If they are healthy, they are not victims either. But the reality is that very few people survive a period of extreme stress unscathed."[5] On top, it wasn't just the war that was to blame, with which Gisolf added a third reason to the spread of the syndrome. Or perhaps better: he lent its distribution, its inkblot effect, a hand. Other terrible events, such as child abuse or frightening and threatening situations in any other phase of life, emphatically including hostage-taking, could lead to a KZ syndrome, or at least to a "KZ-like syndrome".[6]

According to Gisolf, in case the war was involved the syndrome was made worse by the fact that often doctors as well as patients were reluctant to mention the war. "'Not all that ballyhoo once more', the doctor seems to think, and the patient is convinced that the doctor 'doesn't understand anything anyhow'." As a result, for a long time the real causes weren't discussed while due to various complaints the patient was sent from one specialist to another, until finally someone, usually a psychiatrist, brought up the war. Only then the treatment was aimed at talking about it consciously. Only then the patients could learn to live with their war experiences, "because you never forget!"

> Now, for many victims, 32 years after the fact, the problems become more serious. They are "more sensitive" on this point than, let's say, ten years ago. This is why it became increasingly difficult to release the Breda Three. The victims find it more and more problematic to process emotions like these.[7]

Het Parool spent an entire page to the theme too. 'The war still has a profound effect on many humans' was the title of an interview with Hans Hers, who ten years later would be one of the authors and editors of the book *Stress. Medical and legal analysis of late effects of World War II suffering in the Netherlands.*[8] Hers, son of an anti-Nazi GP, was an internist and colleague of Bastiaans at the Leiden Academic Hospital. When the war started, he worked in the Netherlands for British intelligence, was arrested in October 1940, survived six concentration camps, and provided medical assistance to resistance fighters, soldiers, and camp survivors pro bono from

1950 onwards. That they shared experiences played a firm role in this because many of his patients tended to beat around the bush. "I speak their language; they can't cheat me. Because of this I can track down their sometimes-malicious ailments better than their GP can, from whom they have kept so much a secret."[9]

Hers, who was infuriated about the bureaucratic squabbling in the payment of war pensions,[10] had been present as a medical reporter at the international conference on late effects of war experiences organised by the *World Veterans Federation* in 1961. His report, he said, had helped prevent "suspending the Extraordinary Pensions Act because the war had been over for so long. We reported that the number of patients didn't decrease but steadily increase. In those days I gained an important ally: Professor Bastiaans, for whom I have the utmost respect."[11]

It too had been in those days that in total around and about 850 men and women began to visit Hers; men and women of a kind he hadn't seen before. They were highly educated people in leading positions. For a long time, this had increased their resistance, but now they too became overstretched. Now, the physical and psychological complaints of these "forgotten war heroes" manifested themselves. To Hers, this was one of the indications that indeed we all have our breaking point, to them it only had come a little later, around the age of sixty, than usually was the case. For years they had been too proud to ask for help, and most had lived a good life financially. But with age rising, problems arose as well, and with it, financial downturn showed its head. However, he didn't want to call their problems a KZ syndrome. He "very much" hated the term because it had become a collective diagnosis for all kinds of psychological and somatic complaints of which the majority had nothing to do with concentration camps. Therefore, he preferred to speak of a "war stress syndrome because they had been confronted with death every minute, every hour, every day, every month, every year during the war – always, and in some cases for five years in a row."

Contrary to popular belief, this meant that a psychiatrist wasn't always necessary. The stress had physically set itself, for example leading up to a hernia. In such cases surgery helped better than psychotherapeutic sessions. "How many people improved because of my intervention? I think eighty percent of the about eight hundred and fifty that has knocked on my door. But this doesn't diminish what psychiatrists and others do."[12]

17. TWO MORE MOLUCCAN HIJACKINGS: BOVENSMILDE AND DE PUNT

Those who thought that with Wijster and Amsterdam the Moluccan campaigns were over, came home from a cold fair. The passengers in a train at De Punt, as well as the children (who were released after four days) and teachers from a primary school in Bovensmilde – both in the province of Drenthe – were taken hostage from 23 May to 11 June 1977. Two hostages and six hostage-takers were killed during the military action ending the train hijacking. Mulder, in his capacity as the negotiating psychiatrist, was already on the second day able to report on the latter that they had a paternal disorder. Although there was a woman among them as well, because of this they had "a morbid need to show their manhood".[1]

The hijackings rekindled the discussion about the psychological fate of hostages and, especially because of the school children, their relatives. In view of the medical course of events during the previous hostage-takings, usually pictured as too little too late, it was urged to act quickly. The script for helping the children after their release was written within two days. An agreement was made with the nearby Groningen University Hospital that, once the hijackings would be over, all the hostages could go there for observation. Its psychiatry department set up an aftercare centre in the same period of time, the *Begeleidingsgroep Noord* (Northern Counselling Group). Guidance teams were formed for those who returned home. Also, within a few days the parents of the children held hostage organised a mutual emergency service. Former hostages of Wijster played a significant role in all this. On 25 May, in *Het Parool*, professor of psychiatry in Groningen, Wybe Kuno van Dijk, said about them: "They are indispensable." Their input was of great importance. Furthermore, according to Van Dijk, the idea of setting up a number of special educational offices was considered. All this was supervised by Bastiaans' research project group, set up after the previous hostage-takings.[2]

This diligence didn't go unanswered. In the *NRC Handelsblad*, the day after the children of Bovensmilde were released, Rob Lubbers, professor of pedagogy in Utrecht, called upon the psychiatrists not to interfere with (the families of) the children too much. The parents had to be able to meet their children spontaneously, and to treat them as usual. Above all, they shouldn't be overloaded with commandments and prohibitions, as did happen. Predictions about how children will react who experienced something similar, should be avoided also. Because, if a reaction wasn't in accordance with what was predicted, a deviation was thought of immediately.[3]

This view was endorsed in an article published one week later in *Het Vrije Volk* entitled 'The aid workers are besieging the hostages'. It was feared that the 'too little too late'-criticism was taken at heart by aid workers too much. In case such a scenario was repeated, already diverse scripts had been written and protocols drawn up by "committees of soul-searching experts". As a result, more institutions gathered in Groningen and Drenthe than we "may be able to take hostage in the entire decade to come". Masses of aid workers were on stand-by "to talk the first cases back into society". The only thing the hostages had to do was to get out of the train or school alive. Anyone who had enough resilience to handle the event on his or her own ran the risk of not being seen as a "good hostage". "I don't care if you say you're alright. You're suffering from this or that abnormality. It says so in our script." A Red Cross volunteer noted that the parents were already beginning to resist the "'suffering-lechery' of the organised 'trists- and gists-hood'." They felt brought down by the rain and had the idea that, even if nothing was wrong with them, they would be talked into a disorder, so that assistance could start anyhow.[4]

In addition, it wasn't just the hostages and their families who suffered and asked for help. Especially the images of trains and airplanes made minds drift towards the years of war and persecution. As a result, on 1 June, that same *Het Vrije Volk* reported that at the Jelgersma clinic right from the start of the hostage-takings various former camp inmates were knocking on the door for support and help. And Centre '45 had received dozens of calls for assistance too. They suffered from nightmares and had taken tranquilisers. Bastiaans: "One shouldn't exaggerate, because it actually isn't uncommon, but it is indeed clear that these people experience new problems as soon as, let's say, the 'old experiences' are updated."[5]

Bastiaans repeated that suchlike problems had occurred during the previous hostage-takings and the Breda Three discussion as well. Remarkable about the Moluccan hostage-takings was that especially those who suffered in Japanese camps, "'among the blacks', as they say themselves'", relived their experiences. "This we see time and again."[6] Apparently, that the parents of the Moluccan hostage-takers had fought on the side of the Dutch was of little consequence.

Such opinions will have been an additional reason to create some space on television for a conversation with Bastiaans about the possible psychological consequences of hostage-takings. This was regretted by the TV columnist of *De Waarheid*, which may have been the first sign of a slowly developing 'Bastiaans and psychotrauma'-fatigue. The conversation came at the expense of an interview by a TV critic with directors and actors such as Alfred Hitchock and John Wayne about (the consequences of) violence on television and in feature films. Incidentally, in the same piece the Cambodian killing fields were defended implicitly.[7]

For the time being, however, *De Waarheid* was the only paper not eager to get information from Bastiaans continuously. Thus, after the violent ending of the train hijacking, he again was asked to give his opinion, although not only about the victims, his expertise, but about the end of the hijacking itself as well. On the basis of international statistics, pointing out that an average of 14 percent of the hostages died during hostages, he showed that, "if we ignore the hijackers themselves", the death toll in De Punt had been significantly lower.. "Even from this cynical point of view, this proves that the decision makers have done the best they could."[8]

Bastiaans derived his figures from a conference in Evian, France, where, early in June, criminologists, police officers, and medics discussed international terrorism. One of the conclusions was that compensation was crucial for therapy to be successful. It gave a sense of security; the idea of being taken seriously. In war victims this was evident too. If therapy was not supported by material compensation, it wouldn't work. Bastiaans himself spoke in his capacity as a member of the CBOG. This project group, he told *Het Vrije Volk,* encountered two specific problems: the arguments with the ex-hostages in Wijster, and the settlement of damages suffered during the hijackings and occupations. This process proceeded too slowly and in a "not optimal" manner. Because not everyone was insured, some sort of buffer fund had to be created. If the government didn't do this, it "leaves the people out in the cold", which creates "discontent and a starting point for depression".[9] It's a fine example of how possible medical problems in the future can serve as political leverage in the present.

That the hostages of Wijster caused more problems than the others, was the result of their initial treatment "by local neurologists and social workers, who didn't provide the help needed".[10] Also, or because of this, things hadn't worked out between the CBOG and the Northern Guidance Group. The hostages in Wijster therefore set up their own contact group, also to assist Bastiaans in his investigation.[11] It was all the more reason for him to argue that "we'll be ready when another disaster like this occurs, because I actually knew for some time more hijackings would come". He immediately had called Van Dijk in Groningen to tell him: "Do something right now, because you weren't ready last time." As a result of this intervention, Van Dijk organised a reception centre. Bastiaans could imagine that Van Dijk was slightly disappointed after it turned out that everyone just wanted to get home after the hijacking and leave the centre for what it was. After all, he had no experience with such situations. The hostages needed rest, sleep, family. Bastiaans himself didn't mind so much that they went home first, as long as they would come back as soon as problems arose. Nevertheless, they had to be given the opportunity to tell their story as soon as possible, preferably in the presence of professionals. Then they could relive what they endured, "but now without the fear and the threat of death". Clamming up had to be prevented.

> Especially the ones who by nature are in possession of strong personalities sometimes say: "Well, that's it. Let's forget about it and move on!" This is ostrich politics. The emotions, which had to be suppressed during the hostage situation, have to come out sooner or later. The best way to achieve this is by talking to each other.[12]

These sentences were applicable to the treatment of war victims as well, and Bastiaans was aware of that. One of the lessons the war had taught him was that assistance and, if necessary, treatment should begin as soon as possible. Everything "not completely disposed of right away" would "return in an intensified form twenty or thirty years later".

> One of the people held hostage in the Scheveningen penitentiary once said to me: doctor, we were isolated twice. Once in jail and the second time when, after the wave of publicity, we were forgotten and left alone with our problems. That second isolation has to be avoided.[13]

From his words to Van Dijk, it can be concluded that modesty and collegiality weren't Bastiaans' most striking qualities. However, for his COBG-colleague Mulder, who wasn't able to be present in Evian because, as mentioned, he played a mediating role in the latest hijackings, he had nothing but praise.

> At first, he gave the hijackers every possible effort so as not to irritate them even more, but gradually he introduced a kind of dosage and rhythm in the negotiations, which created a basis of peace and security even in this very difficult situation. He did everything humanly possible.[14]

The role Mulder played immediately showed how enormously important it was to make use of trained psychiatrists in situations like these.

> All those policy and decision-making groups, the military, the Red Cross, social workers, the judiciary: these are all groups with some kind of power sitting opposite of each other which creates a tendency towards violent

> decisions. As a psychiatrist, you have to keep on trying to streamline suchlike processes.[15]

Incidentally, the stress to which all these people were exposed, including Mulder, the politicians, and the military, shouldn't be underestimated. They had to deal with this in no small measure too, although usually the usage of the word was limited to victims, *in casu* the hostages. "Amidst all the criticisms, it would be fair to consider this every once in a while." Little was known, however, about the consequences of stress for policy makers and executives, and certainly not about stress among the military. "It's a Defence matter. We don't get access to that easily."[16]

Bastiaans wasn't the only one praising Mulder. In an article in the *NRC Handelsblad,* foreign specialists, like the American director of Mental Health, Frank M. Ochberg, was enthusiastic about the way the Netherlands handled the hostage-takings. The efforts of Mulder could meet with his approval in particular. That he simply maintained contact with the Moluccans by telephone was, according to Ochberg, characteristic of the high level of mental health care in the Netherlands. Abroad, this was still left to police officers.[17]

The *NRC Handelsblad* also consulted Bastiaans because of the Evian conference. Under the heading 'The real hangover is yet to come', the possibility was discussed that the ex-hostages would suffer from nightmares, depression and physical complaints resulting from mental problems. In addition, financial reparation "without the nagging of authorities and officials" was touted as a simpler means than psychiatric help, although of course its importance was not to be discounted. On the contrary. The hostages including their families, had to talk, preferably in a group.[18]

Van Londen was asked what exactly was done at the time of the hostage-taking. He spoke about the "care meant to assist the after-care". Everything that was already done for the victims and their families before the drama was over helped to reduce problems occurring afterwards. For example, with the help of the child psychiatrist Cornelis Rümke, son of the aforementioned Henricus Rümke, anticipatory talks were held with the parents of the children held hostage in Bovensmilde. This meant bluntly speaking about what could happen. "This is of far more worth than the usual chitchat of 'just keep calm, it'll be all right'."[19]

Bastiaans explained that, when assisting the hostages, his experience with war victims came in handy. Although a hijacking seemed less serious than a concentration camp, it too could have a serious impact because of its sudden nature: the surprise, the unexpected threat to life, the uncertainty about the outcome. However, it could well be that, in spite of its violent ending, the train hijacking at De Punt would turn out to be the less traumatising than the one at Wijster, a year and a half before, because all in all, the threat to life was minimal. Also, in general the hostages were young and, therefore, more flexible in processing experiences like these than people who already reached a more advanced age. By the way, speaking of life-threatening situations: it was remarkable that, in contrast to the Wijster hijacking, at De Punt there was no mention of sympathy from hostages for the hostage-takers. Would this, Bastiaans wondered, have anything to do with the fact that, unlike Wijster, there were only deaths when the hostage situation ended, so that thoughts of a possible passing were less present?

> We would like to find out what those mysterious aspects are in the contact behaviour between hijacker and hostage. When does something like this happen? When does the companionship in order to survive turn into identifying with the aggressor, with the one in power?[20]

This identification – dubbed Stockholm Syndrome after a hostage-taking in the Swedish capital in 1973, a name that became widely known a year later because of the far-reaching identification of millionaire daughter Patricia Hearst with her captors – had both positive and negative effects. The positive effect was that it reduced the danger to life during a hostage situation. The negative effect was that after a while a hostage could become ashamed of his or her identification, with all the associated psychologically problematic consequences.[21]

Incidentally, according to the final report of the CBOG, published in 1979 and simply called *Psychological Research into the Consequences of Hostage-taking in the Netherlands,* no typical case of Stockholm syndrome occurred during the hostage-takings. In average, however, the hostages stood neutral, not negative, towards the hostage-takers.[22] It was a conclusion fiercely criticised in *Het Vrije Volk* by the journalist and teacher at the School for Journalists, Piet Heil. In reaction to current affairs TV programme *Hier en Nu* (Here and Now), in which Bastiaans spoke extensively about the report, he wrote that affiliation, “that’s what it’s called in professional circles these days”, is something to be witnessed in all times and all places and that it’s grossly used, or rather misused by governments. Of course, there had been fraternisation. After all, the life of both the one and the other were threatened by possible outsider actions. This outside world became the common enemy and if the enemy of the one is the enemy of the other… It was, he said, yet another fine example of an old wine, merely talked about because it had been poured into a new, scientifically labelled bag.[23]

Despite the emphasis in both *Het Vrije Volk* and *NRC Handelsblad* on the importance of material compensation in order for therapeutic help to be successful, in the latter newspaper Van Londen made it clear that this was quite a challenge still. Moreover, that Hendriks made promises about it was merely a rumour and therefore incorrect. The only thing he did was advising to send every claim to a central point, from which they could be forwarded to the Justice Department. This didn't alter that this department had formal, legal objections to payment. It was difficult the verify the validity of the claims, ranging from a lost coat to a cancelled holiday on the Canary Islands. In addition, compensation could set a precedent. Why should victims of a hijacking receive it and other victims, "for example of traffic disasters, violence and fires", not? Van Londen did expect that eventually there would be some sort of financial compensation, but that it would not be registered as such, and serve more as a confirmation that something happened in which the government was involved.[24]

A few months after the hostage-taking in Bovensmilde and De Punt, Mulder gave a lecture in Israel about his experiences, as well as about the cause and aftermath of the events. It was a Dutch-Israeli, five-day conference. In addition to Mulder, for example, Bastiaans, Speijer and Jaap van Praag, the chairman of the WAC, the Working and Advisory Committee for war harmed, were present as well. Speijer stated that he demanded an unambiguous definition of the concept 'victim'. Bastiaans spoke about 'Control of Aggression and Psychotherapy'. According to the *NIW*, he was the centre of the conference. In total, the Dutch delegation consisted of 32 persons "if the spouses are included". Among them were officials from the Ministry of CRM, charged with the implementation of the WUV. Hendriks himself was present as well. The conference was the result of a request from State Secretary Meijer several years ago. When visiting Israel, he suggested organising a symposium "by scholars and social workers from the Netherlands and Israel about their experiences in the treatment of people who fell victim to persecution".[25] This indicates that the conference itself was devoted to the reception and treatment of war victims. The emphasis was on the Second World War as well as on the generation born afterwards but affected by it as well. That Mulder spoke about the hostage-taking, unrelated to the war, once again shows how much the psychological problems of hostages were drawn into the sphere of the KZ syndrome.

Mulder touched on the long-standing tense relationship between the Moluccan and non-Moluccan population in the surroundings of Wijster, De Punt and Bovensmilde. According to Mulder, this was partly because, when in violation, Moluccans weren't fined by the police out of fear of reprisals. He went on to say that he was surprised that "former hostages expressed their need for attention and security in an extremely materialistic way". He probably had in mind the complaint of a number of former hostages that the amount they received was insufficient to compensate for the damage (*f*3000,- [€1365,-] for the hostages of De Punt and Bovensmilde, less for the ones taken hostage a shorter period of time, and nothing at all for those who fell victim to the hostage-takings in the Scheveningen prison and the French embassy in The Hague in 1974). According to Mulder, the hostages expressed an "obsessive need to be financially compensated" by often aggressively approaching the government, for loss of or damage to property on the one hand and psychological distress on the other. This, he said, had to do with the fact that the government and not the group of terrorists, as he called the Moluccans, was held responsible by many of the hostages for what happened to them.[26]

It was spicy that in his lecture Mulder talked about the plan "to form special units under the responsibility of the Ministry of Defence, to be used in case of hostage-takings". This meant that the armed forces would be trained beforehand for domestic deployment, possibly against Dutch nationals.[27] No wonder the Ministry of Justice was quick to disprove Mulder's story. Two days after his lecture – which led to various parliamentary questions, including about the discrimination against non-Moluccans by the police – the Ministry of Justice announced that the policy on hostage-taking was and remained a matter for the judiciary and the police. Even in case military assistance was requested, like at De Punt, the deployment would take place under supervision of these two. According to the spokesman for Justice, the fuss about Mulder's lecture was based on "one big misunderstanding". As a scientist, he spoke among scientists about hostage situations that, certainly because of the deployment of military personnel, suggested a war situation. This was anything but to say that from now on special military teams would be formed under the responsibility of Defence to act in the event of subsequent hostage-takings.[28]

So, it was a misunderstanding that had arisen out of a talk on aftercare for hostages at a conference about aftercare for war victims. This misunderstanding was not surprising, although it is debatable whether 'misunderstanding' is the right word to use. The armed forces unit, called *Bijzondere Bijstandseenheid* BBe (Special Assistance Unit), was already there, as were a BBe Marines and a BBe Police. They were created after the hostage-taking and murder of Israeli athletes during the 1972 Munich Olympics.[29] However, from a psychiatric point of view the word was appropriate. In those days, the pre-PTSD era, the KZ syndrome was virtually the only frame of reference for psychiatrists, at least in the Netherlands, dealing with problems following the use of violence, whether or not this violence was related to the Second World War in general or the concentration camps in particular. As a result, the views on hostage-related problems were shaped by what was known from literature dealing with the KZ syndrome.[30]

Bastiaans, Hers, Van Londen: they all emphasized the importance, materially as well as psychologically, of benefits being awarded without too much fuss. In their eyes, it was of little concern whether this payment was called compensation, pension, or confirmation. But the simple fact that this already created difficulties with recent hostage-takings shows that in the case of a war decades in the past, hassle was insurmountable. A persistent and over time increasing problem was that it became more and more difficult to prove whether an application for a war pension was justified; the Eibert Meester affair served as proof. So not only the number of applications was still increasing, the number of rejections was as well. This was reason for *Het Parool* to consult Arie van Namen, the man who was one of the leading figures in the resistance magazine *Vrij Nederland* during the war, and one of the founders of what rather optimistically was then called the Foundation 1940-1944. In addition to being a judge, he was chairman of both the Foundation 1940-1945 and the War Victims' Benefits Council in 1977. The interview confirmed the view that providing benefits under the Extraordinary Pension Act was easier said than done.

Van Namen was not a sweet potato. He therefore protested against reports circulated by members of the former resistance casting doubts on the correctness of some of the benefits given and in which mentioning man and horse wasn't always avoided. As if fraud was the rule. It wasn't, and certainly not out of greed.

> May I first say that I am gradually getting sick of some of the publicity about people who receive an extraordinary pension. People forget that in fact it always concerns people who are ill, usually psychologically ill. This publicity makes them even more sick. Already people have died because of this. Take your objections where they belong. In our legislation, special bodies have been created to take care of this. In an instance, impure elements poison the publicity: personal views, personal ambitions, the need to be recognised as a resistance member. And then there's the issue of invading one's privacy. I don't think all this is very appropriate.[31]

After the war, the foundation thought it would finish making an inventory of the needs of the war victims quickly. After a year, the applications for receiving a pension had to be send in. This turned out to be a bit on the optimistic side. The foundation employed 350 people in 1977. Their most important task was the approval of applications. In doing so, Van Namen said, they worked accurately, critically, and anything but long-suffering. The main cause of the increase in the number of applications was the KZ syndrome. The people who immediately after the war had still been able to work had run out of their reserves, physically, psychologically and (thus) financially. Often, it wasn't hard to indicate a relationship between their past war experiences and their present problems, for instance in the case of concentration camp survivors. For those who, for example, 'merely' participated in the resistance, without being imprisoned, let alone were detained in a concentration camp, it was an entirely different matter altogether.

> We are placed before extremely complicated situations. We have our standards, but they aren't clearly visible in legal formulas. That's the problem. In fact, for over thirty years now we've been constantly changing those standards, making them more applicable to present practice.[32]

However, there was another cause: the publicity about assisting other victims. Van Namen explicitly mentioned the discussion about the Breda Three, but the hostages irrevocably come to mind also. Among a number of people from the former resistance this publicity led to a "narrowing of consciousness of sorts". They had come to think that the pension law served as an acknowledgement, as a kind of reward for resistance work, when in fact it was a law to support those who had become psychologically or physically entangled as a result of their war work to such a degree that they could no longer function in a normal way. However, this hasn't been emphasised enough. As a consequence, the meaning of the word 'dysfunction' was stretched considerably. For example, in the Breda Three discussion there were former resistance members who said they no longer were able to adapt to a society in which the release of war criminals was seriously discussed. "Now, you will have to take care of us."[33]

The latter turned out to be an example of a broader phenomenon: the cry for help in case of some adversity resounded more often and was agreed with more often. Voices were raised in the CBOG to expand its field of activity. It no longer had to take care of the victims of hostage-takings alone. Victims of any violent crime, air crashes, and perhaps even traffic accidents, had to be eligible too.[34] Apparently, the resulting problems were the same and treatable in a similar manner as well, although in most cases the cause had become far removed from the concentration camps and resistance work with which support started in the 1950s.

The result of all this was a reinforcement of an idea that at the time of the hostage-taking gained weight: the idea that no longer helping victims but providing work to caregivers had priority. Psychiatrists who initially focused on a specific group, the hostages, allowed this group to expand. An organisation started to assist this group, now wanted to lend a hand to victims of all kinds of other things also, even if no crime whatsoever was involved. On New Year's Eve, 1977, in a retrospective entitled 'If only the psychiatrists hadn't interfered', *Het Vrije Volk* recalled the post-hostage-taking warnings against "the experts" and the sneers "about the 'lustfulness' of men in white coats impatiently kicking in academic care shelters". In short, the reception had been "too pompous".[35]

It was criticism the psychiatrists, Mulder and Van Dijk first and foremost, obviously didn't agree to. Yes, mistakes had been made. Naturally. Mulder's remark to British television that "among the train passengers were 'some unstable subjects' who posed an increasing risk", among them the two who died during the military intervention, was a clear example for which he later apologised. But barring such mistakes, the psychiatrists were convinced they did a job well done, especially when considering how, after previous hostage situations, society in general, and the government in particular, was accused of abandoning the victims. In 1975 it was thought that anyone getting into trouble would come forward. This didn't happen, which is why the proactive method used at De Punt and Bovensmilde could indeed be called successful. For example, experience had shown it was prevented for certain that many would still develop problems. What, Van Dijk said in *Het Vrije Volk,* do "those journalists, what does my pedagogics colleague (the Utrecht professor Lubbers. LvB) know about these matters? Recently, reality taught us differently. I don't mean to be unkind, but I can be brief and clear about this."[36]

Not all hostages agreed.[37] According to another article in *Het Vrije Volk*, they were "constantly put under the skin of 'pushy' aftercare workers". Again, they expressed their resentment that it was seen as a sign of abnormality if someone said *not* to have complaints. Clockwise or counterclockwise, you were sick, and you would be helped. What changed since then was that none other than Bastiaans – who, as described earlier, had already indicated that the hostages shouldn't be seen and treated as patients immediately – had let it slip that the assistance of former hostages was too much of a psychiatric nature. This criticism was supported by others, including Ochberg, who previously had spoken highly of the Dutch approach. *Het Vrije Volk* concluded that the "hangover from the hostage-taking is yet to come. But probably in a different sense than the professional shrinks intended, when shortly after the June hijacking they stated that aftercare 'will take at least another two years'."[38]

The criticisms of the hostages themselves mainly concerned the reception centre set up by Van Dijk. For example, one of them – who had the idea that ever since the hostage situation he was merely a study object for care workers and that his only reason for living was to stroke the egos of Mulder and Van Dijk – hadn't immediately allowed himself to be conducted there. Nor did he want to stay overnight and disqualified the train-style windows in the lounge, "supposedly to letting us get used to our freedom gradually", as utterly ridiculous. His ironic remarks, so he said, were interpreted as a desire to suppress his feelings. According to Van Dijk, it was clear that he still had a few things to process. He himself said about it:

> Maybe my somewhat grumpy attitude has annoyed them a bit, but they really didn't leave you alone. I couldn't even cry side by side to my wife for a few minutes without some psychiatrist running along to stand next to me. I thought this was rude. Even some normal decency was too much to ask.[39]

His conclusion was that without this immediate relief attempts, and if he hadn't been harassed for months by all kinds of aid providers, he would have processed things long ago. Precisely because of the aid given, he remained "on the train" far longer than necessary.[40]

18. Right and wrong

The science correspondent of the *Nederlands Dagblad* brought up the discussion about LSD as a remedy for the concentration camp syndrome early 1978. In general, the Dutch newspapers were rather lenient towards the psychedelic, certainly as compared to parts of the government and the medical establishment. Their attitude can be summed up with the words: 'Bastiaans is a doctor. He knows what he's doing. Medicinal usage is not the same as fun tripping.' Contrary to what many expected, the conservative-Christian *Nederlands Dagblad* was no exception. According to the newspaper, the number of KZ syndrome patients was "still" estimated at "about 100,000" (the same number of people of whom a year earlier it was stated that they only needed short-term social support). Some of them improved "visibly" after LSD treatment. The careful use of words made clear that the article's author feared that parts of his orthodox Protestant readers wouldn't share this liberal attitude even in case of a purely medical use of the drug.[1]

The reason to write the article was the increase in the number of chemical products influencing human behaviour. In the near future, the magazine wrote – or better: warned – there would be drugs directly affecting and changing the mental state of human beings. This applied to the mental state of former resistance fighters, concentration and internment camp survivors and their families, especially their children, as well. It prompted the newspaper to inquire about the administration of LSD in the Jelgersma clinic.[2] Bastiaans then indicated that he was "not a champion of the therapeutic use of LSD". But this didn't alter that in certain cases, if applied expertly and carefully, it could alleviate psychological suffering.[3]

However, this positive attitude towards LSD care for war victims, wasn't the same as a generally positive attitude towards psychotropic drugs as such, and certainly when used more generally than solely for a very specific target group. For this, the *Nederlands Dagblad* wrote, its dangers were far too great, both for the individual – sick or healthy – and for society as a whole. "Creepy results" of scientific research into chemical substances couldn't be ruled out. Manipulation methods, including the use of LSD, by, for instance, the American and Russian secret services were already in practice. And then there was the danger of a general change of mentality by man himself, without external, malicious influence.

> For example, a mentality like this can easily take root: "If you have a toothache, take an aspirin. And whoever has a bad mood or walks around with feelings of guilt, takes a cheering pill." Revolutionary new "medicines" don't cure. They contribute to a situation in which man doesn't live but is being lived.[4]

The references to America and Russia didn't come out of the blue. The American experiments on Vietnam soldiers are mentioned already. Criticism of the abuse of psychiatry in the Soviet Union and of the drugs and methods used by psychiatrists in that country were around since the conference of the *World Psychiatric Association* (WPA) in Mexico in 1971. At the time, this was skilfully brushed under the rug by the Soviet delegation. However, this postponement turned out to be no adjustment. *Amnesty International* published the report 'Political Prisoners in the USSR' in 1975. It was followed by a report from the WPA itself in 1977. This in turn led to an accepted resolution at the WPA conference in Honolulu the same year. It condemned the Soviet Union for the use of psychiatry for political purposes. Due to ongoing criticisms of human rights violations, the country eventually left the WPA in 1983 (to re-join it six years later, after the Iron Curtain was pulled open).[5]

In Honolulu, the Netherlands had backed up the WPA report. This was discussed at the annual conference of the Dutch Psychiatric Association in April 1978. Initially, it hadn't been part of the programme, but had become so at the insistence of the Hague psychiatrist Cees van der Kroef, chairman of Amnesty International Netherlands. His motion was passed unanimously. It said it was disturbing that seven psychiatrists were fired in the Soviet Union shortly before for refusing to "treat mentally healthy dissidents as psychiatric patients". Two of them were subsequently admitted as psychiatric patients themselves. In a following interview, Van der Kroef addressed that other form of abuse as well, namely that of physicians "who don't use certain treatment therapies for the purpose for which they are designed". He pointed out that some psychiatrists were employed by the KGB. Meanwhile, all this attention had international consequences. A WPA committee was set up to investigate all abuse of psychiatry in any way and "all around the world", words, undoubtedly, added to avoid critique of being biased. Bastiaans was the psychiatrist who filled the committee's Dutch seat. Following the publication of the *Amnesty* report, he had already spoken at a conference, organised by Amnesty Netherlands in November 1975, "about the weapon of declaring political prisoners insane".[6]

While in this debate distinction between right (dissidents) and wrong (doctors instructed by the state), was clear, at the same time it slowly began to fade in the Netherlands. After all, even people who had been on the wrong side of history during the war could develop psychological complaints because of what they had done or had failed to do.

A year after the first time in 1977, Gisolf reiterated his full-page focus on the KZ syndrome. He converted the *approximately* 100,000 victims the *Nederlands Dagblad* talked about a few months earlier, into *more than* 100,000. Times certainly had changed since Bastiaans was told not to exaggerate when assuming "there had to be thousands of people with post concentration camp syndrome".[7] Gisolf agreed with those who were'nt puzzled by this ever-increasing number. He too pointed out that the ones experiencing the war more and more reached the phase of life in which tension decreased, physically and mentally. He quoted Hugenholtz:

> As they grow older, people tend to forget and forgive less easily. The panache diminishes. The impact of events from the past increases. The reckoning is coming. In order to function, they have to push aside daily disruptive factors, their past's burden. This decreases as time goes by. The more grievous, the more slanderous the past, the more threatening old age.[8]

Because of this process, instead of slowly disappearing behind the horizon the war gradually became more topical. Every day people broke down with illnesses unexplained by usual medical examination. If this happened with similar symptoms to different people with some regularity, a syndrome was born. The actual cause of such a syndrome, Gisolf continued, was of no importance. While people with a past in a Nazi camp were considered typical for a long time, hence the terms KZ or (post-)concentration camp syndrome, now many groups more threatened to become victims of past events as well. He thought in the first place of "those who were in Japanese camps in the Indies". But also, people who had been in hiding or military veterans could be mentioned, certainly if their lives had been in danger. Moreover, the victims of the hostage-takings were added. And there was yet another group of people that, until now, was never mentioned at all. People who didn't seem to exist but nevertheless were very much out there: "The Dutch who sided with the occupying forces during the war. People of whom it is said they were *fout* (evil; wrong). Many of them fought on the eastern front as SS, became POW of the Russians and finally ended up in Dutch camps on their return to the Netherlands."[9]

The resilience of those who were 'wrong' during the war began to diminish as well. They too began to suffer the consequences of the hardships they endured. And perhaps these consequences were even more serious than those who hadn't been 'wrong'; those who had been *goed* (good; right). They may have felt guilt; guilt because they were part of the perpetrators instead of the victims during the war and/or because they concluded after the war that the Nazis behaved much more brutally than the communists they detested. They had to keep their mouths shut for three decades, and still they had to. "Because don't think we're ready for forgiveness yet."[10] Again Gisolf quoted Hugenholtz. "The gap between good and evil, right and wrong, was never bridged. And it was impossible to bridge. They are and will be detested their entire lives. Even after they served their legal sentence, the human sentence is here to stay."[11]

That forgiveness was difficult and perhaps even impossible was apparent in the trial against Dutch war criminal Pieter Menten held at the same time, a trial that probably was the reason for Gisolf to address the forgotten group of 'wrong' Dutch (wo)men. Menten was a member of the SS during the war. He was charged, and eventually convicted, for his part in executing dozens of Jews. In June, the Supreme Court ruled that in a previous case against him mistakes were made that had to be corrected. The Dutch journalist who played a major role in unmasking Menten, Hans Knoop, commented in the *NIW* that undoubtedly this did justice to Menten. But it also, be it unintentionally, brought new suffering to the war victims. Forgetting that interests of victims differ from rights of defendants and certainly of suspects, Knoop wrote:

> The problem surrounding the Menten affair is in principle identical to that of the release of the Breda Three. Proponents of release believe that justice must be done even if the defendant is scum. In itself, looking at the rule of law, there is not a pin in between. But can a civilised nation do justice to the Breda Three without considering the consequences? In other words: can simultaneously justice be done to three war criminals and thereby injustice to their victims? I was among those who immediately changed opinion from proponent of release to opponent when it became clear how much extra work time release would mean for Prof. Bastiaans. For me, the interests of the victims outweigh those of the convicted or suspects.[12]

However, Bastiaans himself was ready, maybe not to forgive, but certainly to forget. This became apparent after the parliamentary debate, following the investigation by journalists in mid-1978, of yet three other war criminals living in the Federal Republic of Germany. Of them, one even applied for *and received* a Dutch benefit. Together with Joop Wolff, communist MP and editor-in-chief of *De Waarheid,* Maarten Schakel, former resistance fighter and MP for the *Christen-Democratisch Appel* CDA (Christian Democratic Appeal), asked to establish a special department at the Ministry of Justice to investigate war criminals. Pointing out that it was the massive public attention and investigative work of a journalist that ultimately determined the decision-making about the Breda Three and the Menten case, he stated that it should be avoided that the Dutch people began to think that the justice system really didn't care about the whole issue of war crimes; that the department had no interest whatsoever in tracing and convicting war criminals.[13]

Lou de Jong and Bastiaans, the two most prominent Dutch figures at that time when it came to the Second World War, were thrown into the fray. De Jong denounced the Justice department and expressed his appreciation for the journalistic investigative work.[14] Contrary to De Jong, Bastiaans turned out to be the main witness against the accusations at the department's address. He wondered if, after more than thirty years, the time of statute of limitations hadn't come. Moreover, recently the department had to give a fair amount of attention to other matters, "terrorism in particular, which is of importance too".[15] It's an attitude reinforcing the impression that it weren't so much changed personal convictions that had caused him to switch sides during the Breda Three discussion, as simple fear of the consequences if he persisted in his graceful position.

A few weeks later, he extensively explained this position in *de Volkskrant.* In short, it came down to seeing more benefit in helping victims than in tracing perpetrators. Most striking was that the call for prosecution was medicalised. Not for nothing the headline read: 'How sick are those who cry for persecution?' The sensitive nature of this subject was apparent from the very beginning of the interview. Bastiaans didn't want to start until an employee joined to attend the conversation. He thought this was safer. When she arrived, he set off "in a pedantic tone". That, in 1973, he told the government to be careful about releasing the Breda Three was mainly prompted by the fact that indeed there were three. It had little to do with the individuals themselves. At their age, they really couldn't do any more harm. In the past, several people were released already but only one at a time. This had all gone smoothly. However, by wanting to release a number of them simultaneously severe unrest among a large part of "the affected" arose. Those who already received good psychiatric treatment hadn't had such a hard time with the release. They no longer suffered from nightmares or depression. But there was a much larger not (yet) or not sufficiently treated group as well. The government had to take the consequences of release for them into account also. Bastiaans estimated this group consisted now of about 110,000 people. So, he added, the 40,000 he talked about in 1973, were anything but an overestimation, as was said at the time.[16]

After these and some other outflanking moves, Bastiaans got to the heart of the matter. He opposed an active investigative policy. Because, to get hold of one single man, all kinds of misery would be stirred up again "in people perhaps only indirectly involved".

> When we physicians talk to people who were involved in crimes, it's done in a therapeutic setting. The questions are directed at what we think they can gradually process. But police interrogations are much harsher and stricter. The calmness and the time to do it our way, are absent.[17]

In order to catch a war criminal, the entire judicial system had to be set in motion of as well the investigating country as the country in which he was detected. This would cause so much psychological damage that the benefits far outweighed the drawbacks this process would have for many of the Third Reich's victims. In Bastiaans' opinion, a country, a group, a person was healthier and more balanced the less the need to identify scapegoats was felt. A sick man, however, always needed someone to blame. You could already see this within the war victims themselves. Many of them could become very jealous "if someone mistakenly had received too high an allowance or pension".

> All this screaming. Now we have to persecute again. It makes me think, how sick are those asking for it? As a physician, I can never argue for the promotion of an aggression and revenge strategy. Of that I say, it's a symptom of a disease.[18]

This is also why the government had to invest its energy in treatment options, all the more so because the hostage-takings added new victims. Above all, it should not spend millions tracking down those who were wrong during the war just to satisfy the sense of justice of those who were right. Investments like these were far better used by the medical profession treating the numerous victims.[19]

De Waarheid, Wolff's newspaper, was not amused. Bastiaans and *de Volkskrant* couldn't be farther away from the truth in stating that those wishing to prosecute were ill. It was the West German justice system that was sick. It was "sickened by former Nazis and by revanchism". Sickening was the prevailing view in ruling circles of the Federal Republic of Germany that it was time for a "'general amnesty' for and rehabilitation of war criminals. But the Dutch sense of justice in these matters is very healthy, arising from healthy anti-fascism and healthy vigilance!"[20]

This comment was more or less an annex to one in which Minister of Justice Van Agt was the actual one in the doghouse. In a subsequent article in *De Waarheid,* which spoke of "the syndrome of 'social counsellors'", the focus was on Bastiaans, the psychiatrist who "liked to be 'in the news'". He was like that already when he said he was in favour of releasing the Breda Three a couple of years ago. He was like that when, after it became clear that his position wasn't supported by a majority of parliament, he changed position and suddenly was in opposition of release. And he still was like that. Apart from the interview with Milikowski, it was the first article, and a voluminous one on top, dominated by criticism of the man who until then could do little wrong in former resistance circles, including the communists.[21] *De Waarheid* itself dedicated many a positive line to him.

It's clear that Bastiaans' view that persecution was a symptom of illness and that he would rather see aid to victims increased than the investigation of perpetrators, created bad blood. *De Waarheid* wondered whether this last statement shouldn't be called a political statement sooner than a medical one. It was not barter. The one shouldn't go at the expense of the other. Assisting victims and tracing perpetrators could go hand in hand. The second could amplify the first even. In fact, one couldn't do without the other. Moreover, *De Waarheid* wrote, resistance fighters never thought they could benefit from their war work, and they still didn't think this way. All they thought about then and what they thought about now was what was best for country and democracy (which ill-wishers will have found a rather strange argument for *De Waarheid*). So, the Nazi criminals of old weren't to be left alone. They had to be tracked down, convicted, and put under lock and key. It wasn't appropriate to call an essential element of protecting society from the possible repetition of past horrors a symptom of mental disturbance. By retroactively labelling resistance as a disease, a criticism Milikowski already spouted earlier, Bastiaans no longer helped to cope resistance fighters suffering from what they had experienced, with their problems. Quite the contrary.[22]

De Waarheid didn't become more lenient about Bastiaans, which had to do with his forgiving attitude towards politician Willem Aantjes, who was exposed as "having been wrong".[23] It was revealed, early in November 1978, that the until then widely appreciated, progressively minded CDA party leader had been a guard in the Port Natal penal camp near Assen during the war. He allegedly also joined the *Waffen-SS*. De Jong in person past the verdict whereupon Aantjes had to withdraw from politics. However, an especially appointed committee ruled that he was sacrificed on the altar of indignation too quickly. Certainly, he made some questionable choices, but he never was a member of the *Waffen-SS*. That he was a member of the *Germaansche-SS* (German SS) in the Netherlands wasn't mentioned in the report, probably because it couldn't be demonstrated that he actually behaved badly as such.

The report forced De Jong to admit that he judged prematurely indeed. He was accused by criminal law scholars of having acted as a prosecutor rather than as a historian. This led to a new wave of sympathy for Aantjes.

The information about him, some said, should have been checked first and only then released. Bastiaans was one of them.

On the radio, Bastiaans, "as a doctor", said that he was of the opinion that Aantjes had been treated inhumanely, comparable to a public hostage-taking of him and his family. Because he hadn't had the opportunity to respond promptly to De Jong's conviction, he became the victim of a people's tribunal. Bastiaans also knew how this all happened, although he never had Aantjes on his sofa. That the man undeniably skated crookedly during the war was caused by a problematic upbringing. "Aantjes must have been a lonely figure as a boy. I get the impression of a rather difficult childhood situation, of someone who stuck to the formulas and ideals that were forced upon him in his youth. Faithful to God, faithful to the government."[24] Aantjes' later political career was, in Bastiaans' view, an outgrowth of a "vigorous attempt to 'be someone'".[25]

It's striking that many of the articles on this subject only briefly mention Bastiaans' views but did use his name and views as salutation. The article in *Trouw,* for example, was almost entirely dedicated to the opinion of professor of law August David Belinfante. Nevertheless, the title was 'Prof.dr. J. Bastiaans on the Aantjes affair' and not 'Prof.dr. Belinfante on the Aantjes affair'.[26] It once again shows that editors knew that the name 'Bastiaans' in the title generated attention. However, there was yet another reason which was explained by Peter Hofstede, media sociologist at the University of Groningen. Bastiaans, he wrote in the *NRC Handelsblad,* was one of the few Dutchmen with enough weight to compete with Lou de Jong.[27]

Even apart from *De Waarheid*, Bastiaans' position wasn't appreciated by all. The authoritative editor-in-chief of *Het Vrije Volk,* Herman Wigbold, thought that those who wrote mildly about Aantjes and who used harsh words about those who exposed his past, were turning things around. Aantjes had rightly left politics, because in any case, he was with the SS; *Waffen* or German was irrelevant. Moreover, he kept quiet about this after the war, while making a political career as the social conscience of Christian democracy. "Eternal apologists like Prof. Bastiaans" got a slap in the face from Wigbold. He probably used the plural form because another well-known psychiatrist at the time, Jan Foudraine, also emerged as an Aantjes defender. Like so many others in the late seventies and early eighties, this author of the then popular, critical book *Wie is van hout... Een gang door de psychiatrie* (Which one of us is made of wood... A stroll through psychiatry), turned to guru Bhagwan Shree Rajneesh, dressed himself in red and was called Ma Deva Amrito. Foudraine said he deeply felt sorry for Aantjes for being "relentlessly slaughtered by television". According to

Wigbold, however, it was Bastiaans, who by denying personal responsibility, went too far with his remarks about a public hostage situation. "Anyone wishing to use this appalling terminology – and certainly from a psychiatrist one should expect some caution – must say that it was Aantjes who took his voters hostage, voters who only now were able to free themselves."[28]

Naturally Aantjes himself agreed with Bastiaans and Foudraine. He felt that he was treated disgracefully and in an undignified manner. He acknowledged having made mistakes, but they were minor. Therefore, after having been given an ineligible place on the CDA list, he, in vain, tried to return to parliament via preferential votes in 1981. The *Leeuwarder Courant* was highly surprised at the lack of insight this action displayed. But this hadn't been the worst thing.

> The worst thing is that, according to Prof. Dr. J. Bastiaans, a return of Aantjes to the Second Chamber would be mentally and emotionally unbearable for many former resistance members and war victims. By continuing to strive, frozen and blinded, for his personal reparation over the backs of resistance fighters and camp syndrome sufferers Aantjes will lose his honour completely and definitively. His return to politics will damage the cause of democracy, the reputation of parliament, the name of the CDA, and not least Aantjes himself. After all, his comeback would inevitably turn out to be a public and personal drama, a failure through his own fault entirely.[29]

Bastiaans first took sides with Aantjes, but in his attempt to return to the Chamber, a few years later, he stood beside the resistance and the camp survivors. This has an agreement with his twist in the Breda Three discussion. He ultimately opted for what his supporters, the former resistance, in majority wanted.[30] However, the atmosphere was much less emotional during the Aantjes-affair than during the Breda Three period, making a similarity between his two positions at the time of the Aantjes affair striking. At first, he saw Aantjes as the victim. When he attempted to return into politics, this applied to the war generation.

The Aantjes affair of 1978 was the culmination of a year in which the Second World War was in the spotlight once again. The discussions flared up with the Menten affair, the localisation of some war criminals, and the arrest of another one. Why hadn't this been the case in previous years with similar affairs, or at least less so, *Het Nieuwsblad van het Noorden* asked some specialists in December? Differing answers were given. For example, according to Hans van der Leeuw, former resistance fighter and employee of De Jong at the NIOD, there was a need to look back from the current confusing times to a period in which everything seemed black and white. There was right and there was wrong. There was good and there was evil. End of discussion. One of the other answers, he said, stemmed from the KZ syndrome. Many who had been young in 1940-1945 reached the age in which the past began to play up. Bastiaans, who was interviewed as well, supplemented this answer which amounted to a repetition of his 'lust for detection is a symptom of disease'-reasoning; a widespread disease on top, because still many weren't treated for the KZ syndrome they undoubtedly suffered from.

> The increased aggression and calls for punishment and prosecution of war criminals is determined by the fact that most victims are in phase 4 of the KZ syndrome, the so-called exhaustion phase. The exhaustion allows the aggression, hatred, and revenge to emerge uninhibited.[31]

1978 ended in style. Not only were the hijacking victims in the news once more because of the impossibility to reach a decent financial agreement,[32] moreover the KRO broadcasted a radio play with the rightly criticised horror title *Met het hoofd tegen de hekel lopen of hoe iemand die aan een concentratiekamp-syndroom lijdt, leeft* (Walking with your head in a grudge or how someone suffering from a concentration camp syndrome, lives).[33] Also, a few days after the interview and to the dismay of Bastiaans, Menten was released (only to be sentenced definitely two years later). Bastiaans publicly wondered whether the court, quoted the now consenting *De Waarheid,* had taken the rights of the victims into account. He feared this would throw many of the people he treated back a long way.[34]

Like his protest a few years later against Aantjes' attempt at a political return, this criticism confirms that – since his Breda Three U-turn – Bastiaans was against the prosecution of war criminals because it led to medical problems and in favour of the detention of already imprisoned criminals because release would lead to medical problems. To him, the mental ups and downs of the victims, and not so much their rights, the word he used unjustified, stood above the rights of perpetrators. 'Right' preceded 'wrong'. 'Good' went above 'evil'. Also when medical assistance was in order.

19. The *Holocaust* TV series

1979 began like 1978 ended. Firstly, Hans Keilson, a German psychiatrist, poet, and novelist who fled to the Netherlands in 1936, published his study *Sequentielle Traumatisiering bei Kindern* (Accumulation of trauma in children). It was on (the assistance to) Jewish children who, like himself, survived the war by going into hiding and almost always grew up as orphans. Keilson argued that talking to war victims about their past opened up old wounds simply because they lived with the past all day long.[1] Only years later, at the age of 100, he would become really famous for his novels about the war, first internationally and then in the Netherlands as well. However, his dissertation was praised instantly. It was a study called a chronicle of human life and suffering by the *Leeuwarder Courant*; and according to Van Overeem in the *NRC Handelsblad,* it supplemented the work of scientists like Bastiaans. "His conclusion that the (social-psychiatric) caretaking after the war was able to heal a large part of the psychological wounds inflicted, makes the reader long for a kaddish for everything that in the post-war period didn't come to life due to neglect of the victims."[2]

Secondly, a fierce quarrel broke out among the "old war heroes" of the BNMO about how to spend the tens of millions of guilders intended to assist its target group. This sum, some complained, just stood still on a bank account waiting for a destination, while many war invalids could really use some hard currency. Moreover, the president of the BNMO, the banker and bearer of the Military William Order, Willem 'Bib' van Lanschot, would have benefited himself and his bank with those funds to a large extent. The union's fifteen departments, however, kept supporting the BNMO's board. It made *De Telegraaf* remind an old saying of Bastiaans: "War invalids often are at their ugliest when fighting each other."[3]

Thirdly, *Het Vrije Volk* published the story of a woman who, years before, was dismissed from civil service because of a mental disability and who protested against this to everyone. She refused to undergo a psychiatric test, not even by Bastiaans to whom she was referred.

> "I went to Oegstgeest, and there he was, that mountain of a man Bastiaans is, and he said: so, you are that lady they all fear so much. Yes, Professor, I said, and waved with some of the letters I had written to the Queen and to the Home

> Office. Without asking, he picked up those letters and walked over to one of those transcript machines. He wanted to take me in for medical investigation. Well, at that time I was terribly loyal to the government, but I wasn't that crazy that I wanted to be sedated and hospitalised." She leaves without being researched by Prof. Bastiaans any further, who writes down and passes on the impression she had made on him. "The person concerned makes an extremely disturbed impression", Bastiaans wrote. Years later, he deeply regretted this.[4]

And fourthly, CRM Minister Til Gardeniers suggested in a letter to the joint television broadcasters to observe some rules when making programmes involving the war, because "damage to the physical and mental well-being of those involved and their immediate environment often turn out to be the unintended result". Before writing the letter, Gardeniers contacted Bastiaans. He pointed out to her the increasing need for immediate help in case suchlike programmes are aired. Therefore, prior to the broadcast viewers had to be informed that they were going to watch shocking images which could lead to emotional reactions, certainly among the war harmed. After the broadcast, one or more telephone numbers had to be made public which could be dialled by people who, as a result of the broadcast, experienced serious stress. Incidentally, shortly before, at the request of the ministry, this was already done by the *Televisie en Radio Omroep Stichting* TROS (Television and Radio Broadcasting Foundation) during the broadcast of the short series *Voor Koningin en Vaderland* (For Queen and Fatherland) about the England sailor and resistance fighter Erik Hazelhoff Roelfzema. Thus, in practice Gardeniers' letter would change little. The *Evangelische Omroep* EO (Evangelical Broadcast) also announced that already it used suchlike guidelines. The broadcasters therefore regarded the letter as an appreciation of the ministry for what already was implemented by them.[5]

Perhaps Gardeniers decided to write her letter because of the broadcasting of a series on the *Englandspiel* (England game), a German operation in which the codes of captured Dutch secret agents were used to send false information across the channel. In any case, the NCRV made known having received a multitude of reactions. And it immediately announced it expected this certainly would be repeated in case of the broadcasting of *Holocaust*. This series not only marked the definitive breakthrough of actress Meryl Streep, who shortly before already had a small role in the Vietnam film *The Deer Hunter* and who would shortly afterwards play the lead character in the concentration camp syndrome drama *Sophie's Choice.* Although the term – only used sporadically for the Nazi persecution of the Jews up until then – was fiercely criticised because it referred to a spirit of sacrifice, *Holocaust* popularised it. It was a series that caused quite a stir. It won many prizes, but also raised eyebrows because of simplifications and romanticisation.[6] The Dutch broadcast was scheduled between 23 April and 3 May.

The question central to the *Englandspiel* was (and is) whether the British Special Operations Executive was aware that Germany knew the codes and played doubles, or whether all signals pointing in this direction simply were put aside. Anyway, many newly dispatched agents were immediately arrested. Resistance fighters as well as pilots fell victim to it, the latter because their flight plans were known. In the series – which led to a committee to establish a memorial to the victims of the *Englandspiel,* which included Bastiaans as member of the recommendation commission – some of the surviving victims were interviewed. In particular they spoke about the feeling of being abandoned by society and the lack of governmental respect, for example because awards were obtained only after much difficulty, if at all. It's not for nothing that *Trouw* spoke about "heroes without glory". Trix Terwindt, for example, only returned to the Netherlands after a long period of recuperation. According to the *Limburgsch Dagblad,* complete incomprehension of what she had been through was the only reaction she experienced. No one took her physical complaints seriously either. It cost her a lot of effort to rebuild her life after the war. "Had I been taken care of right away, she said, I would have been normal now." Caretaking wouldn't come for years. Bastiaans was responsible for it to come about at last. According to *Trouw,* he was going to inform the viewers of the last episode of the *Englandspiel* series "that there are still thousands of victims like her, victims for whom the war remains unfinished. He believes that certainly in the case of the *Englandspiel*, society is hardly able to imagine what it means to be just a pawn in such a dirty game, in which you are betrayed immediately after the drop."[7]

From the phrasing used by *Trouw* a certain Bastiaans fatigue seems to bubble up. This fatigue also began to characterise (some of) the victims. The time they benefitted, seemed to have benefitted, or thought to have benefitted from openness and public attention, started to become a thing of the past. At least, this can be deduced from the *NIW* article 'Feelings'. In it, among other things, the letter by Gardeniers was critically examined, even though it received full support of organisations such as Pelita, JMW, and other war and resistance victims' organisations.[8] Like a protest by Meijering against the broadcast date of *Holocaust,* to be discussed later on, according to the *NIW* this letter was indicative of the way in which the feelings of war victims were dealt with. "They have to read and hear about their feelings so often, they are mothered so often, that they must be getting over their heads by now. Their feelings have become a slogan."[9]

The magazine – or at least the commentator – still was happy with Gardeniers' willingness to take the war victims' feelings into account. Therefore, it was not without trepidation that the magazine wondered whether it wasn't simply getting too much. Ever since the discussion about the Breda Three, the sensitive psyche of war victims was brought up time and again. At the time, this was completely justified because, indeed, all those fallen victim to war and persecution were wounded to their souls. It seemed as if the government was giving "the feelings" of the three – not their rights – more weight than those of their victims. But now, the *NIW* wrote, it seemed as if the government misunderstands the suffering. Contrary to Gardeniers' message, it wasn't the images the war victims couldn't take. For their sake, she didn't have to make a call to censor or even stop broadcasts.[10]

However, time and again, the *NIW* sighed, the victims' feelings were thrown into the fray. Then this wasn't allowed and then that. Professional caregivers were guilty of this mechanism as well. They too had to let themselves be guided by their profession a bit less. TV images certainly didn't touch the victims. Firstly, they envisioned the images of the horrors on a daily basis, worse than ever could be shown on television. Secondly, if necessary, they knew where the on/off button was. They suffered from the condescending treatment they experienced much more, however unintentional. Taking their feelings into account wasn't achieved "by withholding or denying what actually happened". The victims weren't helped by silence but by recognising what they had gone through. For this, showing the horrors was a useful step; a step towards the acknowledgement of "having endured an unbearable suffering". In addition, such broadcasts could contribute to increasing the knowledge of the "generations who don't know" and the "generations who don't want to know".

> The broadcasts can arouse understanding for the war victims. They time and again and increasingly can lead up to the government showing that it recognises the suffering. That is what taking feelings into account really is. That is what the counsellors should strive for.[11]

This comment on the pampering of war victims wasn't yet published when on advice of the WAC in its final report published shortly before, State Secretary for CRM Jeltien Kraaijeveld-Wouters announced the foundation of the *Informatie- en Coördinatieorgaan Dienstverlening Oorlogsgetroffenen* ICODO (Information and Coordination Body for Service to War Harmed), mid-February. Or better: the foundation was already in operation for six months but was now assigned a building in Utrecht of its own, at last.

Establishment and housing resulted logically from the revived interest in the war. Because of this, Kraaijeveld-Wouters said, society became more aware that a multitude of problems still haunted the war generation. The former resistance urged its establishment. Not without reason ICODO was chaired by resistance hero Pim Boellaard, survivor of Natzweiler and Dachau. People who didn't know to whom to turn with their problems, both material and immaterial, now had a place to go. As a result, they no longer came between two stools, which, according to director Ineke van Oldenborgh, had often happened in the 34 years since the war passed. In any case, according to her, the problems were still underestimated and unrecognised, also because many care providers had little or no knowledge of how to deal with them. But even in case the problem was recognised, help was not forthcoming because of the often-unclear laws and regulations. As a result, the victims were sent from pillar to post, be it unintentionally. ICODO translated the official documents into plain Dutch for them, so they at least would know why they didn't receive a pension. It also looked at whether there were other ways of aiding. It wasn't just about helping recognised victims. All who thought they were affected by the war one way or another and still suffered from it, were welcome. In short, the intention was to put all "on the right track" who had got stuck in the assistance labyrinth. All? No, not all. All except, at least for the time being, former members of the Dutch *Nationaal Socialistische Beweging* NSB (National Socialist Movement) and their children.[12]

In an interview with *Trouw,* Van Oldenborgh also spoke about the media interest in the war, more specifically: the series about the *Englandspiel*, that had just been shown, and the planned broadcast of the *Holocaust* series which had premiered in America, in April 1978. Van Oldenborgh manoeuvred diplomatically between the *NIW* commentator and Gardeniers. Of course, she said, it was very important that the information delivered about what happened during the war years, was valid. Yet, she too wondered whether it indeed should all be stirred up again. "The war victims themselves often say: people have forgotten about it all. On the other hand, such broadcasts can provoke strong reactions sometimes. There is quite a bit of contradiction in all of this."[13]

However, it also was impossible to spare and protect everyone all the time, if, indeed, they were in need of protection. After all, not everyone is equally vulnerable. There were those who cried their way through the 4th of May and as a result can stand it for another year. According to Van Oldenborgh, there was the case of a man who wasn't bothered by anything until, on a beach in Spain, he suddenly heard someone speak German. He jumped up furiously, scolded the German tourists, and went about his business. "However, it's possible that these are the exceptions, while the majority of war harmed still can't cope. And perhaps never will."[14]

Immediately after the establishment of ICODO, the *NIW* expressed its expectation that the information centre would be in for a real treat when *Holocaust* got on television. Such were the lessons learned from previous broadcasts about war atrocities.[15] It was an expectation repeated a few years later, in 1985, by the Rotterdam professor of psychiatry George Ladee. At an ICODO conference he made a stand for curbing the number of television broadcasts on the subject of war. They "irrevocably lead to re-traumatisation".[16]

The *NIW* looked upon all the fuss and initiatives with some dismay. It was too little, and it was too late, it wrote following the publication of the WAC's final report on intangible aid.

> In 1979, people who experienced the horrors of war personally are softly surrounded by television warnings when a programme about the war is broadcast, by protests when something happens that might affect them. Thirty-four years after the war, an information centre for those harmed by the war is opened. A centre that receives 100 requests per week starting immediately after opening. More than thirty years after the war, a ministerial commission delivers a report on immaterial aid provided to those harmed by war. The word 'victims' was removed from the glossary; the euphemism 'harmed' replaced it. This happens when aid services have found a new target group.[17]

Too often the assistance workers, and especially the psychiatrists, saw themselves as the experts, while in fact the victims were the real experts. The reporting by aid workers often took place over the heads of the victims, which gave a feeling of being patronised. As a result, the only thing all the misery had left them, their experiences, and their knowledge, was "taken away from them and labelled as a disease".[18]

Nevertheless, the *NIW* also saw some positive sides to all the attention, which, according to the magazine, would not diminish any time soon. After all, 1980 promised to be a key year in which many who experienced the war reached the revival stage. Quick action, therefore, was even more necessary, instead of soft words and kind intentions. The WAC report provided necessary tools for it, like setting up an information centre. Moreover, suppression of the problem seemed to have come to an end, which would work out rather well for the cultivation of understanding.[19]

On the occasion of the publication of the final report, the *NIW* provided ample space to Henk Leliefeld to have his say. He was the general physician who served as assistant psychiatrist at the *Joodse Geestelijke Gezondsheidzorg* (Jewish Mental Health Care) and who, as advisory secretary, had been the voice of the WAC for three years.[20] Subsequently, at the *Nederlands Instituut voor Preventieve Geneeskunde* NIPG (Dutch Institute for Preventive Medicine) he started research into the consequences for concentration camp survivors of the Second World War. Among other things, the question was discussed whether the so-called Polish solution could offer solace for the Netherlands also. It involved encounters between war victims in small, purpose-built venues in their own hometown. They really seemed to benefit. However, Leliefeld didn't think it would make any sense to transfer this method to the Netherlands. Quite apart from the fact, he said, that the number of war victims in Poland was many times greater – in fact involving the entire population –, special buildings in the Netherlands would only enforce the already existing isolation. [21]

Such objections applied to more solutions usual in other countries. Aid had to fit the culture of the country in which it was given, otherwise it wouldn't work. Contrary to the general assumption, often expressed by the *NIW* as well, Leliefeld didn't think the Netherlands was lagging behind in the field of aid. Organisations such as Centre '45, Jewish Mental Health Care or the Sinai Centre were unique in Europe. Moreover, there were encounters in the Netherlands similar to the Polish solution, although here they rather served as a last resort for finding understanding. Care providers could join existing meetings and, in this way, strengthen the trust. This could lower the threshold and was successful, for example, after the hostage-taking in the Indonesian embassy. Bastiaans provided lectures on it. "In this way, other aid workers can delve into the problems of war victims too, lowering the threat they often pose to those affected. This also applies to general caregiving, increasing the possibilities to have it involved in the reception of the war harmed."[22]

As said, the first episode of *Holocaust* aired on 23 April 1979. However, the discussion about it had started months before. Immediately after the TROS announced that it would broadcast the series, at the end of January, Jungman wrote in *Het Parool* that he was "only looking forward to the series in fear and disgust".[23] It was a judgment he would partially retract two months later.

> I could list a lot of objectionable things about this TV show. But what I can't deny is that this made-up series, with fake victims, played by well-fed extras on an hourly basis and with allowances to compensate for overtime and inconvenient circumstances, apparently produces some effect and makes people think.[24]

That it was a TV critic who wrote this shows that the discussion was largely dominated by the quality and credibility of the series and the good intentions of the broadcaster that was going to air it. They were doubted by many because the TROS almost entirely aimed at light-hearted entertainment until then. Although the Protestant NCRV had the first rights, it announced it cancelled its plans after its management watched the series at the Cannes Film Festival half a year before. Such a "film made with commercial intentions by an American production company about the murdering of Jewish by Nazis" could not with good intentions be presented to the Dutch public. This already indicates that, like in Germany, opinions about the series differed. *Holocaust* was called a sitcom in the Second World War, deprived of any context. Lou de Jong talked about "a miserable product". Also, for example by Leo Derksen in *De Telegraaf* and in agreeance with the NCRV, there was talk of a commercial monstrosity about an event from which all commerce should stay away from for "no greater devaluation of human suffering could be imagined". However, others including the Dutch Auschwitz Committee, thought the series had lots of merits. And then there were groups and individuals who, despite strong objections to the series itself, thought broadcasting was a good thing because it did focus the public's attention on the *Final Solution* and thus combated the ignorance existing about it.[25]

Apart from the cinematic aspects, the discussion was dominated by the emotional reactions the series was expected to elicit from those who experienced the war.[26] Next to the Dutch past itself, this expectation was based on the reception in West Germany. The broadcast of the series there, January 1979, sparked a heated and emotional discussion involving historic heavyweights.[27] Even transmission masts were blown up, most probably by neo-Nazis, to make broadcasting impossible. Besides the discussion, the organisation of the German relief efforts was closely monitored as well.[28]

Because *Holocaust* was a television series, the worst was feared by some. For instance, Sunier, the director of the Sinai Centre, abhorred the series calling it "licking at suffering". And, moreover, this abhorrence was administered to mankind by means of the most intrusive medium possible: television. "For the sake of education, victims and children are hurt. While as a psychiatrist I know that moving, coloured images have a tremendous impact. Visual thinking is the last to stand, we notice this in our clinic also."[29]

Suchlike critique led the JMW to advise to not watch the series alone if one wanted to watch it.[30] The *NIW* went even further. A few days before the broadcast of the first episode, it simply said: don't look.

> One doesn't need to continue unnecessarily to drink from the chalice of persecution and to draw on the grief. The grief one carries with oneself is heavy enough as it is. One doesn't have to continue tormenting oneself with

> insomnia at night and miserable memories during the day. *Holocaust* was neither made for those who felt the horrors themselves, nor for the second generation. Don't hurt yourself. Don't look. The series is not for you. You even know better. Leave your device dead.[31]

According to the *NIW*, the series was "a harrowing event, especially for those who had to experience the harsh reality". No doubt, its purpose was to increase the number of people who, because of their war experiences, had to frequent psychiatrists and other professionals, "unless they can resist the urge to look. Unless they use their mind."[32]

According to a telephone sample conducted by the *NIW* following the broadcast of the first episode, the Jewish community appeared to have followed the 'don't watch'-advice *en masse*, unless, of course, they had no intention to watch anyhow. Nevertheless, many were in favour of broadcasting, but only because they hoped others could learn from it. They didn't have to see the series for themselves. Surely, they knew what the camps had been like.[33]

The fuss gained momentum in early February. Meijering, the director of Centre '45, saw the series on German television and liked it a lot. However, he considered the timing of the Dutch broadcast to be extremely tasteless and would certainly cause emotional reactions. Early in May, everything that might evoke stress should be avoided as much as possible. Especially the date of the last episode, 3 May, the day before the commemoration of the war dead, was chosen extremely badly. In fact, Meijering wrote, "you can't make it any crazier". Broadcasting a series like *Holocaust* on a day like that turned it into a kind of warm-up for the commemoration which was absolutely unethical. As Meijering already expected, the TROS immediately announced it didn't adhere to his critique. The dates were discussed with several authorities and most of them felt that it was precisely during this period that there was a great deal of interest in what had happened during the war. However, it was decided to abandon the original intention to start with a double episode on 28 April for this would mean that, because of the Sabbath, some groups within the Jewish community wouldn't be able to watch the entire broadcast.[34]

A few days later, various newspapers reported that after each episode the TROS would provide aid and guidance. This, possibly, was even more necessary now the decision was taken, by popular request, not to broadcast the series in the original English, but in the German dubbing that many considered to be more realistic.[35] This, with a probability bordering on certainty, is a unique event in Dutch television history.

Preparations for the accompaniment already started at an early stage, in fact immediately after the broadcaster took over the rights from the

NCRV in mid-1978, although it was feared that the reactions could hardly be predicted. Part of the informative and social guidance plan was that the TROS would send all 3247 secondary schools an information package about the Second World War mid-March. School newspaper editors and teachers were invited to an information day. It was a second unique. Never before – and probably never after – the Dutch educational system was so closely involved in the preparation of a television programme. After each episode, there were forum discussions on the radio. Telephone numbers were provided, both in Hilversum, the centre of Dutch radio and television, and the several provinces. The intention was to answer viewer questions for two hours. Furthermore, there were introductions on both radio and television and a viewer's survey into the effects of the series and the attitude towards the war among the generations too young to have experienced it themselves.

The TROS was assisted in the telephone sessions by the Jewish Mental Health Care, the JMW, the Radio-Television reception project group, the Foundation 1940-1945, and the so-called Foundation *Korrelatie*, established in 1965 for helping with psychological and social problems. Especially in relation to aid and guidance, the broadcaster received help from ICODO, the general pedagogical study centre, the Anne Frank Foundation, the CIDI (Centre Information and Documentation Israel), the Interdenominational Contact Israel, the Jewish Historical Museum, the Dutch-Israelite Church Association, the Ministry of CRM, the Ministry of Education and Science, and Leliefeld, the aforementioned secretary of the WAC, which since was abolished. Both these lists were preceded by the words 'among others'. Yet, the absence of the Dutch Auschwitz Committee in the explicit enumeration is striking. After all, according to the *NIW,* it was this organisation that, like no other, consistently stood up for the victims of the persecution and tried to gain recognition for what was done to them. The NIW wasn't alone in this. The committee itself was surprised as well that it hadn't been invited to the series' previews for aid-workers and counsellors. Nor was it asked to play a role in the supervision. This can't have had anything to do with the communist character of the committee for something similar was true for the anti-communist Expogé. It then contacted the TROS in order to be able to play a role in the care of viewers in need. However, it was feared that there was little left to change.[36]

The *NRC Handelsblad* found it remarkable that, in the person of its former secretary, the WAC was involved in providing aid as well. After all, chairman Van Praag sent a letter to the TROS in August 1978 in which he urged the broadcaster to seriously reconsider broadcasting. It was extremely doubtful, he said, whether "this not very realistic film" could contribute to the understanding and insight of the post-war generation about Nazi barbarism. Rather, he feared that "newly emerging fascistic tendencies" would be provided with ammunition to downplay the atrocities. Together with the free cooperation of so many other organisations, the turnaround of the WAC proved, according to the *NRC Handelsblad,* that "people in our country have now also gained confidence in the way the series pictures the Holocaust and in the way the TROS has provided guidance".[37]

The *Leeuwarder Courant* and *Het Nieuwsblad van het Noorden* presented a full page with an interview with Leliefeld and Hans van der Elsen, social worker at the Sinai Centre, early in April. More importantly, they also were two of the aid-workers of the support team during the broadcast of what the paper called the "most baffling television series in years". The word 'baffling' certainly wasn't meant in an entirely positive way. Coincidentally, in the week prior to the article, in Germany a book was published glossing over Nazi activity in the Second World War – unfortunately the title wasn't mentioned. It was a book German historians blew to Kingdom come. "Compared to the utter distortion of the facts in which this work excels," the newspaper wrote, "the kitschy holocaust is an informative cartoon about Nazi Germany." Yet, precisely because of the absence of direct horrors, viewers were able to identify with the victims and continue watching at something that in reality would have been impossible to watch. In Germany, the result had been that many had started to emotionally discuss their "horrifying piece of history".[38]

The expectation was that this would happen in the Netherlands as well. Therefore, preparation to lend assistance was necessary. For example, the 17,500 Jewish survivors were doing quite well only seemingly. Yes, the ambulatory care in Amsterdam and the JMW supervised 'only' 2000 of them and the Sinai Centre had 'only' about a hundred patients. However, those figures didn't give an accurate impression of the real need and not just because those hundred were a snapshot and that in reality, over a longer period of time, it was hundreds. Leliefeld: "It's a well-known misconception that only people with problems go to a clinic. There is a large group struggling with great difficulties but not reached by professional care."[39]

There was another reason yet. Leliefeld and Van der Elsen already revealed some scenes that could very well irritate camp survivors. For example, there were images of camps where women walked around with beautiful long hair, when in reality they had been bald. In other words, the series was too beautiful in many ways. Essential points were missed, but, Van der Elsen said, now that it was there, it could have positive effects such as providing information to the young and self-examination of the elderly. If they wanted to look, the latter had to ask themselves why. Doing so "things had to be sorted out" which could be of "benefit to an affected person". The TROS, they were convinced, had organised it all perfectly, and this also applied to the helpdesk.

> The TROS made the mistake not to sufficiently check whether enough supervision could be organised. When, after the purchase of the series, this question was raised in life size, the answer did come, but with a lot of pain and effort. I have to say that the TROS didn't run away from its part in this task, although it required a lot of time and effort.[40]

To those who said it was all a lot of hassle for a marginal group at best, Leliefeld and Van der Elsen said they had to have a look at the WAC's final report. It stated that this group was anything but a small minority only to be treated by specialist psychiatrists. There were still 71,500 people whose lives were profoundly and negatively determined by their war misery. About 20,000 of them were in urgent need of help. They could call, as people who, because they had or thought they had fallen victim to some form of oppression, felt "very much a 'Jew'" as well. And then there still were phone-calls from former NSB-members, either because they felt guilty, or because they wanted to say that the series exaggerated the horrors. The latter were listened to, but a discussion wasn't started. Former SS-men who "mop the floor with us in unexpurgated language" would even be cut off by saying there were ten others waiting.

> But I hope that the silent middle will react too. For 90 percent of the people, the war has been little more than an unpleasant event largely passing their door. I am very curious to see what process the series will initiate in them. Do they become aware of a certain guilt, or do they leave their own attitude and that of their family completely out of discussion?[41]

Two days before the first broadcast, 23 April 1979, *de Volkskrant* was a lot more negative. It printed a multi-page denunciation entitled 'They can never tell the truth, never'. In line with the *NIW* advice, one of the interviewees said: "'Oh no boy, don't worry. I don't watch Holocaust. Oh no, oh no.' A sweet smile." The article was intended to denounce the commercialisation of the Final Solution of which *Holocaust* was said to be a sign.

> *Holocaust*: raked paths and well-fed American ladies and gentlemen in neat striped attire. "A film can never portray how horrible Auschwitz was," one survivor says. We are printing her testimony today. And that of the person in hiding who escaped the gas chamber. "I feel guilty because I'm alive. Do you know there never was one green leaf in Auschwitz? Never a bird has whistled. *And then you have to see in Holocaust how beautiful it all was.* Beautifully green. Nicely landscaped paths. Clean clothes. While we… God, those filthy

> clothes. Someone else's shit in it still." She watched Holocaust on German TV. She was disappointed that in the debriefing nobody said that we should remain *vigilant* against fascism. In Holocaust you see a few women sitting peacefully on a *Heizung* (heater. LvB). In reality, this was impossible. You simply were knocked off. In Holocaust you see women sleeping with guards. It will have happened because everyone wanted to survive. But you don't see how we fought like beasts for a pan of food. When you met a man, he was hideous, just like you. You don't see that in Holocaust. That whole commercial thing: that love story, they can never tell the truth, never, neither can I.[42]

The number of reactions turned out to be far lower than feared, at least after the first episode. Certainly in comparison to Germany, and Austria as well, where the average perspective had been that of people feeling guilty and responsible, they were much less violent and emotional than expected. Although *Het Vrije Volk* wrote that the telephone wires were overheated, according to that same newspaper the Netherlands received *Holocaust* in a controlled manner. The TROS received approximately five hundred telephone calls; 170 to a radio forum it organised and the remainder at the telephone helpdesk set up in accordance with Gardeniers' guidelines. They were equipped for 1000 reactions. The duration of the interviews varied from two minutes to half an hour. However, the TROS thought that not everyone had been able to connect. Only a small number of responses had been highly emotional; among them one suicide announcement. The woman hung up before an aid-worker had the chance to talk to her. Especially in the beginning, most reactions were negative because people didn't expect misery but distraction from the "normally always so pleasant" TROS. The complainants didn't want to be confronted with the war. Five of them cancelled their membership. The other responses were questions for further information mostly. It also was predicted that the series would fuel hatred against the Germans. *Het Parool* commented: "Not everyone was opposed to this." For example, it was announced that a vigilante group would be formed that in the summer would act against German tourists visiting the beaches. Another, however, thought the series was a devious ploy to foment discrimination and more specifically anti-Semitism.[43]

A single former NSB-member complained about the treatment he and others like him had to endure. A child of an NSB-member, 13 years of age in 1945, also complained about the completely unjustified social treatment he had received. Because of this, he too still suffered from the effects of the war. A former SS-man reported feeling guilty about the suffering in part caused by him. All in all, though, the twenty first responders who manned the phones hadn't the predicted busy, gruelling evening. They did say that they thought this would change after the next episodes – covering less the run-up to and more the Final Solution itself. But this expectation could have had to do with a threat that had been received also: "If the TROS broadcasts Holocaust on 3 May, it won't be around for much longer. The consequences will be horrific."[44]

Of the seventy patients in the Jelgersma clinic, where Bastiaans advised those who had experienced too much not to watch, twenty gathered in front of the television. According to Bastiaans, there was little comment afterwards and the outpatient clinic hadn't received any reports the morning after either. The JMW, which helped by telephone as well, also received few responses, fifteen in total. Of these, social workers had been sent to two people because of their acute nature. "According to a spokeswoman for the JMW, in general the tendency of the reactions was opposite to that of the participants in the TROS radio debate: people were in favour of re-exposing the issue."[45]

Still, it's not correct to say that the broadcast of the first episode went by fairly quietly. The building of the TROS was heavily guarded, because of bomb threats in the afternoon before as well as after the broadcast.[46] A busload of people who just returned from a carefree TROS holiday in the south of France and had to leave the bus at the TROS building, was kept separated by the police from those who had come to pick them up. Amazement, indignation, and name-calling were the result. The word 'fascists' fell.[47]

Indeed, the relative calm of the first broadcast turned out to be uncharacteristic. The aid-workers were right. As the series progressed and the death toll mounted, the number of comments rose. For example, after the third episode the *Algemeen Dagblad* headlined: 'Telephones rang off the hook'. The Hilversum telephone central was disrupted for a while. It provided the emergency services an unsolicited but not entirely unwanted rest in an otherwise hectic evening. There even was a call on the radio not to ring anymore. It's remarkable that the cause of this influx was not so much sought in the series itself, as in the documentary about Auschwitz broadcasted afterwards. It wasn't the only documentary linked to the series and it was especially because of these documentaries that, for example, Abel Herzberg praised the TROS. In any case: the 1500 responses, 600 of which for the care providers who, on average, also spent more time per conversation than on April 23, are indicative of the increased desire to contact a professional caretaker. What stayed the same was that even now the need for a conversation exceeded the demand for actual help. And what stayed the same as well: because of renewed threats, in both the second and third episodes the TROS building was hermetically sealed off from the outside world.[48]

It was a trend that continued with the final episode, as said, on the day before Commemoration Day. Then, there even were massive calls already prior to the broadcast and, to be able to process the flood of responses, the aid-workers had to start earlier than planned. This also because many callers hadn't been able to get one of them on the phone the previous evenings, despite several attempts. *De Waarheid* concluded that this growing influx of responses made it clear that the series deeply impressed millions. This was apparent from the trend in the responses also. Were they partly negative after the first episode, a few episodes later almost everyone said it was a good thing the TROS had decided to show the series. However, the gradually rising number of phone calls doesn't alter the fact that viewed over the entire series, their total number was below what was expected. And this also applied to the emotional content of the conversations.[49]

The broadcast of *Holocaust* took place almost simultaneously with the publication of Cohen's *De Negentien Treinen naar Sobibor* (The Nineteen Trains to Sobibor), an, according to *Trouw*, astonishing book about an extermination camp that had been wiped off the face of the earth and therefore at the time not too well-known, despite Gitta Sereny's *Into that Darkness*, published a few years earlier.[50] However coincidental, of course these events were linked. *Trouw* pointed out that Cohen's book perfectly described the triptych the Shoah actually was: firstly, the destroying of evidence and the killing of witnesses; secondly, the selection of accomplices among the victims themselves, blurring the difference between perpetrator and victim, and, thirdly, the mechanical method of destruction. "Cohen's work may lead to elucidation of Jewish criticism of Holocaust, because (as far as I am currently informed) in it the middle panel is omitted, a, in Jewish eyes, unjustifiable reduction to reality."[51]

The Nineteen Trains to Sobibor was presented by Bastiaans in the Amsterdam Historical Museum. He said that despite the broadcasting of *Holocaust* and various documentaries, many still denied the Shoah, even in today's Germany. He said the book was "a monument in which, in a grandiose manner, Cohen describes the processes of depersonalisation, suppressing or denying of feelings, becoming egocentric, living in a state of narrowing of consciousness, while the biologically founded desire for survival persisted."[52]

Cohen – who, due to illness, wasn't able to attend the presentation himself – was a general practitioner in Arnhem until his retirement. Afterwards, he mainly treated war victims diagnosed with KZ syndrome. Despite all the horrors performed, the book was, as the reporter for *Het Nieuwsblad van het Noorden* wrote, "not cruel, but real". It was the result of conversations Cohen had with fifteen of the thirty Sobibor survivors.

According to the *Het Nieuwsblad*, they represented about 800,000 deaths in a year and a half. (In fact, there were 200,000. Sobibor was bad enough even without exaggeration.) Of the thirty survivors, one was a Dutch woman, and one was a German Jewish woman who had fled to the Netherlands in the nineteen thirties. Two survivors from the Netherlands out of about 35,000 deportees. And they survived only because of a major uprising that marked the literal end of the camp in October 1943. Nine of the 15 interlocutors, Cohen had said in an interview with *Het Nieuwsblad van het Noorden*, "were diagnosed with post concentration camp syndrome to a greater or lesser extent".[53]

Het Nieuwsblad van het Noorden took advantage of the presentation to honour Cohen as the man who, not long after the war, 'discovered' the KZ syndrome and who allegedly gave it its name. (However, it doesn't appear in his thesis on the medical effects of the concentration camp and sometimes De Wind is given this honour as well.) *Het Nieuwsblad* further pointed out that according to Cohen the main lessons of the war were that everyone should abhor dictatorship of any kind or direction, and that democracy, that is, democratic control of power, should be embraced no matter what, however flawed it sometimes worked in practice.[54]

20. THE CAREGIVING CRITICISED

The report from the CBOG, the Committee on Guidance and Reception of Hostages, was published in June 1979 and it was no less than 400 pages thick. This was due to the ample quotations from conversations with 168 victims of all hostage-takings between 1974 and 1977 (the schoolchildren of Bovensmilde weren't involved in the investigation). The committee stated that it became clear that the duration of a hostage situation made little difference to the nature and intensity of the complaints. Bastiaans said that even a short-term hostage-taking made an indelible impression on the unprepared hostages.[1] Moreover, it was concluded that hostages preferred immediate and active help. At first, help had to be delivered by the GP. But this didn't mean other aid-workers could rest on their laurels. They too had to be active and shouldn't wait for a former hostage to ask for help. This would prevent that, due to lack of attention, those who returned to society felt being taken hostage for a second time. When handing the report over to the State Secretary for Health, Els Veder-Smit, Bastiaans said:

> The victims of hostage-takings and disasters are all too often neglected or even completely ignored. They are left alone at their homes to come to terms with the damage inflicted. This only increases the sense of isolation and in fact continues the hostage situation.[2]

Had, at first, because of disinterest the camp taken seat in the survivors' brain, now the train threatened to do the same, and disinterest was to blame once more. As a result, hostages ran the risk of being liberated in a physical sense only.

Bastiaans' view that care providers shouldn't give assistance-seekers the feeling that they were ill, was considered crucial. They shouldn't be approached as a doctor who approaches a patient, but as one individual to another. The problem with this was that half of the GPs and other care providers involved in the various hostage situations, indicated that they didn't have the relevant expertise. Hence, the CBOG advised to organise theoretical and practical training courses.[3]

According to *De Telegraaf*, the report contained "a number of conclusions and recommendations worth considering with regard to the psychological consequences for victims of violence".[4] Be this as it may, *Het*

Vrije Volk called it compulsory reading for every aid worker. This partly because some of the interviewees – in the newspaper reports ranging from one third to almost half – spoke of positive consequences. This includes a closer family bond as a result of co-processing, as well as increased self-confidence from having endured the trial. However, in most hostages – here the numbers ranged from two-thirds to almost all – the negative consequences were paramount. Mentioned were tension, concentration problems, insomnia, physical complaints, anxiety, and an increase in family conflicts. To enable better research, and thus improve treatment, Bastiaans argued for more attention to 'victimology' during the report's presentation. In other words, to 'victim science', an, according to him, internationally emerging branch of science which, certainly in the Netherlands, was in its infancy still and therefore desperately in need of further development. As the KZ syndrome had first been extended to hostage-takings, and although the report was on hostages, Bastiaans emphatically extended the scope of activity to disasters (and *Het Vrije Volk* even to violence in general). Vaders, former hostage and editor-in-chief of *Het Nieuwsblad van het Noorden* – and a veteran of the decolonisation war – therefore preferred to speak of catastrophology, accident science; undoubtedly unintentionally turning the Shoah into an accident as well. However, Bastiaans thought this really went too far.[5]

In terms of terminology, Bastiaan's appeal was successful. A little over a month later, in an article that was prompted by a horrific event a year before, *De Telegraaf* called him "the only 'victimologist' (victim expert) in our country". That event took place in the summer of 1978. Over two hundred people, including eleven Dutch, were killed when a tanker exploded at the Los Alfaques campsite in Spain. In the article a few paragraphs were devoted to the excellent and selfless assistance provided by Spanish doctors in the hours and days after the disaster. It earned them awards from West Germany, France, Belgium. "No thanks from the Netherlands yet…"[6]

The reason for the article was that the only Dutch person who, although badly burned, survived the inferno of Los Alfaques, decided to return to the campsite. Bastiaans thought this to be very sensible. As described in the introduction, he regularly recommended such a 'back to the scene'-therapy to war victims. Gratitude was often an asset. "It's corrective. It is noticed that disasters don't always happen there. This works self-healing. As a result, the horrific image of the past can perhaps be replaced by the better image of today."[7]

Bastiaans was asked to give his opinion on the Los Alfaques survivor's journey just a few days before caregiving experts were criticised for saying all sorts of things in public, in a subsequent report on the hostage-takings. Of course, the authors stated, in part this was unavoidable, even good, but it was excessive. In addition, the information given turned out to be only partly valid. The report was the result of a study into interviews with 25 of those experts in the period May-June 1977. It was written by two of Bastiaans' colleagues at Leiden University. Among them Henk van der Ploeg, who later became professor of medical psychology at the Free University of Amsterdam. According to them, the statements in the press resulted in the hostages being labelled as psychiatric patients in need. Family and acquaintances were "imposed with the expectation that the victim's behaviour would show certain more or less negative characteristics". They derived one of the clearest complaints about this from a study by Bastiaans, probably referring to the CBOG's final report. The comment came from the wife of one of the former hostages. "The first weeks were terrible. I kept looking at him and watching him expecting to see abnormal behaviour. Because everyone had said they would come home half crazy. But this wasn't the case. He didn't seem to have changed at all."[8]

In fact, the report by Van der Ploeg and his colleagues came down to criticising the double flywheel that pushed up the numbers of victims ever further in the past.[9] Firstly, anyone who experiences something bad must experience psychological problems. If not, they still are in a phase of denial. Secondly, the ever-increasing expansion of the groups of victims, or groups allowed to use the term victim, or: harmed, who were considered to suffer from the KZ syndrome. From a word pointing at a specific group, the syndrome now turned into an umbrella term. This not yet translated into criticism of Bastiaans specifically, at least not in the public sphere. As noted earlier, personal criticism, or better: criticism on his use of LSD, had been going on among physicians for at least ten years. In the autumn of 1979, several new critics joined them and they too targeted Bastiaans' use of LSD.

In September Bastiaans had to appear before the medical disciplinary court in The Hague and Amsterdam. He was charged by the *Nederlands Comité voor de Rechten van de Mens* (Netherlands Committee for Human Rights), a three-person group in affiliation with or even directly subordinated to the Scientology Church, Bastiaans treated a woman suffering from obsessive-compulsive neurosis with LSD somewhere around 1970 (one report speaks of 1968, another of 1970 and 1971). The treatment hadn't been successful, so Bastiaans had sent her on to three neurosurgeons, who wanted to cure her neurosis by destroying certain brain cells using electrodes. Again, without success. They too were charged. According to the committee, the woman's continued disorder was "due to the very dangerous LSD treatment". It "had destroyed her". Moreover, both Bastiaans and the surgeons failed to provide information and aftercare. Bastiaans, who said not to remember the patient, defended himself by saying that the LSD treatment was intended to prevent surgical intervention. Therefore, the charge seemed to him to be quite exaggerated. Only in exceptional cases a patient was referred for brain surgery. Articles on the case furthermore emphasised that Bastiaans was the only one allowed to use LSD. Arendsen Hein had retired in 1977, although on a few occasions he continued to provide LSD privately.[10] Moreover, Bastiaans had extensive experience with its use, always using it with the utmost care. On top, he only used it when nothing else helped.[11] It was clear on whose hand the newspapers were. They would see their preference legally confirmed.

During a public hearing, because the case was considered to be of general interest, all charges were dropped at the end of 1980. Scientology especially had flown in the American professor of psychiatry Thomas Szasz as an expert witness. He was a leading proponent of so-called antipsychiatry and known as a social and science critic. However, his summary of the disadvantages of LSD treatment and neurosurgery failed to impress the court. His objections were considered irrelevant because they were "balanced against the seriousness of the case by a, in this field, highly skilled team". Incidentally, someone who only read the headlines of the newspapers will have had the idea that the complaint was directed at Bastiaans only. Apparently, that the neurosurgical team was charged and acquitted as well was considered less interesting. Their names were no public knowledge.[12]

The acquittal didn't mean that the criticisms disappeared too, although no longer aimed directly at Bastiaans and his method. It also came from a less suspicious side than a religion/cult usually labelled as quite odd. Having the aftercare of the hijackings criticised by one of the hostages themselves was a different matter entirely. In October 1979, George Flapper, a psychology student held hostage for three weeks, announced that he recovered well. There was no use in whining and complaining. After all, something bad happens to everyone every now and then. "But hay, if you've been held hostage, you need to see a psychiatrist. Well, in that case psychiatrists will get an overload of work to do. Since, isn't the whole world actually being held hostage? Because of nuclear weaponry?"[13]

Flapper criticised the aftercare from scratch and saw his criticisms confirmed in the report *Nazorg Gegijzelden. Verslag van het projekt nazorg gegijzelden van de treinen bij Wijster en De Punt* (Aftercare for Hostages. Report of the project aftercare of the train hostages at Wijster and De Punt). It was published by the Centre for Mental Health in Drenthe in October 1979. This report confirmed his ventilated view that hostages were perfectly normal people who experienced something bad. Therefore, it was necessary to prevent their experience from settling in the mind. In other words: prevention. Instead, they immediately had to put on the coat of a psychiatric patient. In doing so, he focused on Van Dijk in particular. Of course, Flapper said, there were people suffering mentally after the hostage-taking experience. However, the question is, was this caused by the experience in itself, or had the experience been the trigger only, releasing already existing tensions? In other words, was something else going on with them already before De Punt or Wijster?

> That's why I keep yelling: psychiatrists, don't interfere. The whole psychiatric rampage was curiosity pure and simple. Totally useless. There has been no real aftercare from that side. And scientifically it had been mere castles in the air. Do you know what a colleague of Van Dijk said to me? "If I'd been taken care of like that, I'd have started screaming right away."[14]

In this umpteenth report on the hostage-takings, hard nuts were cracked about aftercare indeed, especially its psychiatric component. As already stated in Van der Ploeg's report, hostages are no patients, and certainly not psychiatric patients. Nevertheless, they were seen and treated as such. Exactly this made them in need of help, in the eyes of their loved ones and society in general as well. "As was always claimed, the public thinks that the ex-hostages are 'damaged' and acts accordingly. As a result, disruptions occurred in existing and new contacts and in relationships of the hostage victims."[15]

Although they didn't name names, it was clear that the researchers in the report weren't only directing their arrows at Groningen, but also at Leiden, at Bastiaans, although he too emphasised that hostages shouldn't be treated as if they were mentally ill already. Immediately, in newspaper articles, he saw the word 'expert' after his name surrounded by quotation marks. He was accused of having generalised the condition of the hostages on a par with that of concentration camp survivors. Of course, being held hostage could be a traumatic experience, but it was really going too far to immediately label them with 'KZ syndrome'. In *Het Vrije Volk* it was explained why. "In the first place, the concentration camp experience was of much longer duration and, moreover, the camp victims were confronted not only with fear for life, but also with hunger, exhaustion, and atrocities."[16]

Two weeks after the publication of this report on aftercare, it was announced that Bastiaans was going to participate in a meeting in Leiden, organised by the conservative Christian *Nederlands Artsen Verbond* NAV (Dutch Doctors Association). The theme was the finally relaxed abortion legislation, after years of struggle by women arguing they alone were masters of their womb. Psychiatrist Harmannus Blijham, a fierce opponent of abortion and euthanasia, gave a lecture on what he called the post-abortion syndrome. Bastiaans acted as co-referent because the organisers saw similarities with the KZ syndrome.[17] Even though he supported an appeal to broaden abortion legislation a few years earlier,[18] because of this he was fiercely criticised by Van Overeem in the *NRC Handelsblad* already prior to the meeting, in an article that, according to *de Volkskrant,* considerably boosted audience numbers.[19] He and the other doctors, in the, with three hundred visitors, indeed well-attended gathering, would, Van Overeem said, not bring the flanks of the debate – the defenders of the damsel in distress versus the defenders of what they saw as God's commandments – any closer. It was inevitable that the meeting would drive "these individual females with their unwanted pregnancy, into the corner of sinners" even further.

> "Madam, if you terminate your pregnancy, you will receive the same mental problems as those who were imprisoned in Auschwitz, Dachau or Sobibor." This, gentlemen, seems to me to be moral blackmail of the most infamous sort. That a physician and psychiatrist of justifiably great fame as Prof. Bastiaans lends himself to this, makes me gasp for breath from astonishment.[20]

How could he allow himself to be abused like this by the NAV and their sticking of unscientific labels? It was beginning to look like he could no longer see the world other than through a KZ lens. In itself, there wasn't anything wrong with this. The whole world was bursting with concentration camps and man was wolf to man making other's life hell. The ultimate hell was called KZ.

> But, professor, in that case put the KZ label on *all* misery. Don't reserve it for women coming to your doctor's office after they had an abortion. You know they are a selected small group. You also know that in the Jelgersma clinic you have neither the time nor the manpower to do anything but treat some of the symptoms. You know that no psychiatrist is able to pinpoint exactly where *the* cause of mental disorders lies. Unwanted pregnancy is often the straw that breaks the camel's back. Professor: You know that you can't point at the straw and call it cause, don't you?[21]

It was a frontal attack that could not go unchallenged. Two days later there was an article in the *NRC Handelsblad* about the meeting. Bastiaans distanced himself from the concept attributed to him. In fact, according to *de Volkskrant,* he immediately called *NRC Handelsblad* to say that the NAV made the supposed connection without consulting him.[22] He spoke of a misunderstanding, born out of his expertise in the field of war trauma and the general theme of the evening of problems occurring after an abortion.

And this was combined with the statement that some comparisons between the two could be detected. This was not to say that after having an abortion women developed some kind of KZ syndrome. And indeed, Bastiaans had to admit to Van Overeem, the two cases Blijham discussed hadn't exactly gone through life unscathed prior to their abortion. Nevertheless, according to Blijham it was the primary cause of their psychological problems. This was why, Bastiaans said, on the night itself he spoke about two women who got into trouble because they had *refused* to have an abortion. The only thing he wanted to point out was that there was a general law for situations that can't be processed. After an "external wounding experience", people could go through various phases, namely shock, alarm, adjustment, and exhaustion or… recovery. This was seen in road traffic victims, abused children, victims of natural disaster or hostage-taking, and indeed, in some women who had an abortion. This was compared to KZ syndrome by Blijham. Exactly because of such unfounded and 'over the top'-comparisons, Bastiaans himself, in imitation of his colleague Hustinx, preferred to speak of EESS, the existential emotional stress syndrome.

> The specificity of the KZ syndrome lies in being constantly busy processing the inhumane experience war victims have gone through. Day and night thinking of torture, of having been confronted with death. That specific after-effect is incomparable to the memory of an abortion, a traffic accident, or a natural disaster.[23]

However, this statement doesn't alter that the symptom of stress, being a consequence of certain experiences, came to play a more important role in the psychiatric diagnosis and thus for the treatment method than the experiences themselves. This could not remain without consequences, not even for the diagnosis and treatment of problems that did arise from the experience called concentration camp.

A few days later, the comments about EESS also made it into the report that the *Nederlands Dagblad* made of the evening. It stated that not only according to Blijham, but according to Bastiaans as well it was clear that in many cases in the alarm phase notable similarities could be detected between patients with KZ syndrome and those with post-abortion syndrome. However, further research was needed to establish with certainty that after an abortion "the ees stress syndrome (sic) will occur".[24]

The difference with the report in *de Volkskrant* could not be greater. It first mentioned Blijham was a tough pensions' examiner who sent a lot of disabled people back to work. Moreover, it stated he defended the position that KZ syndrome was little more than a severe form of EESS and that many women developed EESS after an abortion. Bastiaans distanced himself from this, and from Blijham and the NAV general, "in full length and weight (both quite considerable)". After a repetition of the arguments also given in the *NRC* article, *de Volkskrant* concluded that Bastiaans didn't want to say in the least that the KZ syndrome had anything to do with "the EESS syndrome" (sic) and therefore certainly not with a possible post-abortion syndrome.[25] And so Van Overeem had been right on at least one point. The medical discussion about trauma or not, syndrome or not, hadn't led to any connection in the abortion debate. The KZ syndrome had become a political instrument used by both sides, embodied by the Christian conservative *Nederlands Dagblad* on the one hand and the secular progressive *de Volkskrant* on the other.

21. THE STORY CONTINUES

In 1980 the Second World War was a thing of the past for 35 years. It was also the year in which an enormous pile of books about the occupation years rolled off the press, such as the novel *Ga Maar Rustig Slapen* (Go Sleep Peacefully) by Louis Frequin. He was the former editor-in-chief of *De Gelderlander* and the man who sent his reporter Wennekes to Oegstgeest to study Bastiaans' LSD treatment years earlier. This resulted in the book *All wretchedness, all misery* and lifelong mental problems for the author because his book, hailed at first, was retrieved from the bookstores. In *Go Sleep Peacefully* Frequin wrote about his resistance activities and subsequent time in concentration camp Vught, as well as the psychological problems the war had had in store for him. The foreword was written by Bastiaans.[1]

In addition, many TV and radio programmes were made about the period 1940-1945 and the time around 4 and 5 May was loaded with commemorations or other war-related gatherings. One of these was the second Israeli-Dutch symposium, which took place in the little town of Dalfsen from 15 to 19 April. At least one of the presented lectures, 'The Inability to Listen', dealt with acquired syndromes and attempts at coping. It was given – and later turned into an article for the *NRC Handelsblad* – by professor of sociology Abram de Swaan. The lecture dealt with the survivors' unspoken and unheard stories. They weren't told by the one because the other couldn't listen to them and/or they weren't heard by the one because the other couldn't speak about it. It was the core and cause of the syndrome. However, there was something else.[2]

De Swaan argued that the survivors' problems became a psychiatric syndrome only after, and because of, the fact it was named, or rather: was given different names, from KZ to survival, and from EESS to disaster syndrome. Camp survivors recognised themselves in the descriptions and rang the psychiatrist's doorbell. The political history of the six-million-fold murder of Jews was in this way degenerated into a series of separate medical histories, to be discussed between doctor and patient. As a result, their stories remained outside the war's historiography. Its common core, the political-racial background, disappeared from view. Because of this, psychological care was turned into a buffer zone between the private and the public domain, between "the private survivors and the society of their contemporaries". In this way the psychiatrists protected individuals against rudeness and incomprehension on the one hand, and society against expressions of individual emotions that were deemed too disturbing on the other hand. However, when it comes to the Shoah it couldn't and shouldn't stop there. By keeping these stories within the safe environment of the consulting room, public statements about the genocide seemed to be about a world far beyond our own too often. No consequences for today's society needed to be drawn from them. But only through public discussion and drawing consequences for today's society the real processing came within reach, on both a societal and an individual level. Processing wasn't just a personal process, but a social one as well.[3]

De Swaan hit the nail on the head. The war victims told individual stories about individual psychological problems, for which individual help was sought, provided by individual psychiatrists. The social response, see for example ICODO, was also fully focused on this. Of course, this was necessary, but there was too little awareness that this was a social problem as well, requiring both social reflection and processing, and even then, it often didn't go any further than a single reference to the Vietnam War and/or fascist regimes or regimes called fascist.[4]

It will certainly have contributed to the phenomenon that those stories hardly changed in content since the mid-1960s. The victims still focused on the story that acknowledgement wasn't forthcoming: acknowledgement of their victimhood, acknowledgement of their suffering, acknowledgement of their deeds, acknowledgement of the social amnesia, acknowledgement that support was lacking. They were forgotten and their misery was unknown to many. Still, and more often, former victims found themselves in financial and/or psychological distress. This became apparent, for example, in an interview with the board of the recently established *Nederlandse Vereniging van Oorlogsslachtoffers* NVO (Dutch Association of War Victims) in *Het Vrije Volk* in December 1979. According to the board, it wasn't surprising at all that the numbers were still rising. The war generation had wanted to forget the war and had been busy rebuilding the country. This generation was retiring now and had time to think and reflect, and they noticed they had to lead a meagre existence. The cases of Menten, Aantjes, and the Breda-Three had raked up the past.[5]

The NVO was established to ensure that individual victims didn't fall between a rock and a hard place when they applied for support. This often happened because of the mentality, referred to by the organisation as typically Dutch, to neatly classify all kinds of groups and label them. If you didn't fit into a box exactly, a bureaucratic Procrustes would say 'no'. In other words, ICODO was created with exactly the same intention earlier that same year. However, the NVO had nothing good to say about ICODO, or any other governmental institution, for that matter.

> They're all small bureaucratic clubs. We have received letters from people who have given up, who after two years still haven't received an answer to their letter from the authorities. You sometimes get the impression that all those foundations are just set up to create jobs. Jobs that take advantage of war victims. Sometimes it seems like they want to postpone the payment of benefits until there are no more war victims left. But we'll try to put a stop to that.[6]

Acknowledgement was also the theme of a special edition Aart Gisolf made of his tv programme *Artsenij* (Doctoring), called 'Unfinished Past'. In it he denounced the "hype" to open telephone lines after every programme that broached a sensitive theme. All too often this only served as a band-aid for all the bleeding that was caused by the programme makers. Furthermore, there was a fair chance that the really bad cases couldn't get through because they would be pushed aside by all kinds of people who thought they had a story to tell as well.

Basically, the programme was about people who had experienced a life-threatening situation in their youth and as a consequence suffered from a disaster syndrome, "also called the 'concentration camp syndrome'". The fact that he didn't use the chronologically justified phrase 'KZ syndrome, also called disaster syndrome' is typical for the gradually fading away of the specific cause related terminology, in favour of a more general terminology. Maybe Gisolf just followed a generally accepted feeling. However, by accepting this without any question marks, he also further strengthened the expansion and the broadening of the KZ syndrome into the disaster syndrome. This becomes even more obvious from his statement that he wants to stay away from applying labels himself. He preferred to speak about "the consequences of life-threatening stress" that, overall, even transcends the disaster syndrome.[7]

Gisolf's show was proof that, after having filled the columns of various newspapers and magazines regularly for more than a decade now, the KZ syndrome became the subject of tv programmes as well. In response to 'Unfinished past' the *Nederlands Dagblad* wrote nevertheless:

> It's *gradually* becoming more and more known that people who stayed in a German concentration camp during the Second World War can begin to experience the physical and mental consequences years later. However, this belated reaction, concentration camp syndrome, can also occur after other life-threatening experiences. Hence the current name 'disaster syndrome'.[8] (Ital.: LvB)

The war was the starting point of Gisolf's broadcast. But because the symptoms of the problems many war victims came to suffer from, were similar, or rather: were called similar, to those of people who endured other traumatic events, Gisolf wanted to go beyond the war. In his broadcast he, therefore, didn't only speak about a Jewish man who went into hiding during the Second World War or about a man who was in a Japanese prisoner of war camp. It was also about a woman who lost her family during the flood disaster in the provinces of Zeeland and South-Holland in February 1953, and about one of the Wijster train hostages. The first three all had problems. The fourth didn't really have any recognisable symptoms, but the event did start to negatively affect his everyday tasks. The message: everyone had to be aware, or even assume, that experiences like these would lead to problems later in life. Talking about your emotions helped, but wasn't enough, Gisolf said. According to *de Volkskrant,* he showed in his documentary that "the only thing that really liberates you is acknowledgement of the suffering that happened to you".[9]

Of course, Bastiaans was also interviewed by Gisolf. They discussed the various aspects of the interviews. Bastiaans emphasised that even though the timespan after which the problems manifested themselves differed, the cause always lay in an unprocessed past.[10] Therefore, repression needed to be avoided above all else, as the *NIW* also advised its readers after a modern psychiatrist, by which it almost certainly referred to Bastiaans.[11]

The opinion shared by all was that 'Unfinished Past' was an interesting and important documentary. There were, however, some cautious caveats. In his review in the *Leeuwarder Courant,* critic Cor van de Poel, in a previous journalistic life chief foreign affairs of *Het Vrije Volk*, once again referred to the history of the KZ syndrome. He pointed out that it became widely known in the Netherlands nine years earlier because of the TV broadcast of Van Gasteren's film. The problems experienced by former resistance fighters and inmates of German camps were seen more and more in other groups as well from then on. Although he thought this broadening was a good thing in itself, he also questioned it. Not that Van der Poel was troubled by the fact that by replacing KZ syndrome with disaster syndrome, the concentration camps turned from a politically and ideologically inspired atrocity into, indeed, a disaster. What did trouble him was that as a result the complex history of psychotrauma was in danger of being hidden and forgotten.

> Unfortunately, I felt that the KZ syndrome as a legacy of the German camps was deliberately underexposed, making this TV product seem a bit unbalanced to me. I can kind of imagine this choice because what is more obvious than comparing qualities of suffering? Of course, there is nothing worse than the

> German camps, but this clouds the view on the consequences of several *other disasters*. The personal consequences differ according to the nature, time, place, and quality of the experienced disaster. The most serious disaster doesn't always have to have the worst personal individual consequences. This makes the collective treatment of the problem in all its diversity difficult. Any group can feel underestimated.[12] (Ital.: LvB)

Maartje van Weegen, one of the Dutch media's famous ladies at the time, also spoke with Bastiaans in a special episode of her radio programme *Ratel* (Rattle). She had invited several programme makers, including Gisolf, to discuss the large or even excessive amount of Second World War related television programmes in the days around 4 and 5 May. It was an annual ritual that tempted Gisolf to coin the phrase Animal Day Syndrome. Just as animals received extra attention only one day a year, while they needed care all year round, the problems of war victims didn't just exist at the beginning of May. Bastiaans advised people who had experienced the war that they should look selectively at war themed programmes. According to him, the programmes only made sense if they carried a deeper message, such as: "people have fought for human values and have found a solution to their problems." The crux of the radio show was that the programme makers discussed whether their programme met Bastiaans' postulate. In any case, according to both Gisolf and Bastiaans, it was certain that even war programmes of poor quality and/or not meeting the professor's guidelines, could contribute to talking about the war. And talking about the war was and remained a dire necessity.

> There are those who suffer in silence and are afraid to talk about their fears. Because of the attention in the media more and more people now know what it's like to have experienced events like these. Moreover, the sufferers begin to realise that they can't deal with their fears all by themselves.[13]

This already shows that Bastiaans continued with his story also, and this applied to the hostage story as well. In a big interview in *Het Parool*, following the then two-month hostage-taking of Americans in the embassy in Tehran after the Islamic revolution of 1979, he maintained that, despite the criticism of psychiatric care after the Dutch hostage situations, hostages would suffer scars that were likely to necessitate psychiatric aid. This was especially true for the Tehran hostages. As a consequence of the constant alternation of the guards, they had no chance of getting any kind of human contact with their hostage takers. As a result, feelings of safety that could have emerged otherwise, didn't materialise. Most likely there were also attempts at indoctrination and brainwashing; a suspicion that was confirmed a few months later when some of the hostages confessed to being spies.

How invasive this could be, was known from American POWs returning from Vietnam. They had come to believe the Vietnamese view of matters completely and sometimes continued to do so. Therefore, Bastiaans was convinced that the hostages would still experience problems for years to come after their release.[14]

However, there was also a change of mind. From a certain perspective, the Netherlands was fortunate to be a country that systematically gained experience with both the short-term and long-term consequences of hostage takings. Naturally, hostages wanted to go home immediately. It became clear that this was a good thing. To be cared for in special centres shouldn't be a hard and fast rule. They just needed to be left alone for a few days. Have a nice and peaceful sleep. Nevertheless, there was a fair chance that after a few days or weeks at home they would be confronted with incomprehension resulting in conflict. The emergency services had to be alert to this. According to Bastiaans, too few experts tackled these kinds of problems immediately, and that led to double isolation. As the hostage situation moved further into the past, the attention, including from the press, waned, while at the same time the problems grew; problems within themselves, with their families and other loved ones. However, too often they had to solve these problems all by themselves.[15]

However, the belief persisted that the problems the hostages would face didn't differ that much from the KZ syndrome, especially if it lasted as long as in Tehran. In an interview with Peereboom, Bastiaans said that the treatment could be the same as well. Like war victims, the hostages in Iran had to be given the opportunity to talk about everything and let of steam after their return, possibly with the help of narcoanalysis or hypnosis.

> These techniques were applied with a certain verve in England and America on soldiers who returned from the Second World War, but this knowledge has been lost completely since that time. They actually look at it in a brand-new way now, repeating the mistakes made in the Netherlands. The talks psychiatrists have with them are usually too superficial.[16]

Instead, the hostages had to be pinned down to the suffering they endured. Like the concentration camp survivors, they had to relive the inferno. They had to be asked what they had experienced, what they would do differently next time, and whether they were ashamed of certain behaviour. These kinds of matters had to be discussed "expertly, focused, humanely and informally". Otherwise, talking was pretty pointless.[17]

To prepare the American psychiatrists for their task, Bastiaans urged them in a number of American TV programmes not to make the same mistake the Netherlands made after the war. Above all, they shouldn't rely on the care in the victims' immediate circle too much.

> Intervene, offer help, no matter the resistance you may encounter. Because in the Netherlands, armed with all our experiences with war misery, we said to the media from 1975 onwards: we have to be ready in time. What happened? There was a wave of protests along the lines of: what are these psychiatrists and psychologists thinking? That our boys, that our kids who just got out of embassy, school, or trains, are crazy? It's precisely among those involved themselves and especially among their relatives that you'll find a large group of people saying: treatment isn't necessary, we can cope ourselves.[18]

If this happened in the USA as well, it would inevitably lead to psychological setbacks among many of the hostages, as was the case with the Dutch war victims, although this could take twenty to thirty years to happen. The barrier, that had been taking care of repression, would have been broken after that time, and "the unprocessed remains of this experiential situation would present themselves in nightmarish forms". After that, any assistance from relatives was too little, too late.[19] The implied message was clear. Although he himself always emphasised that a violent event as such didn't have to lead to trauma, while pointing out the role of a failed upbringing and problematic childhood years, all the hostages who said they didn't need assistance would be knocking on the doors of the psychiatric consulting rooms around the year 2000.

And then there was one more story that sticked around: the critique on the use of LSD. Bastiaans continued to defend the drug fiercely and newspapers continued to support him in his fight against this criticism. In spite of the fact that charges were dropped against him and the three neurosurgeons, over treating a woman with obsessive-compulsive disorder, Scientology believers didn't rest. Similar to the *Pro-Life* demonstrators at abortion clinics today, they organised gatherings in front of the Jelgersma clinic, during which pamphlets were handed out about the degrading things that happened behind the doors. This didn't miss its negative effect on those treated there. Moreover, the editors of newspapers were regularly bombarded by the aforementioned Dutch Committee for Human Rights with reports and telephone calls about Bastiaans' treatment method. However, according to the *Leeuwarder Courant,* he managed to refute the committee's claims in a conversation with that newspaper and with the help of a large amount of documentation. Until she fell into the hands of that so-called human rights committee and thus into the hands of Scientology in 1975, things hadn't gone so bad for the woman, who left Bastiaans before he was able to finish the cure,[20] which contradicted, by the way, his earlier statement that he referred her to Amsterdam because of little success.

LSD, the *Leeuwarder Courant* repeated, was an excellent drug. There were no grounds for questioning this. Within a few sessions it accomplished what used to take much, much longer when using only psychoanalysis. And the fear that all war victims were being treated with LSD, spread in part because of the film *Do you now understand why I cry…*, was unfounded also. It was only administered when the usual psychotherapeutic methods failed. LSD was an internationally recognised treatment agent, that didn't pose more risk in expert hands than other drugs did, according to the newspaper quoting Bastiaans. However, it was difficult to talk to dogmatists and so he feared that he was far from being free from the committee. "I deeply regret that a method having healed so many, is discredited. These LSD treatments are performed with the utmost precautions and with the best supervisors."[21]

It seemed the criticism began to tire him out. For the first time Bastiaans openly indicated in 1980 that he wanted to take a step back. But for this to happen, it was necessary to find someone to follow in his footsteps so the Bastiaans method could continue. However, there was no suitable successor yet. And this was anything but strange. "It isn't the unwillingness of young doctors, but the fact that they are unable to sense the problems of former camp inmates and others who suffered under nazi atrocities."[22]

It's an understandable, often heard and often repeated argument. Indeed, it's far from easy for doctors born after 1945 – or, for that matter, for anyone born anytime or anywhere – to imagine places of horror such as Auschwitz, Natzweiler, Treblinka, or Sobibor. However, at the same time it's a strange argument, not to mention the fact that it makes it impossible for others, including doctors, to develop a critical attitude towards traumatised individuals.[23] Physicians are confronted on a daily basis with people whose psychological ailments (and often their physical ailments as well) they don't completely comprehend, or understand the reasons that caused them. Nevertheless, they treat them anyway and often successfully. Bastiaans knew this. So it seems very likely that it was just an argument he could use for saying he wanted to stop, but nevertheless didn't, because he couldn't. Therefore, there was no question of a farewell, not medically and not as far as public appearances were concerned. For example, he was one of the speakers on a conference in Utrecht, on 15 August 1980, where the definitive ending of the Second World War was commemorated, and where an exhibition about 'The Netherlands East Indies in the Second World War' was set up (in *De Waarheid* the words 'Netherlands East Indies' were put between quotation marks).[24] As said: the story continued.

22. The East Indies camp syndrome

There weren't only commemorations in May 1980. As mentioned at the end of the previous chapter, there was one on 15 August as well, and it marked the breakthrough in attention for the group that was responsible for the greatest numerical increase of people labelled, or wanting to be labelled, with the camp syndrome, in their case the *Oost Indisch kampsyndroom* (East Indies camp syndrome).[1] The Dutch and Indo-Europeans who spend the war in one of the Japanese camps were experiencing mental distress as well. They visited the Jelgersma clinic before and they had some newspaper attention before, but this wasn't translated into a several pages long article entirely devoted to the situation in Indonesia during the Japanese occupation until 1979. Or rather: to the *Dutch* distress that arose from it. The camp residents in the archipelago were, at most, presented as one of the groups whose members were likely to suffer, or almost certainly would suffer from KZ syndrome prior to that time.

This article, published in the *NRC Handelsblad* of 25 August, showed many similarities with articles that appeared about the German camp syndrome some twenty years before. Again, it was all about suffering and incomprehension. Those who hadn't endured the camps wouldn't and couldn't understand. But something was added: even though there were people who said that indeed the German camps were a degree worse than those in the Netherlands East Indies, many victims of these latter camps felt disadvantaged to those who survived the German ones. Society had paid much more attention to the latter and had shown much more understanding for them, and this was still the case on an almost daily basis. Disinterest and neglect perpetuated and exacerbated the suffering of the survivors of the Japanese internment camps, although they also took a look at themselves. Before turning to the government for material aid many of them waited until the mid-1970s. According to W.C. Lemaire, former member of the WAC and director of the Pelita Foundation, this was the result of "the Indonesian mentality: waiting until they find themselves in dire straits".[2]

Pelita, as mentioned, the organisation for the relief of the material, moral and social needs of the victims of the war with Japan, now wanted to engage in immaterial assistance as well. Perhaps, Lemaire said, the flood of material aid requests from several years earlier would repeat itself with immaterial aid if Pelita's tasks were expanded in that direction. The government was asked for funding, but a decision was still pending. Pelita itself offered no assistance. The already existing institutions were far better equipped to fulfill this job. "Our task will have to be to identify possible needs and in case of a referral keep a watchful eye. Our concern is: those social institutions need to know what the particularities of persecution in the archipelago were. Pelita can advise them on this."[3]

After this article silence returned, a silence that was rudely broken by the article about the East Indies camp syndrome mentioned in the introduction, written by Rudy Kousbroek and published in April 1980. Kousbroek spoke about the syndrome for the first time in the last episode of a series called 'Back to Negri Panerkomst' in the *NRC Handelsblad*. It dealt with his childhood days in the Netherlands East Indies. While writing this episode, he saw an article in the medical journal *NTvG*, called 'The Japanese Camps, not yet a thing of the past', written by a general practitioner and a psychotherapist. Both spent the war in a Japanese camp and had therefore not written solely on the basis of literature, that an increasing number of their fellow sufferers dealt with "psychological and somatic problems associated with their camp experiences".[4]

Kousbroek raised his eyebrows. In any case, when he thought about psychological traces of the past, his thoughts didn't go back so much to his camp years than to his entire youth in the archipelago; to having "a thousand memories of something that never existed": a time of bliss in the so-called Emerald Belt.[5] "The camp syndrome. Does that concept really apply to the former Indonesian internees? I have often wondered, and it will probably not come as a surprise to anyone when I write that, in principle, I am quite sceptical about it. Maybe I'll come back to it later."[6]

Kousbroek did come back to it. He published 'The Camp syndrome' as a follow-up to his series less than a month later.[7] In it he stated that indeed he had serious doubts about the existence of an East Indies camp syndrome. Existing problems should be called country-of-origin syndrome. It caused a lot of criticism. He was particularly blamed for adhering to a hierarchy of suffering.[8] A woman interviewed in *De Telegraaf* said that until then she had been able to live with her nightmares. She wrote them down but hadn't intended to ever do anything with her writings, until she read Kousbroek's article. Angrily she decided to turn them into a book. "They aren't made up; they are as real as this room around us. And that's not normal, so many years later, is it? The war will never be over for us."[9]

The *NRC Handelsblad* itself gave room to an extensive rebuttal by Corina Engelbrecht, who grew up in Indonesia and who played a major role in the commemorations of the Indies' past. She bundled her articles about this and the late psychological consequences of the Japanese occupation in her book *Wie niet herdacht wordt leeft niet voort – 70 jaar Indisch herdenken van 15 augustus 1945* (Those who aren't commemorated don't live on – 70 years of Indies commemorations of 15 August 1945) in 2015. Yes, she wrote, Kousbroek was right when he spoke of a country-of-origin syndrome. But the war experiences did add an essential experience to this, without which the problems of the Indies people couldn't possibly be explained. It failed to convince Kousbroek, especially because of the inadequate 'first this and then that' reasoning that kept popping up. First there was the camp, then mental problems occurred. Conclusion: the problems were caused by the camp. Moreover, Engelbrecht didn't ask, let alone answer, a crucial question: "to what extent did the syndrome exist because there was a word for it." He concluded with the sentence:

> I don't know if there's a 'medical' reason to distinguish between reality and myth, but this doesn't change the fact that, against our better judgement, the East Indies camp syndrome comes down mainly to a stubborn adherence to untenable myths – myths about the colonial period, about ourselves, about the internment and about the Japanese occupiers.[10]

Kousbroek's criticism failed to prevent – most probably even contributed to it – that the commemoration of 15 August 1980, and the run-up to it, marked a breakthrough in attention for the victims of the Japanese internment camps, even though an article that was published three years later reiterated that they weren't able to cope with their camp suffering yet and that, as a result, they became the stepchild of the Dutch decolonisation process.[11]

First there was the article 'Prisoners of Peace', again in the *NRC Handelsblad,* again written by Engelbrecht, published on 23 July 1980. In it the calculation was given that the WAC had presented in its interim report of 1977 on the number of Indies/Indonesians that were war harmed, as said, the word that had pushed its predecessor 'war victims' to second place. Their number was estimated at 127,500 in 1975, extrapolated to 106,300 in 1985 and 66,900 in 2000. About 10,000 of them were classified in the so-called H-category: high-risk. This meant that they had endured above average hardships. Much larger, almost 40,000, was the number of people who applied "for acknowledgement and reimbursement of medical expenses" in the 1970s. When the then State Secretary Meijer opened the benefits act WUV for victims of the Japanese camp as well, there was a rush. Of the 10,000 applications since then, 1000 were granted by 1980. The amount of 40,000 was two-thirds of the total demand for war related material aid in the 1970s. The WAC report also stated that every request for such support "contains a potential demand for some form of immaterial aid".[12] In other words: the number of people who would seek out a social worker, psychologist or psychiatrist could well exceed the H category number in time.

The 15 August commemoration, with the purpose of a better societal understanding of all camp victims,[13] would be followed by the five-yearly special commemoration of the women's camps' victims two weeks later. Engelbrecht wrote that both remembrances mainly arose from the need to do justice to the people who were forced to spend the war in a Japanese camp, after which they became "prisoners of peace". Because of the extremely unsafe situation following the Japanese surrender, the violent so-called Bersiap period, liberation only took place in theory. The camps couldn't be evacuated. The Japanese guards remained at their post, only not as the enemy now, but as protectors against the violence of the Indonesian youth shouting 'Bersiap', be vigilant. In the Netherlands, both the war against Japan and this time of 'un-liberation', as Engelbrecht called it, were often ignored. According to her, little was known about what had happened in the former colony, in the camps and the time thereafter, and just as little was known about the consequences this time had had and still had on those affected, even as late as 1980.

> Lack of interest and also of historical awareness led to the disregard of the very intense feelings of a large group of compatriots from the East. Many of them came to feel cut off from the past and this got in the way of processing their experiences. They remained prisoners of peace.[14]

The Dutch policy was aimed at integrating those who came to the Netherlands after the war. From a social point of view, this integration could be called successful, but, Engelbrecht wrote, the problems they carried with them were neglected as a result of that policy. This changed slightly with the WAC reports, but these failed to reach a general public. This applied also to the figures mentioned therein. They showed that a large, unexpected group of war victims began to come forward: the former Japanese camp children. According to Engelbrecht, they often held a severe grudge, also because they had to constantly show their gratitude for the shelter they had received. As a result, it was impossible for their scars, incurred in and as a consequence of the past, to heal.[15]

And those scars were real. "Disintegration of existence, decline, powerlessness, loss of home and sometimes of work, expulsion from familiar soil, arriving in the Netherlands as a have-not – all that was certainly humiliating." The Dutch public at large failed to understand this and thus the East Indies camp syndrome grew into a reality. Everything brought forward by Bastiaans about the causes of the German camp syndrome, also applied to the Netherlands East Indies variant and he stated "that the Japanese occupation was an expression of perfidious, destructive aggression as well". Engelbrecht:

> Many who tried to fit in or adapt seemed to really succeed for a time after the war. But, especially in the face of a hostile, usually unreceptive outside world, they also kept a real low profile to such a degree that, superficially seen, there didn't seem to be a major problem in their behaviour caused by unprocessed war experiences. But only too often this was misleading, which is why their inner unrest and inner tension, still just as camouflaged as they were in the camps, weren't spotted. The result was that the victims ended up in a vicious circle: even more isolation, even more repression.[16]

In order to be able to process these problems, understanding was necessary and that required proper information, in addition to good will. However, until that moment information was stuck in comparisons between one camp and another, emphasising the differences rather than the similarities. Many of those similarities didn't lay so much in the camp time itself as in the consequences this time had had for life afterwards. Understanding and acknowledgment of the suffering in the former Dutch colony lagged behind that of the German camps. Yes, many books were written about the Indies 1942-1945, good and bad, distant and emotional. However: "even the good ones" never generated the same interest in the Netherlands as, for example, the numerous published volumes of the series by Lou de Jong, that mainly covered the experiences on Dutch soil.[17] In other words, there was 35 years' worth of reporting and gathering of knowledge to catch up on. "The most important things still have to be mentioned. Talking and listening should provide the solution. Because those days haven't gone. They still live on in a large group of Dutch people and their children as long as their liberation can't be *celebrated.* With others."[18]

Engelbrecht's article was followed by others,[19] such as 'Forgotten camp victims' in *Het Parool,* in the week before the general commemoration. It was subtitled 'We Indies people are continuously discriminated against' and discussed a woman who, while under LSD treatment by Bastiaans, dared to talk about her experiences "in the Jap camp" for the first time since her arrival in the Netherlands. Bastiaans wrote to a colleague that she was "one of very many cases of returnees from the camps", who should have received "effective assistance immediately after that stressful period. Because this hadn't been possible, we are now, so many years after the war, often seriously burdened and confronted with therapeutic tasks that can only be brought to a successful conclusion with great difficulty".[20]

The woman was lucky because regularly help could be delayed for quite some time. When, according to an ICODO employee, the Indies people, numbed by their camp experiences, the post-war incomprehension, and lack of interest, visited the information centre, there were only a few psychiatrists close by who were able to understand their problems. And these psychiatrists had too many patients. A referral to Bastiaans hardly helped, because he often had to tell people as well that there was a waiting period of nearly a year. "That's a new blow. And these people already have such a hard time talking about what they've been through."[21]

Around 10,000 visitors attended the 15 August commemoration. Among them Queen Beatrix, Prince Claus, and various members of government and parliament. One of the speakers was Gerhard Sietse Vrijburg, chairman of the organising committee and author of the book *Een Ereschuld Ingelost* (A debt of honour paid), written on the occasion of the 25th anniversary of the Pacific war's end in 1970. He told his audience that Dutch society was too preoccupied with the war against Germany to be able to listen to stories about the suffering and starvation in the Japanese camps.[22] A second speaker, Nicolaas Beets, professor of psychology at Leiden and a former physician in Japanese POW camps, said that a grave injustice was done to the former inhabitants of the Netherlands East Indies after 1945. Until a few months ago, it wasn't acknowledged that they had done nothing but serve the Netherlands. After their return they were "treated shamelessly".[23] "The indifference with which they were received in the Netherlands, the carelessness with which their interests were judged, the actual denial of the sacrifices they had made; it all deeply shocked their sense of justice."[24]

Bastiaans, as often happened mistakenly called the director of Centre '45,[25] took the words 'isolation and liberation' as the theme of his speech. These also became the title of a book he published about the KZ syndrome and his treatment method, in 1986.[26] He recalled that tens of thousands of the 300,000 internees had succumbed and asked his audience therefore to pay more attention to the, relatively unnoticed, horrors of the Japanese occupation of Indonesia. These Indo-Dutch people were part of the thousands who were never fully liberated in the Netherlands either. They also were still trapped "in a traumatising past, in the horrific powerlessness of those days". On their return – which, by the way, in many cases wasn't a return at all, but an emigration – they arrived in a society that first and foremost focused on the nazi horrors, and this made them feel misunderstood. It led to a forced adaption, that took a heavy toll on them.[27]

The lack of attention, Bastiaans continued, had taken on such proportions that former inhabitants of the Netherlands East Indies no longer dared to talk about their experiences. This further perpetuated the lack of psychological liberation.

> The isolation they had experienced in the camps continued in Dutch society. For them the Japanese camps didn't become a thing of the past, because misery you can't talk about continues to exist. And it turned out that the children from the camps of those war days, still bear the scars as well.[28]

According to the *Nederlands Dagblad,* the East Indies camp syndrome was officially acknowledged with these words. And judging by a testimony about "the Jel" of the woman who underwent Bastiaans' LSD therapy, those scars were considerable.

> What I've seen there. Nine out of ten patients there are Indies people, and most are younger than me. They are the so-called baby children, the children who were four or five years old when the war ended. They survived all the hardships, they lived through all the fears, but they haven't consciously experienced what happened. There are about twenty to thirty thousand of them. There is an unbridgeable gap between my mind and my feelings already, and I feel very aggressive already. But they have a hatred, a hatred, unimaginable. I've seen it, in their eyes, this hate, horrible.[29]

23. THE AFTERCARE UNDER FIRE AND THE HOSTAGE-TAKING IN TEHRAN

Meanwhile, the American hostages were held in Tehran for a year. Therefore, it was high time for the media to ask Bastiaans, "expert in the field of aftercare" (marks before and after 'expert' had disappeared again), to shed some light on the possible consequences. Besides appearing on television once more,[1] he was interviewed by the *Algemeen Dagblad* at the end of October 1980. This resulted in the article 'Hostages threatened by camp syndrome'. Although, at the very least, the hostages were "pushed around in an unbelievable way" – free, not free, etcetera – it was still anybody's guess what consequences the deprivation of liberty would have on them, also because the outside world was deprived of new information about their physical well-being for quite some time now. "Are they brainwashed, physically abused? Questions we don't know the answer to." Nevertheless, without a doubt their situation was serious.

> Gradually, I am comparing these Americans more and more with the people who were in concentration camps during the Second World War. Living between hope, fear and resignation destroys people. The tensions will be enormous. It depends on the personality of the individual in what state he gets out.[2]

However, the camp survivors of the Second World War, be it in Europe or in the Pacific, were no longer the only frame of reference. The soldiers of the Vietnam War were added. Veterans dealt with psychological problems, the *Vietnam Veterans Syndrome,* and recently they were joined by returned American POWs, who frequently showed antisocial behaviour as a result of the alienation that resulted from their deprivation of liberty. Adaptation became impossible. Crime and/or alcoholism were just around the corner. Suicide occurred frequently as well. Moreover, probably due to mistrust, misunderstanding, and alienation, marital problems started to arise. An absence that long will almost certainly disrupt relationships. This was also due to the fact that the only thing the veterans thought about was survival. Other needs, such as sexual pleasure, disappeared into the background. "The sex function", Bastiaans explained, was "unconsciously switched off" and couldn't be switched on again that easily.[3]

Bastiaans was convinced that the Americans had sufficient expertise to arrange the hostages' aftercare as soon as they were set free. He did play a part in this. He was, the newspaper reported, "widely appreciated" for "his pioneering work" with patients with KZ syndrome and because of that he had been a regular guest on popular American tv programmes in recent months, "in the interest of the United States", as he himself stated. It also wasn't inconceivable that he would be asked to cross the ocean again, if it, unexpectedly, turned out that the expertise in the field of aftercare proved to be insufficient, nonetheless. In any case, he was asked to remain available in case of such an event. According to Bastiaans he had already given one piece of advice, an advice that arose directly from the lessons learned from the hostage-takings at De Punt and other places in the mid-1970s.

> Based on our own experience, I warned against bombarding the hostages with interrogations. The most important thing is that they get as much rest as possible in the beginning and that they can re-establish contact with their family. Only when this is done, researchers can be let loose on them.[4]

That lessons were learned from the aftercare of the hostage-takings turned out to be no superfluous luxury; criticism of it was growing. Especially Vaders vented his heart more and more, for example in an interview conducted by his own *Nieuwsblad van het Noorden.* For the hostages of Wijster, he said, the aftercare had started too late anyway, not before the hijacking situation in De Punt, almost two years later. "If you don't provide any help right after a hijack, you don't have to help at all." In fact, he said, the hostages of Wijster were completely left out in the cold. Moreover, the few attempts at assistance there had been, had "the speed of a snail". Vaders was all the more hurt by this because he and the other hostages felt like substitutes for the state since the hijacking wasn't directed against them but against the Dutch government. To add injury to insult, the care by the local health authorities for the victims of the simultaneous hostage-taking in Amsterdam had been good.[5]

Following Bastiaans' advice, the government did decide that in Wijster aftercare had to start immediately after the hijacking ended. This led to the formation of the Working Group North. Vaders:

> Well, that didn't go unnoticed! Those people seemed to just have meetings and only concerned themselves with competence issues. The only thing I've noticed is that some well-meaning social worker knocked on my door one fine day, but that didn't do me any good.[6]

The problems the Working Group encountered after Wijster, made them get in touch with and thereafter join the CBOG. That committee drew up a policy plan on how to act in case of future hostage-takings. According to Vaders, it proved useful in the hostage situation in De Punt. A social-medical centre was established and working groups of experts were formed to deal with the hostages' aftercare. At that time some of Wijster's hostages were helped also. They previously organised a number of aftercare meetings themselves, to which they invited Bastiaans, among others. Meanwhile, many of this group's members "ended up in a second isolation because their friends and relatives were unable to imagine what had happened in that tin drum and why the hostages had reacted so and so". For example, the public envisaged a strict division between good and bad, between angel and devil, between victim and perpetrator. As a result, Vaders argued, it had no eye for the real, diffuse, and vague boundaries.

> When people are brought together in a stressful situation, relationships develop, even between hijackers and passengers. A process of mutual influencing takes place, a struggle for psychological supremacy. The terrorists tried to convince us of their RMS ideal (*Republik Maluku Selatan* or Republic of South Moluccas. LvB). In turn, the passengers tried to reverse the methods by which the terrorists tried to reach their goal. No more killing of innocent people, but the greatest possible publicity.[7]

Vaders – who, in a later column, made it clear that in his eyes Bastiaans was the exception that proved the rule –[8] was still shocked about the way in which politicians and doctors acted after five years.

> Doctors advised: take some tranquilisers, dig up your garden, while all we wanted to do was talk. We were looked upon as mentally damaged patients. Th then Minister of Justice Van Agt thought so too. A blunder of the first order. We had a conversation with him later. That turned out to be a huge failure as well. Completely pointless. Van Agt hid behind his ignorance. It was embarrassing.[9]

Interest was below par, except for the scientific interest. According to Vaders, they were guinea pigs for the scientists. Apparently, he joked, the horrific experiences he and his fellow hostages had endured "were good for some interesting dissertations".[10]

The scornful nature of Vaders' last comment is striking because a review of two university studies about media interest in the hostage-takings was placed adjacent to the interview. The reviewer had nothing good to say about one of the two, which had the reporting of *Het Nieuwsblad van het Noorden* as its research topic. According to this paper the two researchers from the Leiden University Centre for Research into Social Contradictions insinuated, in a confrontational manner, that the newspaper's above-average interest in the train hijacking in Wijster was solely due to the fact that Vaders had been one of the hostages. It further concluded that the articles had added to the suffering unnecessarily, and that they had come at the expense of the coverage of other important news items. Proof for any of this was lacking. The other study was conducted by a psychologist from Leeuwarden. Precisely this research concerned a dissertation, and precisely this research was discussed sympathetically, in spite of the fact that the conclusions drawn were anything but pleasant for the Dutch press. A large part of the hostages and a big majority of their family members were negative about the press publicity. Journalists, for example, were called pushy, although this did depend on the degree of contact. The more often they had been in touch with a journalist, the more positive their judgments.[11]

Vader's negative opinion about the aftercare for the Wijster hostages was confirmed by another hostage, Truus van der Giesen-Rosenhart. The hijacking certainly had had a positive impact on her life, only not because of, but in spite of the aid given. Since there had been no immediate assistance, the hostages had started organising everything themselves. That commitment and togetherness was blissful and gave them a nice feeling. But once you returned home from meetings like these, you were alone again. She agreed with Vaders that it wasn't until after the hijacking at De Punt that "some official psychologist" arrived. The hostages had been left on their own for too long. "After returning home an expert should have spontaneously come in to have a chat. This didn't happen. You did talk to those around you, but they didn't understand you. If you said you didn't hate those South Moluccans, they thought you'd gone mental."[12] As a result of failing care and misunderstanding – "Well well, did you receive 3000 guilders (€1365) in compensation? That's a nice bonus." – Van der Giesen fell "into a second isolation" as well. Most liberated themselves from it on their own, like she did. Most. Not all. One of the youngest hostages "ended up in a psychiatric clinic".[13]

And then, after 444 days, the 52 hostages in Tehran were finally released at the end of January 1981. It was the inauguration day of Ronald Reagan, the 40th president of the United States. It was indeed decided to use the POW script. This meant that at first the group was kept together, in order to process their first emotions in the presence of family and friends. At least, according to Bastiaans, who was interviewed together with Van Dijk, about the release by *de Volkskrant.* The hostages were kept under medical observation for several weeks in preparation for a return to normal life. Factors that, according to the two psychiatrists, could negatively influence the consequences were, firstly, the extreme length of the hostage situation and, secondly, the fact that it had happened to the hostages despite their diplomatic status, "which until that moment was a sacred principle in the relations between nations after all". A third factor was the constant yelling and screaming by the Muslim youth outside the embassy. This will have come across as threatening and thus constituted an aggravating factor for psychological distress. Then again, they were able to associate with each other fairly freely for a while, within the borders of the embassy, although this ended after a failed liberation attempt, by the end of April 1980, at the cost of eight American servicemen's lives.[14]

That the article was entitled: 'Prof. Bastiaans on "Tehran": "Hostages seriously disrupted"', suggests that Bastiaans had let go of his earlier reticence about the consequences, although, contrary to earlier expectations, he wasn't directly involved in the debrief and shelter of the hostages. Neither was Van Dijk, although he was asked by the Americans about his experiences with and knowledge of hostages' caretaking. According to Bastiaans, the situation of the Americans resembled that of the Dutch elite hostages in St. Michielsgestel, near Den Bosch, during the Second World War. This meant they too would probably suffer from issues like mental instability, anxiety, difficulties to adapt, as well as sleep, concentration, and/or memory disorders.[15]

Het Nieuwsblad van het Noorden emphasised that indeed there definitely was some genuine Dutch aid. After all, Bastiaans, Van Dijk, as well as Mulder, the negotiator during the most recent Dutch hostage-takings, had repeatedly advised American colleagues. Contrary to what was reported in the *Algemeen Dagblad* a few months earlier, in *Het Nieuwsblad van het Noorden* Bastiaans said that treatment of the hostages had to be started as soon as possible and without relatives present. Moreover, without expert aftercare, let alone no aftercare at all, the complaints would persist for years. It was also reported that the Leiden psychiatrist was ready to travel to Wiesbaden, where the hostages had their first stopover on their way home. It was emphasised that, because of his television appearances, he had become a well-known figure in the United States. There he had warned the relatives that, mentally speaking, their loved ones would have trouble finding their way home again. After a while, they would withdraw into self-imposed isolation because all the attention wore them out. Furthermore, he had impressed upon them that the definitely necessary and lengthy psychiatric treatment didn't mean that their loved ones were mad.[16]

In addition to dyke monitoring, dredging and impoldering, trauma relief had become a Dutch export product to be proud of as well. According to *De Telegraaf,* the Ministry of Health even suggested to Bastiaans they could present his services to America on his behalf. Bastiaans politely but decisively declined. "I am convinced the Americans have arranged their aftercare very well. They don't need the experiences of a small country like ours."[17]

This was all ridiculed by a columnist in *Het Parool.* He mocked that, in addition to Van Dijk and Bastiaans, his socio-therapeutic neighbour had also received a telephone call for help from the Americans. At a hefty hourly rate, he had explained, among other things, how long a period of 444 days was and that emotions were hidden very deep in the human body, especially if they were repressed. Because, evidently, the Americans themselves weren't aware of all this.[18]

The columnist could have republished his ironical article a week later, with just slight changes like ignorant Dutch people instead of Americans as the direct object. Apparently, the time had come to publicly rekindle a message, known for years, but somewhat faded. On the same day that CRM Minister Til Gardeniers announced that in Westerbork, the place in the East of the Netherlands where the trains left for Auschwitz and other camps, at last a monument would be erected for the Jewish war victims,[19] the Amsterdam *Psycho-Analytisch Instituut* PAI (Psycho-Analytical Institute), of which Bastiaans had been the director before his departure to Leiden, published a report that was ordered by that same ministry. It, once again, stated that aid to war victims isn't just a medical matter, but a political and financial one as well, the latter for both government and care workers. It also showed that from time-to-time scientific reports don't appear entirely by chance at a moment that is convenient politically; reports shouting out their main message: we need more money!

The subject of the report was the damaging effect of war experiences on persecuted people and resistance fighters. The conclusion was that these experiences had a "long and deep" effect on them, so that many of them weren't able to hold their own in society. Often, they themselves refused to see the connection and doctors and other care workers were "still not focused enough on this denial of suffering to be able to properly respond to requests for help".

> The need for help is increasing. It's still impossible to say how extensive the need of war victims and their children is. There appears to be a great threshold fear among the victims. The feeling of having to be strong, and experiencing it as an offense to still have to look for help and not knowing where to look for it, have created an insurmountable obstacle to many.[20]

The researchers, who had been tasked with investigating the extent to which psychotherapeutic care and treatment was possible, were quite aware they hadn't come up with revolutionary findings. According to De Wind, who was one of the researchers, the research not produced anything new scientifically. However, this too wasn't without importance, because from this they concluded that shelter and treatment was desirable in many cases, but not always possible, although this was less due to the problem itself than to the lack of financial resources of the care providers.

> Institutions such as the Psycho-Analytical Institute and the institutes for psychotherapy have recently been financed on the basis of a fixed budget by the Health Insurance Board. According to deputy director Dr Folkert Beenen of the PAI, this means that these institutes can't expand the scope of their activities. "In fact, the Health Insurance Council has cut 3.5 million on our institute's current budget of 11 to 12 million."[21]

But even if finances are left aside, psychotherapeutic care was a complicated matter. Firstly, it wasn't easy to determine in advance whether outpatient care would be sufficient or whether hospitalisation would be in order. In addition, it had to be kept in mind that the two clinics eligible for admission, the Jelgersma clinic and Centre '45, had long waiting lists. And on top of this, a new group with specific problems was knocking on the therapist's door: the now adult children of former Dutch national socialists. They reported complaints they themselves often didn't associate with their parents' war history and the societal response to it. Nevertheless, they evidently suffered "from shame and from a feeling of 'belonging to the scum of the earth, no matter what'". An additional problem was that it wasn't an easy matter to get them involved in the research. This was "politically unfeasible", according to the chair of the research group, Mario Montessori.[22]

As *pars pro toto,* the problems of one of the NSB children were recorded in the book *Niet de schuld, wel de straf* (Not to be blamed, punished nevertheless) two years later. The first copy was presented to Bastiaans. On that occasion, he called it astonishing what was done to them after the war. They had become victims of "tremendous mental child abuse". Their experiences were "as bad" as those of children of concentration camp victims. And it wasn't just the experiences. For them as well, the war was still an "unfinished period". Their problems also surfaced after almost forty years. Until then, they were tucked away in a life of hard work, which hadn't prevented that most of them "turned out badly in the end".[23]

A few weeks after the publication of the PAI report, (child) psychologist Henri Benders was given a full-page opportunity by *Het Nieuwsblad van het Noorden* to place the psychological problems resulting from hostage-takings, such as those in Tehran, in a broader perspective. Benders had been involved in the debrief and shelter of hostages and their families in Wijster and Bovensmilde, as well as in a short but bloody hostage-taking in the provincial house in Assen in March 1978. It resulted in a piece filled with quotations by Ivan Illich, a then popular philosopher, social critic, and liberation theologian.

Benders started by asking questions. He argued that the major problem with psychological complaints was that it was difficult to get any real certainty about their existence. Did the victims indeed have them? And if they had, were they fully the result of the hostage-taking? There also was the problem of proportionality: which complaints were logical and acceptable, and which were disproportionate, implying the need for treatment? And, should it always be assumed that complaints would emerge and that those complaints, therefore, had to be dealt with by 'experts' (quotation marks by Benders)? He emphasised that in no way he wanted to downplay the possibility of delayed complaints, nor to create the impression that it was never necessary to have psychiatrists deal with them. However, this didn't mean that their performances weren't in need of critical comment. For example, the statements made by Bastiaans and Van Dijk after the Tehran hostage crisis shouldn't be left unanswered because they encompassed several, unproved aspects: "the prediction that these people will sooner or later get into trouble, the warning not to leave ex-hostages untreated, the need to initially conduct treatment independently of their family members."[24]

It was clear: debrief and aftercare were necessary and had to be carried out by medical experts, thus closing the possibility of processing among family and friends. In fact, those family and friends needed assistance as well. An erroneous assumption, according to Benders. People should never be deprived of the opportunity to work all of it out together. Those who did, underestimated the possibilities people had to get over their problems by themselves. In other words: they should be given the benefit of the doubt and be left alone until it had become clear they couldn't process their past without professional help.[25]

The broader perspective was that this philosophy of expertise, "which sees itself as the only right one, leaving no room for a different approach", wasn't limited to hostage-taking and the like. This is where Illich came into play. In his book *Tools for Conviviality,* he wrote about how difficult it became for family members to care for their sick and frail loved ones in this modern capitalist society. This resulted in a growing demand for medical assistance. The more that service increased in value, the more difficult it became to provide care in one's own circle. It also resulted in a growing number of medical and paramedical specialisms. Subsequently, those specialists had an existential and financial interest in taking and keeping the right to decide if someone had to be called sick and to get and keep the associated care in their own hands. This, in turn, was accepted by society. Someone was sick only if an expert acknowledged he or she was sick. As a consequence, Benders continued, a person "is forced to seek help from experts more and more". This manifested itself in a multitude of societal areas and, according to him, it couldn't be said loud enough that "the expert society disrupts and turns everyone into a victim".[26]

After this, Benders returned to the specific issue of victims' debrief and aftercare, including the final report of the CBOG. It was clear, he wrote, that this report was written out of the unquestionable belief that expert follow-up care was necessary. Any information that could possibly show the contrary was interpreted from that point of view. Why, for example, did Bastiaans advise to keep family away as much as possible after Tehran, while according to the CBOG report 79 percent of the hostages in the Netherlands hadn't experienced any negative consequences in family relationships and 92 percent thought that one should primarily deal with the hostage situation among loved ones?[27]

Another example was the fiction of the need for a group debrief and shelter, of processing together with fellow sufferers. According to Benders, this ignored the fact that hostages usually form a completely random group, having nothing in common except the hostage situation. Or, as an ex-hostage put it: "Such a company gathers with a bang and shatters with a bang." In such a randomly composed group, irritations and tensions were lurking constantly. What one person thought to be a good thing, another considered worthless. What bothered the one, the other hadn't even noticed. But, as British psychologist and filmmaker David Cohen, director of the film *After the Highjack,* noted: "The trouble is that psychiatrists and psychologists often follow fixed protocols. A person has been taken hostage and therefore has to behave in a certain way."[28]

Last but not least, the report found it striking that many of those involved didn't ask for help – 69 percent of the hostages and 77 percent of the family members – regardless of the fact whether help was offered or not. This was attributed to the notion that those involved often found it difficult to ask for help themselves. Benders: "The idea that people simply don't find it necessary to ask for help doesn't dawn upon the researchers."[29]

24. FINANCIAL AND MEDICAL WORRIES

The experts (with or without quotation marks) continued to stir. Thirty of them, both lawyers and physicians, had united in the *Comité Verzet en Vervolging* (Resistance and Persecution Committee). Among them Bastiaans, Van der Ploeg and Harry Rooijmans, professor of clinical psychiatry in Leiden since 1976 and the new director of the Jelgersma clinic. He is also the author of the book *99 Jaar tussen Wal en Schip* (99 Years between a rock and a hard place), that describes the history of academic psychiatry in Leiden in the twentieth century and was published in 1998. In it, the first twelve years of the Bastiaans' period, the period until Rooijmans' appointment, were characterised by the word 'rudderless' and the following eleven as a time when, euphemistically speaking, discussion prevailed about which course to take. Not until 1987, and only after Bastiaans' farewell, did tranquillity return.[1]

The Committee informed State Secretary Kraaijeveld-Wouters that it didn't bear thinking about that war victims on benefits still suffered from "all kinds of bureaucratic abuses". And about the ones not even receiving benefits, the secretary of the right-wing *Nederlandse Bond van Oud-Strijders* (Dutch Association of Veterans), W. Eleveld, said that enough was enough. It was an utter disgrace that "former resistance fighters, who kept a stiff upper lip for years, but now – due to the consequences of the war – suffered anyway", had a hard time getting financial support.[2]

According to Bastiaans, an absolute low was reached. The dissatisfaction with the rejection of benefits by the official authorities was severe. At least, that could be concluded from the large number of protests that reached the Central Appeals Board. No less than seventy percent of the war victims did so, compared to twenty percent when it concerned other official decisions. According to Bastiaans, this was sufficient proof that there was something rotten in the state of the Netherlands.[3] He received support a few years later, when the large-scale budget cuts of the 1980s also started to affect the war benefits. At an ICODO-conference, a general practitioner denounced the fact that people who had survived the war didn't receive benefits on the basis of their merits but based on the consideration whether or not they suffered from mental problems caused by their former activities; a causality difficult to establish. "As doctors, we should not have taken part in that assessment."[4] In other words: everyone who had survived the war and had problems now, should receive benefits, whether the war had caused them or not.

The same problem afflicted the POWs and internees of the war against Japan. It was decided that the breadwinners among them would receive a one-time *f*7500 (€3410) each in 1980. "Sixty cents per day of camp. A tip, but better than nothing," one of them said.[5] That money, *f*225 million (€102,250,000) in total, was not at hand but, according to Hans Wiegel, the Minister for the Interior, had to be found, nonetheless. This financial assistance was a debt of honour, just as Bastiaans had called medical assistance a matter of honour. The indignation about the small, symbolic amount was huge already and it would become even greater when it turned out that no one had received anything yet after a year. By then, Wiegel had left office already. The cabinet he was a part of had fallen. No new cabinet was formed yet and by the time it was, *De Telegraaf* wrote, the new minister would have other things to worry about than finding out where the money should come from and how to distribute it. Anyway, it would take quite some time and by then, it said cynically, the problem created by the government itself would have been solved naturally already. In that case the government would have saved 225 million and the Netherlands East Indies file could finally be closed. "It's a blow harder than the hardest beating by Japanese camp guards."[6]

Real or perceived lows weren't only felt on the victim's side. This also applied to the side of the care workers. In Centre '45, tensions appeared to have built up between the staff and Karel Ceha, the man who had succeeded Meijering as director two years earlier. In addition, problems had arisen between Ceha and the management of the centre. This couldn't but lead to his dismissal. Chairman of the board Voogd expressly stated that it wasn't the intention to coordinate the activities of the centre with those of Bastiaans' Jelgersma clinic, although this would save a considerable amount of necessary expenditures. Voogd wanted the victims to still be able to choose between two treatment methods. It was an idea Bastiaans rejected. He said he wasn't surprised by the problems his immediate neighbours struggled with and wanted to seize the opportunity to join forces in the interest of the war victims. Firstly, the need was greater than ever, and secondly, "due to the enormous influx of patients" his clinic was "severely understaffed for several years now".[7]

With Ceha's departure, the problems turned out to be anything but over. An investigation published two years later – unfortunately at the same time as the reprimanding of three of the centre's psychologists after complaints from one of the patients, by then renamed as 'guests' – showed that many of them had problems with the day-to-day running of Centre '45.

For example, mention was made of the age difference, or rather: the difference in experience, that often existed between the older patients and the younger practitioners. It was also pointed out that when groups were created, no subdivision was made by type of victim. The latter indicates that there was a hierarchy of misery among the guests. This didn't help the atmosphere either. Nevertheless, the final conclusion of the study was positive. All things considered meaningful work had been accomplished.[8] It was a conclusion that was drawn in a major article in the *NRC Handelsblad* a little later as well. In it, some of the guests were allowed to speak and the reporter wrote that among them he felt a great need to defend the centre against recent criticism. He quoted: "If it weren't for the Centre, I would have killed myself" or, "The Centre is my last straw. At least they understand me here."[9]

25. The book *People at Hostage-takings*

In the debrief and aftercare of hostages, attempts were made to avoid, or rather: to remove, the dividedness that had characterised the aid to war victims. A joining of forces had taken place. In the presence of Johan Manusama, the RMS' president-in-exile, the first copy of the book *Mensen bij Gijzelingen* (People at Hostage-takings), written in response to the Tehran siege, was presented to, the now Prime Minister, Van Agt at the end of September 1981.[1] He considered it a work of great importance "that has much to teach us, as well as many beyond our national borders". As for the latter, he got his way quickly for American and English editions were in the works. Four people had contributed to the book, the psychiatrists Bastiaans (about the hostages), Mulder (about terrorism), Van Dijk (about the hostages and their families), and psychologist Van der Ploeg (about the care workers). According to *De Telegraaf*, they probably were "the best-informed group of experts on hostage-taking, terrorism, and the ever-increasing number of violent crimes that are the bane of the Western world in general".[2]

According to the authors themselves, the book wasn't intended to be purely scientific. However, the reviewer of the *Leeuwarder Courant* wrote that this comment could be taken for granted.[3] And reviewer Sietse van der Hoek even stated in *de Volkskrant* that the book proved the Netherlands had amassed more scientific knowledge about the consequences of hostage-takings than other countries that had to deal with them. In part this was probably due to the special circumstance that the descendants of a formerly colonised people started hijacking trains. But it was certainly due to the person of Bastiaans. He had for a long time dedicated himself to the more general matter of what happened to the psyche in case of violence and was asked to share his expertise internationally, as recently happened by the United States. However, his knowledge wasn't appreciated there, at least according to Van Dijk. Based on Van der Hoek's review, he stated after the book launch: "Those Americans were like, we are a nation with great resilience, the consequences won't be that bad. Now, six months after the hostages' liberation, they are experiencing the exact phenomena we predicted."[4]

The economic malaise and the current social structure led to a strongly increasing "collective feeling of powerlessness and anxiety". So, the foursome feared the number of terrorist attacks would gradually increase and that they would be characterised by a rising level of violence. They also warned that women would play an ever more important role; a warning to which the major role they had played in the German *Red Army Faction* won't have been alien. "She will act more hostile, deal with the victims more brutally, and be tougher in her persistence to achieve the goals they have set themselves."[5]

Due to the increase in violence predicted by the authors of *People at Hostage-takings,* they also strongly advised against playing chess or a game of checkers with one of the hostage-takers during a hostage situation. Because, if the hijacker lost, chances were that he or she would lose control with possibly bloody consequences. All this could be countered only by showing greater understanding and tolerance for migration workers and the Moluccan people, for instance. At the time of the Moluccan hostage-takings proposals for de-escalation, from both the Netherlands and abroad, like sending in "dogs carrying anaesthetic gas" or allowing "trains with hot girls" to drive past, weren't followed up, but according to the researchers they were a sign of social involvement.[6]

But cooperation isn't the same as unanimity. For instance, there was a lot of discussion about whether terrorists shouldn't be given the silent treatment as much as possible, because attention was exactly what they wanted – a discussion that hasn't died down since then. According to Mulder, this was a nonsensical position. Perpetrators didn't want any attention at all. The less attention, the easier it was for them to carry out their plans. Van der Ploeg, however, thought that terrorists did seek attention, that it played into their hands and incited them to further activities. He wondered "whether the Indonesian consulate in Amsterdam would have been occupied if the shortly preceding train hijacking in Wijster hadn't been given so much coverage in the news".[7]

However, there was no disagreement whatsoever that victims of hostage-takings had to be provided with prompt, active and intensive care. They were exposed to an event that would have "largely negative consequences" both psychologically and socially. The life threat was particularly burdensome, although positive consequences were also noted, like the ability to handle the setbacks life has in store for everyone more easily. Added to this was the feeling of powerlessness, which in turn led to apathy. The mistakes made at Wijster weren't repeated at De Punt. There, they were active, but not intrusive, from the outset. "This turned out to be much better for the victims." Nevertheless, the absence of intrusiveness had one disadvantage. Not everyone took advantage of the help offered, although, according to Van Dijk, they needed it.[8]

The book said that almost everyone who was involved in the eight hostage-takings in the Netherlands between 1974 and 1978 – their number was estimated at about 1200 – had subsequently developed psychological and/or physical complaints. Two out of three hadn't gotten rid of this within a year. Naturally, the complaints resulted mainly from the actual hostage-takings and the sense of dehumanisation they had caused. But Van der Ploeg said, in accordance with the report on the aid delivered after hostage-takings he and a colleague had published in 1979, they also arose from societal expectations. An image was created that the hostages had to meet. Based on what they heard from experts, relatives thought that a certain syndrome *had to occur*; that problems *would* arise anyway, if not immediately, then certainly after some time.

> Before he even knows it, he is seen and treated as a person to be handled and approached carefully. The question is how relatives will react if the person in question doesn't want to identify with a patient's image. It isn't improbable that they won't accept this and want to keep him in the patient's role until an expert declares him healthy.[9]

Henri Benders will have read these comments by Van der Ploeg with approval but will have raised eyebrows at an interview Van Dijk gave to the *Algemeen Dagblad.* In it he said that the victims weren't only the hostages, not even just the hostages and their relatives. Anyone who had experienced a hostage situation before, as well as some victims of the Second World War, had also suffered from the tensions created by the hostage situation. The fact that the interviewer, who had been the reporter of the *Algemeen Dagblad* at De Punt, indicated that he had gotten a "somewhat uneasy feeling when reading the book", wasn't strange at all. "It's a general psychological principle that a sensitivity to events that make a big impression on you can continue to exist. This is why several war victims were stressed again by the violent occupation of the train. It evoked associations with their war experiences."[10]

It was striking that Van Dijk didn't mention two groups that also dealt with the aftermath of the events: the soldiers who had put an end to the hostage situation and the hijackers themselves. This was done intentionally. He and his associates kept them out of their shelter activities so they could tell the hostages: "We're here just for you."

> I've heard that some of the liberators have been messed up by the events as well. After all, this action by the Marines was preceded by weeks of tension. Of course, they are trained to kill, but that causes psychological problems as well. I don't know much about the hijackers either. But it's known that one of

> them committed suicide in prison. That certainly is an indication of psychological distress.[11]

This aloofness only applied to the debrief after a hostage situation was ended. Prior to the ending of the hijack in De Punt, a light was shed on the hostage-takers. Mulder, a teacher at the Royal Military Academy in Breda, described his so-called three phase model, which, in the meanwhile, had become commonplace. In the first phase the hijackers were hyper-nervous. At that time, it was of the utmost importance to meet them as much as possible, at least in words, without giving them the idea that a solution was near. The second phase was the one in which the psychiatrist made a psychological profile of the hijackers and tried to force them into a certain routine, such as diet, hygiene and sleeping times. This put the psychiatrist "in a psychologically dominant position" and it enabled him to know fairly accurately what was going on with them. Finally, in the third phase, the hijackers got the idea that they were going to lose, which caused the aggression of the first phase to resurface.

> The psychiatrist now promises them that their wishes will be granted and that they will be victorious. This literally puts them to sleep. They sleep more deeply that night than before, after which the military attack is started in the early morning with an optimal amount of noise, so that there is as much panic as possible.[12]

The general praise for the knowledge of the researchers doesn't mean the book didn't get any rebuttals. Especially Mulder, the author of not only the "longest" and "most spectacular", but, as Van der Hoek wrote, also the "least scientific and most vain prophetic" chapter, was criticised.[13] More in general, the communist *De Waarheid* accused the writers of lumping together terms like 'hostage-taking' and 'terrorism' too easily, while "liberation movements are often dismissed with the accusation of 'terrorism'".[14] It was a discussion that, shortly afterwards, became more widespread because of the film *Het Meisje met het Rode Haar* (The Red Haired Girl), about resistance fighter Hannie Schaft. After all, in the eyes of the powers that be at the time, her resistance activities had made her little less than a terrorist. The film was also accused of wilfully ignoring Schaft's communist beliefs, which made her a potential supporter of the ideological enemy behind the Iron Curtain. So, attention could be paid to her anti-Nazism and resistance activities, but the alternative she had envisioned had to be kept out of the picture as much as possible.[15]

However, something was added to this by Mulder, even if the linguistic creepiness the *Leeuwarder Courant* reproached him with isn't considered.[16] According to Henk Glimmerveen, author of the article 'Psychiatry of the mole corridor. The Mulder Syndrome' in *De Waarheid*, he continued to label hostage-takers as mentally disturbed, something he had also done immediately after the hostage situation had started. This stood in blatant contrast to the other three, who stayed away from labelling and conclusions that were too simple. It was a judgment Mulder took further in the book by saying that, due to their lowered consciousness and narrowing of vision, anyone undertaking actions like these was suffering from 'hyperarousal syndrome'; an accusation the hostage-takers' lawyer threw back in his face. According to Glimmerveen it all stemmed from the position Mulder had taken up in the crisis centre at Assen, a city not far from De Punt. A position that had become so dominant after a while that he even started to interfere with what kind of ammunition had to be used.[17]

In addition to a lot more, like his view that the Vietnam War was purely a humiliation for America, Glimmerveen discussed Mulder's views on world economy, democracy, and the feminist movement as well. According to the psychiatrist, democratic struggles like those waged by the squatters' movement, the anti-nuclear energy movement, and the peace movement could easily degenerate into anarchy. To him, female terrorists were little more than "accelerated forerunners of women in emancipatory development". Fortunately, there was still hope for the female sex because, according to many of their peers, including "progressive women", feminists had an attitude that was "too masculine".[18]

De Waarheid certainly wasn't the only newspaper in which questions were raised about Mulder's contribution, although there were some positive comments as well. For instance, all in all the *Leeuwarder Courant* thought his chapter was valuable.[19] And in *Het Nieuwsblad van het Noorden* Vaders wrote that because of Mulder's article the book marked "a turning point in the thinking about violence in a society like ours". It had made it clear that a social order as a whole could lead to violence, even in the absence of hunger and oppression, and that this was not merely a matter of derailed individuals.[19]

These remarks don't alter the fact that these newspapers as well reached a negative final conclusion. In fact, only the *Nederlands Dagblad* gave Mulder plenty of praise. Like him, the newspaper endorsed the link between the blurring of social norms and emerging terrorism. The newspaper supported him "from a Christian point of view" and complemented him. It pointed out the support liberation movements generally received, despite the fact that they accepted and used terrorist methods. And it pointed out the "radical moral turnaround in our society, as has become obvious in the discussion on abortion". After all, the relaxation of abortion laws meant "that many are willing to sacrifice human lives for what others consider their right – a 'justification of the same quality as used by terrorists'".[20]

Especially Van der Hoek fulminated in his review against Mulder and his ideas about the world in general and women in particular. Mulder apparently thought that, from a "more or less psychiatric point of view", he could sketch the path from activist to terrorist, understand modern society, and predict the ever-increasing violence and the major role that women would play in this. His "all too easy right-wing" views couldn't be disputed hard enough, and not by colleagues alone, but also and above all by polemologists, sociologists, political scientists, and medical laymen.[21]

Peereboom, in *Het Parool*, wasn't in the least impressed by Mulder's reasoning either. In his sketch of society leading to loneliness – and with that to frustration and thus to violence –, the psychiatrist had apparently failed to notice "how many people took to the streets in massive demonstrations to combat immaterial problems in recent years (and in so doing obliterating their loneliness by showing solidarity)". Then, he too put Mulder's predictions about the future of women on the chopping block. His prophecies lacked any factual basis. Therefore, his contribution, especially when compared to the other three writers' valuable contributions, had to be dismissed as mere suggestive writing.[23]

To close, the Protestant *Trouw* briefly summarised the criticism of the Catholic *De Tijd* (published as a weekly since 1974) showing that it was shared more widely than just by the politically left, secular newspapers. The idea that Mulder was an internationally acclaimed expert in the field of the psychological aspects of terrorism was thrown into the trash. He was "a vain man" whose expertise will be doubted even more now.[24] In short: Mulder had covered his political-ideological views under a jumble of psychiatric words to give them a halo of generally accepted scientific scholarship. He had prepared a meal of personal ideas and served it as medical-scientific findings. The days that medics got away with this, were in the past.

26. The Endgame

The publication of *People at Hostage-takings* closed the chapter discussing the aftermath of the Moluccan hijackings. Another chapter was also nearing its end. Born in 1917, Bastiaans reached the retirement age of 65, an occasion seized by the *World Veterans Federation* to honour him by giving him the *WVF Rehabilitation Prize*. However, he didn't want to retire and managed to get an extension from the university. They said that as long as a worthy successor hadn't been found his work was considered too important to end. This coincided with the move of the Jelgersma clinic for his war patients into a new wing. This was something Leiden university wanted, but Bastiaans contested because, in his view, the place was unsuitable. His patients felt most comfortable in their familiar accommodation, the villa. His protest went against the views of his staff. They thought that the villa was completely outdated. Concerning this, the Academic Hospital Leiden gave Bastiaans approval as well, at least for the time being.[1]

Bastiaans' respite didn't last long and he would be replaced as director of the Jelgersma clinic on 1 January 1983.[2] Again he protested. He was of the opinion that the symbolic function he and his work had in the Netherlands wasn't taken into consideration. This wasn't overstating it, he said in *Trouw*. "When the patients see my car in front of the door, they know: 'He's there, we can go see him.'" With his LSD therapy on up to three hundred patients, he had achieved better results than anyone else. The outcome was that, for the time being, he could stay on as professor and could continue to treat war victims in the clinic.[3] But there were some conditions. He had to get permission from the Ministry of Health, and he would only get it if he agreed to move to the new wing. He kept refusing this because the building reminded his patients of a prison. Therefore, relocation would exacerbate their problems.[4]

According to Bastiaans, the actions of State Secretary Joop van der Reijden made it clear how much the government, science, and society as a whole underestimated the problems war victims still had. With the closing of the villa, all his scientific and medical work was put on the back burner. After all, there were no other psychiatrists who could immediately adopt the specialist psychoanalytical method using, for example, LSD. To be able to do this work a lot of knowledge, experience, motivation, and courage was required. Therefore, he was the only one capable to do the job at that moment. It would take him about four more years before he had finished training a suitable successor. That there had to be a successor was evident, because "the number of war victims is growing and growing."[5]

Members of former resistance and concentration camp organisations – and, of course, especially the patients among them – backed Bastiaans up completely. They saw the impending termination of the treatments in the Jelgersma clinic as proof of "the indifference of the outside world to the problems of the war victims", and a committee to promote the conservation of Bastiaans' treatment was set up. Not without a sense of drama – and blackmail – one of them said: "Bastiaans is a beacon to the war victims. He is their support and refuge. When he leaves us, many of us will immediately lose their sense of living. If that would happen, it can't be ruled out that a lot of his patients will take their own lives."[6]

Protest meetings were set up and Bastiaans made frequent appearances in the media to get his revenge and to once again explain in detail why his work was of such great importance and why it had to continue.[7] This prompted Gerrit Komrij to end his column, mentioned in the introduction, by asking the university whether it could continue to provide him with one bed at least. "For the missionary himself? To cure him of his PR syndrome?" He didn't understand the university's attitude, by the way. Why put this "customer lure" aside? Wasn't he "the goose that lays the golden eggs"? On the other hand, he did understand. In his eyes Bastiaans was little more than a man who made up all kinds of things to attract attention, like inviting Queen Juliana to the screening of *Do you now understand why I cry…* Because of this action his KZ syndrome had become a well-known phenomenon. If attention and fame are added up, the outcome is money. "There's nothing you need to tell me about a psychiatrist's tenacity when he smells the flow of money." The result was a laundry list of syndromes, that, once labelled, always find patients.

> Gradually it is possible to compile a twelve-volume encyclopaedia of syndromes, the competition is fierce. There are more promising syndromes than willing patients. Much to the dismay of the psychiatrists a lot of discontent is being suppressed. There is an extensive grief market, but they often consider the trade in it as too lukewarm.[8]

Many readers disapproved of Komrij's column, to put it mildly. They thought that to attack Bastiaans was equivalent to attacking war victims, and to deny the value of his method was equivalent to denying the sufferings the war had inflicted. One of the most vicious letters was written by Terwindt. She worshipped Bastiaans. He was the man who made the lives of war victims "tolerable" and who had brought relief to their "exploding heads".[9] To her Komrij was nothing more than "a sick, hateful curmudgeon, unworthy of writing for a newspaper like the *NRC*".

> When a little boy called Komrij was born, I sat alone in a cell with a bricked-up window, under artificial light, without any contact other than German SD guards, working on my KZ syndrome. I was convinced that I would never outlive this time unscathed, so isolated, and with nothing to do. What bee does Komrij have in his bonnet that he wants to provoke our seething anger with his abhorrently obnoxious article?[10]

The conflict between Bastiaans and the university dragged on for a long time and it affected him not in a small way. "The one who knows the most about traumatisation is now traumatised himself," the *NRC Handelsblad* wrote.[11] Eventually, he was allowed to continue treating his patients until mid-1985. For this, twelve beds were reserved in the Jelgersma clinic; a fact widely reported on in the newspapers.[12] Gisolf, for example, called it gratifying, because of the work itself and perhaps even more so "because, apparently, it's possible to resolve administrative conflicts by simply talking to each other".[13]

But of course, in the long run his departure was inevitable. Prior to this, Rooijmans had already disallowed Bastiaans to admit his patients as observers into student lectures, something he had done for almost twenty years – or so *Trouw, de Volkskrant* and *NRC Handelsblad* wrote. Rooijmans himself denied that this was the case and stated it only concerned some spectators with one specific patient and that it happened before he became the new director. Anyway, it was a sign of the times. Patients were patients and what was prohibited for one category, couldn't be allowed to another category, even if they were victims of war.[14]

A working group that was erected to keep psychological traumatology as part of the psychiatry department at Leiden University wasn't able to undo Bastiaans' departure either. Nor did his cry for help that the number of Dutch people, who had to be treated because of the psychological consequences of their war experiences, continued to increase, lately even sharply. With the coming anniversary of 40 years of liberation this would only get worse. Even the establishment, in consultation with the *World Health Organisation*, of the *Internationale Stichting voor de Slachtoffers van Oorlog en Geweld* ISOG (International Foundation for the Victims of War and Violence) in 1985, which intended to continue Bastiaans' work, failed to turn the tide. The same was true for an urgent request by the *Stichting Samenwerkend Verzet* (Foundation Cooperating Resistance Movements). They asked the government to keep Bastiaans' work outside its budget cuts. Concerns expressed by various MPs about the impending end of his work, especially because continuation for his specific method hadn't yet been arranged, didn't solve the problem either. The university had lost all faith that Bastiaans would find and train a suitable successor, no matter how long the postponement.[15]

Perhaps further fuelled by the attention for all the fuss at Leiden university, the processing of trauma was again in the spotlights in 1985. This was demonstrated by Van der Reijden's commitment to support the expansion of care provided by Centre '45,[16] and by a two-day conference in celebration of forty years of NIOD, entitled 'Unresolved Past?' in Amsterdam on 7 and 8 May. In addition to historians, lawyers, literary scholars, and political scientists, two psychiatrists, De Wind and Musaph, also took part. History professor Ernst Heinrich Kossman argued that immediately after the German occupation only a few people had realised "that serious processing of those five traumatic war years was necessary".[17]

At the time Van der Reijden said he was still trying to accommodate Bastiaans' work in a foundation separate from the university so that it could be continued in the old villa, but it was already clear that Bastiaans would lose his beds in the Jelgersma clinic on 1 June 1985. Van der Reijden also promised that it would be examined whether his successor was allowed to work with LSD again. However, it was obvious from the start that the chance this would be approved, was minimal, if only because the other doctors at Leiden University started to doubt the drugs' usefulness. It wasn't for nothing that the *NRC Handelsblad* already headlined at that time: 'LSD no longer allowed after Bastiaans' departure.'[18]

Bastiaans said goodbye to the Jelgersma clinic at the end of June 1985, and he ended his professorship by delivering a lecture called 'Security, isolation and liberation'.[19] However, he was able to restart his work in the villa at the beginning of 1986, under the organisational banner of Centre '45, albeit as a part-time worker and not as an associate professor anymore. Infuriated *De Telegraaf* called it a widely puzzling degradation for someone with that many qualities and merits.[20]

In an interview with the *NRC Handelsblad,* shortly after his retirement as a professor, he looked back at it all with a mix of resentment and understanding.

> In my own circle there is jealousy that my international fame is that great. Also, I can very well imagine that the aversion against me is due to a generational conflict. The generation that is now in power, is between 40 and 50 years old, younger than in the old days. They say: "The old guys have to go". That's how I used to look at old professors myself, when I was between 40 and 45.[21]

The fact that he was able to continue working at all, was the result of a recommendation by the *Projectgroep Behandeling Oorlogs- en Geweldgetroffenen* (Project Group Treatment of People Harmed by War and Violence), installed by Van der Reijden in 1984. It was chaired by the Jewish professor of general medicine and former communist, senator Ben Polak, who was also active in the *Medisch Comité Nederland-Vietnam* (Medical Committee Netherlands-Vietnam), and in the beforementioned Committee Resistance and Persecution.[22] The name of the project group is typical of the trend of inclusion and expansion that had taken hold of the world of psychotrauma.[23] They wanted to develop "a well-functioning, scientifically sound, coherent system of facilities for persons living in the Netherlands who have suffered severe psycho-traumatic injuries as a result of significant, prolonged torture, hostage-taking or acts of war."[24]

Bastiaans was told that he had to provide his succession before 1 January 1987. By that time there were no fewer than three psychiatrists that said they were ready to step in his footsteps, although he himself had his doubts. These doubts will have increased rapidly because, already before the official date of instalment, one of them was sued for not having a treatment plan. On top of that, none of them would apply the Bastiaans treatment. In this sense, his succession had failed indeed.[25] To make matters worse, he had to find a place to work elsewhere for a while in early 1987, because the villa was on the brink of being torn down while new accommodation wasn't available yet.[26]

A few weeks after he had started, and just when Centre '45 announced that it had formed the three-person treatment team,[27] it became clear that the Chief Inspector of Mental Health, Jan van Borssum Waalkes, had serious reservations about Bastiaans' therapy, especially about the used doses of mind-altering drugs. According to him, they were irresponsibly high. That this also concerned pentothal in addition to LSD still came as a surprise to many newspaper readers.[28] It led to the fact that, almost twenty years after the discussion about the medical use of LSD in the *NTvG,* for the first time the medical reservations against the drug LSD as being incalculable, but nevertheless passionately defended by Bastiaans, were widely reported in the press; criticism that was not appreciated by all readers.[29] Shortly before, *Het Vrije Volk* already noted that in the eyes of many of his colleagues Bastiaans' method was controversial. However, the newspaper didn't respond to that criticism at the time. It only said that, nevertheless, the Bastiaans method was highly valued by his patients.[30]

To meet the critique, an anaesthesiologist was added to the team,[31] but to no avail. Van der Reijden banned the use of mind-altering drugs in newly started psychiatric treatments. Bastiaans was allowed to continue to treat existing cases but was no longer exempted from the Opium Act in the case of new ones.[32] However, after fierce parliamentary protests, he could continue his treatment with some new patients as well. The conditions for this, again disputed by some MPs, were that, firstly, these patients had already been on his waiting list and, secondly, that he cooperated in an investigation into his therapy based on the files of the approximately three hundred patients he had administered LSD to in the past twenty-five years.[33] In *de Volkskrant* the then well-known psychologist Piet Vroon gave vent to his surprise and indignation.

> Here we see a fine example of the confrontation between scientific considerations and social influences. From a scientific point of view, Bastiaans shouldn't be admired. Nevertheless, parliament believes he should be permitted to continue to treat his patients, supported by people who have outlived the war and who think they know that the therapy is beneficial. This type of conflict is epidemic in medicine and is almost always won by societal forces, no matter how bad the arguments.[34]

Even though Vroon feared that the entire Foundation 1940-1945 would fall all over him, he dismissed LSD as an unsound means of processing trauma, in three further columns. For example, it might well have been the case that Eibert Meester's resistance fabrications were the result of LSD use. In his view, Bastiaans' therapy was a classic example of unproved, alternative medicine that was merely kept in use because a group of patients continued to support it fanatically. However, the fact that a group of people claim to benefit from a certain substance is no proof that it actually does.[35]

Because Vroon equated Bastiaans' therapy with the, in his eyes, equally nonsensical psychic catharsis of the early twentieth-century psychoanalyst Josef Breuer,[36] he was replied by Willem van Hoorn, professor of historical psychology at the University of Amsterdam. Bastiaans, Van Hoorn argued, did a lot more than assisting some nervous ladies who didn't know what to do with their time.

> Bastiaans concerns himself with patients weighed down by the serious consequences of war suffering. A good percentage of Breuer and Freud's clientele would have gotten "well" without therapy as well, or just lead a somewhat neurotically coloured life. With Bastiaans it often is about people at the end of their tether and who have pinned their last hopes on him. This is sufficient reason to continue his license.[37]

From time to time Bastiaans kept making the news, for example when *Tsofen E.D'M.A* (English title: Shivitti, a vision) was published, a book on his LSD treatment at Oegstgeest, by the Israeli author, Auschwitz survivor, and former witness during the Eichmann-trial, Yehiel De-Nur, written under the pseudonym Ka-Tzetnik 135633, his camp number.[38] Or when it turned out that the journalist Jaap van Meekren had consulted him before he invited the so-called 'black widow' Florrie Rost van Tonningen-Heubel to have her say on television, to the disgust of many commentators. There had been a lot of fuss when it turned out that she received a pension because her husband, prominent NSB member Meinoud Rost van Tonningen, one of the most fanatical Dutch national socialists, had been an MP. What reinforced the protests was the fact that she not only didn't renounce her husband's ideas, but still endorsed them.[39]

During the time of the belated process against Rien de Rijke, the former "torturer" of camp Erica near Ommen, Bastiaans made it known once again that he considered it a folly to punish war criminals after such a long time. It might well make his victims feel a bit better for a few days, but after a while the problems returned just as hard. It was a statement that the judges said they would take to heart, because, after all, Bastiaans wasn't just anyone. Lou de Jong, however, had nothing good to say about Bastiaans' point of view again. The Menten case had made it clear that war victims wanted their tormentors to be prosecuted. And besides that, it simply is a legal duty of the state to continue to prosecute war criminals.[40]

Bastiaans was also of the opinion that a war benefits embezzler, a former consul in Los Angeles, had become mentally incompetent because of his war experiences.[41] However, it then turned out that his authority was on the wane. The court rejected his report because what the man had done and endured barely deviated from what every average Dutchman had done and endured.[42]

Furthermore, it was a sign of the times that the budget cuts that prevailed in those days of mass unemployment, anti-nuclear weapons demonstrations, housing shortage, punk music, and 'no future', didn't leave the war benefits untouched. It gradually became more difficult to get one, especially for war victims' children. Warnings that trauma and worse would be the inevitable result, didn't help. The fact that Gerard Londo, none other than the chairman of the Foundation 1940-1945, recommended in 1985 that an applicant should prove by him- or herself that he or she had a past in the resistance, because it became too difficult to do this for him or her, didn't do the protest against the proposed budget cuts any good.[43]

The same applies to a report published by an advisory committee for the government that same year. Despite protests from committee member Ben Polak, it advised phasing out the various pensions and benefits for war victims. This was largely substantiated by, again, a reference to the increasing difficulty physicians had to prove a link between the war and occurring psychological problems. The fact that Polak referred to various opposing voices from, for instance, the Dutch Psychiatric Association and medical advisors of the Foundation 1940-1945, was to no avail.[44]

And this certainly applied to a report on the connection between the war and later physical or psychological problems, by the Erasmus University Rotterdam at the beginning of 1987. It was called *Medische Causaliteit bij Oorlogsgetroffenen* (Medical Causality among War Harmed) and was the result of a government mandate to the *Commissie voor de Vereenvoudiging en Coördinatie van de Wetten voor Oorlogsgetroffenen* (Commission to Simplify and Coordinate the Laws for War Harmed) in 1985, which was set up for this occasion only. They had to create unity in the tangle of war rules and laws. The researchers were Lolke Pepplinkhuizen, professor of biological psychiatry, and Willem Joost Schudel, professor of clinical and social psychiatry. In accordance with the advisory committee's report and the same as practitioners had been claiming for several decades, they argued that unless the problems had manifested themselves shortly after the war, a connection between psychological distress and war experiences couldn't be made and wasn't self-evident. The individual assessors were given a lot of space, too much space, to accept or reject a connection. They therefore advised to not process anymore applications from 1995 onwards. Even though the report emphatically wrote 'No *direct* link', it implicitly, but no less emphatically, raised theoretical questions about the new concept of Post-Traumatic Stress Disorder (PTSD), a prominent part of the third volume of the DSM, the *Diagnostical and Statistical Manual for Mental Disorders*, published in 1980. Moreover, it practically placed a bomb under the right to war pensions because the reversed burden of proof formed its foundation. Because of the latter, the reactions by former resistance members and camp survivors were furious.[45]

In addition to a number of angry letters and comments,[46] the report led to an article in *Het Parool* by the Jewish professor of economics Arnold Heertje, who had survived the war by going into hiding. He especially questioned the motives of the two psychiatrists. He stated that they had to provide the Ministry of Health, that was hunting for budget cut possibilities, with arguments on the basis of which war victims could be denied benefits. With this starting point, the conclusion was predetermined. Therefore, he urged them "to take note of Bastiaans' life work, the only work for which one life is too short". If they did, they would certainly reach different conclusions.

> The report is secret. This is probably for the best, because making it public would teach us how direct, how penetrating, how lively the connection is

between what they – the victims – experienced during the war and the suffering they still experience on a daily basis.[47]

Psychiatrists like De Wind, Musaph and, of course, Bastiaans,[48] didn't like the report of their Rotterdam colleagues either.[49] De Wind accused them of merely looking at the registered disease rates and not at the suffering itself. If there were no real complaints immediately after the war, the researchers stated, there was little chance they would emerge later on. Perhaps with De Swaan's words about supply, demand and misery in mind, De Wind wrote that suffering was always present, even if complaints were not. The suffering causes the complaints, directly or years after the fact.[50]

However, no matter how often it was remarked that the outcome of the report did suit the government very well indeed, the seed of doubt was sown. This happened for instance in an article in which the term PTSD was used for war-related problems, probably for the first time without any reference to the Vietnam War.[51] And in another article *de Volkskrant* wondered "Has Professor Bastiaans always been mistaken?", without, by the way, formulating an answer.[52] On top of that, a well-looked at television programme called *Kenmerk* (Characteristic) paid attention to Bastiaans and his work mid-1987, but no longer because they were respectively fascinating and bringing relief. Now the reason was that both man and method had become controversial.[53]

As if all this wasn't enough already, shortly thereafter the, from the point of view of Bastiaans, rather unpleasant outcome of a research into the scientific value of his therapy, was published.[54] In the year before his retirement, it had been conducted, at his own request, by a team led by Van der Ploeg, his Leiden colleague with whom he had written the book *People at Hostage-takings* five years before. Nevertheless, it turned out quite negative, or rather: it failed because Van der Ploeg announced that Bastiaans hadn't recorded enough data of enough patients, which made a thorough research into the effectiveness of his LSD method impossible. Of the 209 files made available to the team from the period 1968-1985, only nine appeared to meet all the necessary criteria.[55] It initiated a dissociation between Van der Ploeg and his former research colleague. He would call LSD a psychological kill or cure remedy ten years later,[56] while citing the medical criticism of it in the *NTvG* discussion of 1968.

This report marked the irrevocable end of the treatment method, although his patients called the report unsound and continued to defend him through thick and thin, and his method even more.[57] However, this sentiment was shared by fewer and fewer people. "Bastiaans falls from his pedestal", *Het Parool* headlined above a lengthy piece concerning the investigation and the report resulting from it. Although heartfelt words were still spoken about the man and his help to war victims in this article, "his downfall was complete". It was clear that the image that thousands had been helped by his special treatment had been false, and that, everyone, from the Leiden medical faculty to parliament, had been sleeping for decades. Remarkably enough, journalism itself was not mentioned.[58]

If there ever had been a chance that at least one of his successors would be exempted from the Opium Act and allowed to start using LSD, this was over now. The (declining) social support could no longer counterbalance, let alone outweigh, the scientific criticism. The definitive 'no' was pronounced shortly before Christmas 1987. One of Bastiaans' three successors in Centre '45, A. Krumperman, did ask for an exemption of six months for treatments that Bastiaans had already started so he could complete them.[59] But even he didn't fully support the treatment method. Shortly after Bastiaans' death, he announced that his method was a fiction. Bastiaans and many other psychotherapists had simply realised that certain drugs made it possible to make the consequences of terrible, repressed experiences "a little bit more manageable".[60] Manageable. Not: heal.

This criticism of the method – of which is unclear whether Krumperman already adhered to it in 1985 or whether it arose in the time between Bastiaans' farewell and his demise – didn't stand in the way of his admiration for his predecessor. Krumperman stated that Bastiaans could never be replaced completely in late December 1985. After all, he and no one else was "the symbol of years of struggle for the acknowledgement of the concentration camp syndrome of war victims".[61] However, Krumperman loathed the guru-like worshipping that characterised a part of the outside world and certainly a part of his patients, that remained devout believers in his method. Krumperman added that Bastiaans himself had never encouraged this exaggerated admiration.

> The man is a fantastic therapist. He really works very well. This isn't only due to his appearance as a large, paternal figure, but also because, as an old-fashioned psychoanalyst, he doesn't stick to rigid rules. He provides a very clear direction, something which is rather unusual in psychoanalysis.[62]

The report marked the end of the battle that started in 1983 between Bastiaans and the medical faculty. But for this book, which deals with the history of psycho-trauma in the time between the emergence of the KZ syndrome and the establishment of PTSD, these internal university problems and the sparring between government, parliament, university, and clinic, don't matter ultimately. It can, however, be concluded that, even if the argument had then been decided in favour of the university – although 'just a little less against' is probably a better description – it had lost the battle for the public's favour spectacularly; rightly so or not is another question entirely.[63]

The many expressions of support indicate that Bastiaans really wasn't only able to continue with his method for so long, because his friends and patients from the former resistance were fanatically on his side – for instance by sending a threatening letter to Rooijmans, whom they saw as the evil genius behind the termination of their medical hero's employment.[64] The reporting in the newspapers, from *De Waarheid* to *De Telegraaf,* much more reflected this support, these patients' stories, than the internal medical and scientific criticism of his treatments did. It reflected that Bastiaans could be a source of information and an oracle, not because the newspapers and the general public saw him as the medical scientist who knew best, but because they saw him as the man who stood up for his patients, the man who stood up for the victims of war. In short, the reporting reflected a focus on the person of Bastiaans, not so much the physician, but on a man with an abundance of knowledge and human whims. And it reflected a disinterest in, or even aversion to, the impersonal university boards, with their meetings, their financial interests, and their political games.

Bart Lulofs, subtly summing up all of Bastiaans' international honorary memberships and doctorates in *De Telegraaf* in 1985, stated in unpolished terms:

> A distinguished man. Far above the childish envy of his Leiden colleagues, who in these days try to end his possible staying on, try to punch the crown off his head, and try to discredit his work with the cackling criticism "that the Bastiaans method is controversial". These professors of psychiatry would do themselves, their department, and the Dutch war victims a better service if they listened to all those men and women to whom Professor Bastiaans gave back a bit of joy in life. All those men and women who could sometimes cry just like that. Crying for unprocessed grief from those days of old and crying with happiness because, in the crisis of their later life, psychiatrist Bastiaans had crossed their path. Thank you Professor Bastiaans.[65]

It was an opinion that *De Telegraaf* kept repeating,[66] and which could at the least also be read between the lines in other newspapers. And it wasn't for nothing that in that same year the *NRC Handelsblad* gave him the opportunity to reveal his average working day at length.[67] And it also wasn't without reason that several reports about the delay in the succession of Bastiaans had headlines such as: 'Treatment of patients with war trauma *in danger*'.[68] (Ital.: LvB)

Vaders said in *Het Nieuwsblad van het Noorden* in 1986 that without any doubt the criticism of Bastiaans' method would make sense now and then, but in fact he couldn't care less. What did interest him was this:

"Despite his buffalo like gruffness, he is a guy with a heart in his body, with compassion and feeling for the underdog. We have an eternal shortage of people like him, inside and outside the medical profession."[69]

According to the *NIW* his book *Isolatie en Bevrijding* (Isolation and Liberation), published in 1987, was written by "a great man".[70] Bastiaans dedicated it to "the victims of violence and those involved in their counselling and treatment"; so in fact partly to his own patients and to himself.[71] In the book he once again and from various sides shed light on his message that some victims of violence were so isolated that without help liberation couldn't be achieved.[72] Following the publication, psychiatrist Los showed his admiration in the *Nederlands Dagblad*.

> Bastiaans is an indignant and rebellious, but above all compassionate person. He is an old man who doesn't want to rest. A fighter and a difficult man, but also a very warm person when it comes to his patients, who were tormented, who were in concentration camps or who were taken hostage, who were mistreated or abandoned in other ways by their fellow humans, even by their own parents.[73]

Judging by the letters to the editor in those years, this 'Bastiaans must stay' sentiment was the opinion of many readers as well. Among those letters was one from Terwindt. According to her, several war victims had committed suicide after the villa had been closed down. She wanted to lay a wreath at the governmental centre in The Hague, out of respect "for all those who ended their lives out of desperation because they had been deprived of the chance to be freed from their KZ syndrome". And she intended to write a book about Bastiaans. Due to her death at the end of April 1987, this never happened; neither the wreath laying nor the book writing.[74]

Of course, the broad support didn't silence the criticism. After the publication of *Isolation and Liberation*, *Het Parool* stated that the man started to look less and less like a psychiatrist and more and more like a Bhagwan-like saviour.[75] Gisolf had a soft spot for Bastiaans personally and he hoped that he would be able to continue his work for a long time, and also that it would be continued by someone else when he no longer could. However, Gisolf also pointed out that the fact that Bastiaans was an internationally recognised celebrity in the field of processing traumas, especially war traumas, didn't automatically mean that his opinions and findings were endorsed by all his colleagues. There were psychiatrists, for example, who refused to see – and therefore diagnose and treat – the consequences of a time in a concentration camp as a separate syndrome, the KZ syndrome, while others criticised the idea that different experiences led to one and the same infliction, the new kid on the block called PTSD.[76]

The latter critics questioned the enormous inkblot effect that resulted from this generalisation. This continued in the 1980s, for example with the arrival of traumatised veterans from UNIFIL, the UN mission in Lebanon (1979-1985).[77] According to C. Borghart of the Military Social Service, the psychological problems of former soldiers hadn't received any attention until the mid-1970s. At that time the BNMO started to research it as well.[78] In an article with the telling title 'The worst is yet to come', *Trouw* reported at the end of 1983 about the Korean veterans, about whom already in 1955, just two years after the end of the Korean War, the dissertation *Over de Gevechtsuitputting* (On Combat Exhaustion) was written:

> "They worry about the dreams they have, they are always preoccupied with them, and they complain about a lack of understanding in their environment," says Professor Bastiaans of the Jelgersma clinic in Oegstgeest. He sees little difference between the psychological damage of these war veterans and the KZ syndrome that he discovered in victims of the concentration camps at the time.[79]

A few years later, it was said about the veterans of the Indonesian war of decolonisation that they wanted support and rehabilitation. This happened in an article in which Bastiaans reported that he already saw many of them in the villa. He didn't doubt there were many more who were traumatised, in part because their problems were underestimated too much in the past.[80]

In addition to this in *Het Vrije Volk* in 1985, in an article about an ICODO conference, the number of people mentally affected by their experiences in 1940-1945 alone, was estimated at at least 150,000. In other words: "25 patients per general practice".[81] This number returned in later publications and Bastiaans himself increased it by another 50,000 in 1987. About 200,000 people needed help. And: "In the coming years there will be even more."[82] It was the reason the press at last dedicated a few critical words to the inkblot effect as well. In *Het Parool* journalist Johanna Fortuin wondered whether Bastiaans often didn't just say something about all kinds of things, knowing the media would pick up on it because he was such an expert on trauma. Because, in other words, he was 'Bastiaans'. How on earth was it possible that in fifteen years the number of people psychologically suffering from the experiences of the Second World War had increased sixfold.[83] Unfortunately, the question was only raised, but again no answer was given. And, consequently, again the role journalists had played in the process themselves was not pointed out.

Although Fortuin was the first journalist to question the inkblot effect, she wasn't the first to call attention to it in a newspaper. The philosopher of science and professor of psychology Jaap van Heerden had criticised it in a

Kousbroek-like article in the *NRC Handelsblad* in 1983. He referred to the memoirs of Yvo Pannekoek, pseudonym of professor of virology Frits Dekking, published shortly before. In it figured a man who was brought up in a strict protestant environment and saw the world in black and white. A few years in a Japanese internment camp had taught him the value of humour and perspective. After the war he lived his life a lot happier. Dekking called it a 'positive KZ syndrome'. And as for the writer himself, who had experienced the pleasures of living in Vught and Dachau, his camp experiences resulted in "great tranquillity and equanimity in thinking about death and suffering".[84]

Certainly, Dekking and the man 'suffering' from a positive KZ syndrome will have been exceptions. Not many will have responded approvingly after reading that Pannekoek didn't consider "being locked up in solitary confinement in a dark and completely empty cell without any distraction or occupation" to be an unbearable, inhuman punishment.[85] On the contrary, he saw it as a "wonderful change after ten months of never having been alone anywhere, not even in the toilet".[86] The vast majority of camp survivors looked back on the war years with anything but a smile. Nevertheless, it did lead to questions. Pannekoek, who, by the way, thought all the attention for the KZ syndrome was completely justified,[87] wrote that he had never read anything about his positive KZ syndrome in the discussions on traumatic experiences. Therefore, Van Heerden wondered how much the general public really knew about things like the KZ syndrome, despite all the information they had been given since at least the late 1960s, with the screening of the film *Do you now understand why I cry…*, the discussions on the Breda Three, and the hostages in Wijster, De Punt, and Bovensmilde. Public knowledge reflected the knowledge psychiatry had, at least insofar as it was made public. At those public manifestations he had noticed that the syndrome was declared applicable to so many, very different kinds of traumatic experience, that "a certain diagnostic rashness" could be detected. Like Kousbroek did eight years later, he gave the example of KZ syndrome in women who had undergone an abortion. "Although I don't envy the fate of an aborted woman, I assume this is a mistake."[88]

Van Heerden was struck by the same unease in the case of the hostage-takings, although some of the hostages had mentioned the positive influence it had on their lives. Without exception, the psychiatrists consulted by the media at the time characterised the mental state of the hostages as KZ syndrome. Even the fact that some said not to have any problems at all, was, according to one of the interviewed psychiatrists, entirely consistent with this diagnosis. Van Heerden: "While I don't want to downplay the position of hostages, I do believe that understanding their fate and understanding KZ syndrome is not promoted by lumping together all traumatic experiences that occur in this world, while neglecting all the differences."[89]

What, according to Van Heerden, psychiatry should have done and should still do was stop emphasising the similarities that lead up to the same diagnosis. Instead, it should "clarify the effect of all the differences". For instance, a concentration camp was set up by a hostile government and covertly aimed at destroying human beings who had been indicated in advance. A hostage-taking, on the other hand, was aimed at achieving a political goal, including open negotiations about the fate of accidental hostages by a government trying to save as many lives as possible. If psychiatrists were of the opinion that differences like these didn't play a role in the resulting problems, they had to explain why. Van Heerden, however, was convinced these differences actually did have an effect on the resulting problems. "I think they lead to a different kind of trauma. Therefore, I doubt that the KZ syndrome can ever be considered applicable to anyone other than those who escaped death in a concentration camp."[90]

Van Heerden won't have been jumping for joy after reading the interview Bastiaans gave to *Het Vrije Volk*, while he was clearing his desk in the Jelgersma clinic mid-1985. In it, he stated that a rotten youth could lead to a kind of KZ situation, and therefore to a kind of KZ syndrome as well.

> The most compelling example is Hitler, who as a result of lousy childhood experiences was so locked up inside himself, so deprived of human contact, that he had to take revenge on the whole world, and, because of a disappointing experience with a Jewish girl, turned the entire Jewish people into a scapegoat.[91]

The ultimate war offender shared the psychological fate of his victims. Once more, this equalisation of perpetrators and victims, as had already happened when answering questions on the kind of patients Centre '45 would treat, and when confusing war syndrome and KZ syndrome, is clear evidence that for the diagnosis of the syndrome or disorder the cause was increasingly outflanked by its symptoms; a development that culminated in PTSD in 1980. All that was needed for this diagnosis were psychological problems occurring sometime after a shocking event. Bastiaans himself, according to, among other things, his comments about the Dutch East Indies veterans, had apparently thrown overboard all reservations about equalisation that he still had in 1973, during the discussion of the war syndrome. But even if, as for example in the discussion of the Breda Three, it was said that the rights of the victims took precedence over that of the perpetrators, their psychological problems fell into the same category. Or rather: from a psychiatric point of view, they had turned into victims too.

What had been Bastiaans' intention when he said that Hitler suffered from a KZ syndrome as well? Did he want to indicate that perpetrators are not inhuman, not animals, and therefore not fundamentally different from the all-too-human victims everyone sympathises and identifies with? Was he implying that the Shoah wasn't an action of monsters, but of humans, humans like all of us? Or that it had indeed been an action of monsters, but that anyone could turn into a monster under the 'right' circumstances? If this was the case, it wasn't understood. His point of view raised the same questions as the belief of some psychologists and psychiatrists that Hitler was who he was because, allegedly, he had but one testicle.[92] Why, the question was, did only one of so many sexually frustrated men end his life as a mass murderer? Or how could it be explained that so many other mass murderers were in the fortunate possession of both testicles? The same here. If a rotten youth and the rejection by a girl explain Hitler's actions, then why weren't there thousands of Hitlers? How could the genocides and pogroms be explained then, that were carried out by or under the orders of people who hadn't come across any such grief? Whatever the intention, the extreme Hitler observation makes it clear that psychiatry had already formulated the answer to Van Heerden-like criticism. The generalisation of the diagnosis was embraced, and the name of that diagnosis could no longer refer directly to war or any other specific cause.

Due to the desire to be inclusive, the letters K and Z had been erased and replaced by letters referring to indistinguishable events such as E, E, S and S and shortly afterwards P, T, S and D. A shift had occurred in thirty years, leading up to the fact that the cause of trauma was no longer reflected in the name of the diagnosis. Surely, this was conceivable in part, since the cause of the problems lay in the past. That makes the ultimate cure, in the sense that the cause is removed, impossible by definition. This too made the symptoms leading in the treatment and, by extension, in the diagnosis as well.

What happened to the PTSD diagnosis in the public domain after this, reflects the history of the KZ syndrome thirty years earlier (and the one of shell shock forty years before that). Even though, as an official psychiatric diagnosis, it's only one of the problems that could possibly arise from violent events, it became a collective name for every problem, big and small, arising after an event that is either traumatising, is experienced as traumatising or is presented as traumatising. It's noteworthy, however, that nowadays the term most often refers to the problems soldiers experience after having exerted or witnessed violence (the war syndrome) and only to a lesser extent to the problems of those who are victims of persecution and the infliction of violence (the KZ syndrome). Once again, the hierarchy has turned, but whether the cause determines the name of the diagnosis (KZ) or whether the symptoms do (PTSD), the inkblot remains.

CLOSING REMARKS

The Dutch newspapers have closely followed the advance of war trauma from the mid-1950s onward. But after a period of relative calm and almost entirely when current events gave reason to do so, many articles were written about the debates on psychological problems that resulted from traumatising war experiences, certainly from the mid-sixties onwards. The time division that Withuis identified in her study *Acknowledgement*, about the discussion within the psychiatric community itself, can also be found in the newspapers. Denial was followed by acknowledgment, after which, because of the more general, more inclusive terminology, it changed into denial of the uniqueness of the concentration camp experience.[1]

The players in the field, especially the psychiatrists among them, were frequently interviewed. In those interviews they were given anything but a hard time. The steadily rising figures that were presented by them, were uncritically accepted until the mid-1980s. Any nuances the interviewees added themselves were put aside often and quickly. 'Maximal' changed to 'approximately', 'approximately' changed to 'minimal'. This reinforced the upward trend the psychiatrists themselves had initiated, even further. It was typical of the reporting that the problems of the victims were generally regarded as underestimated, and that support was always inadequate. Medical scientific questions about the treatment were secondary to the patient's stories. Who are journalists to doubt the word of a patient who claims to benefit from his or her treatment? The attending physicians were hailed and believed, also because their patients backed them up completely. Especially criticism from trauma experts who didn't treat victims themselves, was considered irrelevant, no matter what the scientific content was.

Perhaps even more important, though, is that the idea had changed by 1970 that there was a direct relationship between the wartime past of former resistance fighters and camp survivors and their psychological problems in the present. From an elusive medical theory, it turned into an undeniable fact, and that fact was disseminated by psychiatrists and shared by politicians. Many psychiatrists told journalists, that those who weren't sick yet would definitely be so soon, unless they died in the meantime. Again: why would journalists doubt that, even more so because their own newspapers' medical employees usually supported this view? Those who did ask questions were treated with suspicion and were thought to be deniers of the Nazi atrocities. They could expect strong criticism: from psychiatrists, from patients, and from letters to the editor writers (who sometimes were patients themselves). Added to this was the tendency to think, that the statements made by the interviewed psychiatrists were by definition scientific statements. ‘Said’ became ‘proved’.

In particular, the former resistance papers such as *Trouw, Het Parool* and *De Waarheid,* supported the former resistance fighters and camp survivors and took their complaints and the relationship they demonstrated with their war past seriously. They therefore supported the psychiatrists who endorsed that relationship and treated them. *De Waarheid,* for example, reported positively about Bastiaans' dissertation in 1957 and about the conference on the consequences of imprisonment and deportation in The Hague in 1961. Piet Maliepaard, a prominent communist and former Spanish Civil War volunteer, spoke highly of Bastiaans and his therapy that he had undergone as well. It's therefore only partly true that the Dutch communists questioned the psychological war trauma. That it was problematic for a communist to be bothered by it indicates that the hard nuts *De Waarheid* cracked from time to time, also on the use of LSD, weren't medical so much, as political ideological in nature. The criticism had little to do with doubts about the syndrome itself or the method of treatment used to cure it. It arose from an ideologically determined hardness (in themselves) and the political context in which, or even through which, the traumas (in others) arose or aggravated at the very least, for example during the time of the Breda Three discussion.

Firstly, victims were those people who were taken away without (a possibility of) resistance. Former resistance fighters, and certainly those who already agitated against fascism in the interbellum, were, by definition, not to be called victims.[2] From this arose the second objection. The war survivors resisted and/or fell victim to fascism and Nazism. Although the battle against Nazi Germany was victorious, the battle against the reprehensible ideology behind it was far from over. The syndrome arose at least from that, according to *De Waarheid*. The struggle continued, with government and psychiatry often opposing each other, rather than standing shoulder to shoulder with anti-fascists. The use of LSD could help individuals cope with the problems that arose from the atrocities committed by fascists in days gone by but could also lead those former resistance fighters and camp survivors to be rather loose lipped to people that were not to be trusted. It's an opinion that fitted in with *De Waarheid*'s paranoid view on humanity and society. However, the newspaper was already too marginal and sectarian in the mid-1970s to give any social significance to this critical voice on psychiatry and LSD use. That this criticism would become more commonplace ten years later should therefore be separated from this.

De Telegraaf was entirely on the hand of the war victims and their therapists as well. This wasn't without significance, since it was by far the largest newspaper in the Netherlands in the 1970s. Paradoxically, one reason for this support may lie in the fact that a large proportion of the non-subscribers characterised it as a former *anti*-resistance paper. *De Telegraaf* supported the German and Austrian occupying forces and its Dutch NSB companions. By fully supporting the victims of the occupation and persecution, as well as the psychiatrists treating them, that stain could be brushed off somewhat.

However, despite all the differences regarding their political views on humanity and society, in general newspapers such as *de Volkskrant, NRC Handelsblad* and *Nederlands Dagblad* also supported the victims and their claims to acknowledgement, pensions and medical aid. They too had little regard for the medical criticism that arose in professional journals, in particular concerning the treatment with LSD. The patients' stories that supported the syndrome and the therapy were found to be more credible, more important, more interesting, than the scientific question marks. As a result, for a long time criticism came solely from those journalists that were free to write what they wanted: the columnists. But if they did, they knew in advance that furious letters to the editor would be the price they would have to pay.

Individual issues and social context

Guest authors, letter to the editor writers, and a rare interviewee were also responsible for another point of contention: the underlying cause of the psychological trauma; not to be confused with the immediate occasion, such as the discussion about the Breda Three. Was this cause partly to be found in a strict upbringing and/or troubled youth, as psychoanalysts put forward and, therefore, Bastiaans as well? Were the horrors of the Second World War completely to blame as the cause, as was the common view? Or should fingers be pointed at the post-war experience at least as much, as De Swaan, Milikowski, Cohen and Boas, with all their differences, argued? In other words, was the delayed revival of problems, observed by psychiatrists from the late 1960s onward, not, or at least not only, the result of a waning resilience, but at the very least also of the changed social circumstances of secularisation and democratisation, resulting in psychologisation?

Milikowski, and with him *De Waarheid,* thought that all resistance stemmed from an anti-fascist, anti-racist, ideological enthusiasm. According to him, the emergence of trauma had everything to do with disappointment about the fact that fascism and racism hadn't perished together with the Axis powers after 1945. In this ideological statement he, firstly, disregarded (or simply didn't believe) that some experiences are really too horrible or are experienced as being too horrible to just live on afterwards, mentally unscathed. Moreover, the concentration camps weren't merely inhabited by resistance fighters. On the contrary. Also, not just resistance fighters were diagnosed with KZ syndrome, far from it, and the behaviour of communist camp inmates towards non-communist, but equally anti-fascist, fellow sufferers regularly contributed to the problems of the latter.[3] Furthermore, people were also diagnosed with KZ in the 1970s who had nothing to do with any camp at all, a development that philosopher and psychologist Van Heerden deplored. According to him, such large, causal differences couldn't and shouldn't lead to the same psychiatric diagnosis.

In addition, resistance wasn't only the result of a communist or even of an anti-fascist conviction. Many chose to resist the occupying forces out of an urge for adventure, the desire to be seen as important, love for the use of violence, out of an attempt to escape boredom, and above all: out of nationalistic fury at a foreign occupation, regardless of the political persuasion of both the occupier and the resistance fighter. Among the nationalist resistance fighters, anger, or disappointment at the unjust post-war society riddled with wars and military dictatorships, played no part in the development of the syndrome. And this was especially true for the people who came back from Indonesia and who had endured the period of the internment camps and the Bersiap. Generally speaking, their ideological convictions had little to do with anti-racism and anti-fascism, let alone anti-colonialism.

In their references to Israel, where, according to them, the KZ syndrome was at best a minor problem, Boas and Cohen forgot that not everyone prospered in the celebrated kibbutz system, and that the creation of that country was entailed by the departure of hundreds of thousands of people to less prosperous refugee camps. In addition, they wrote their contributions on this subject after 1967, the year in which Israel fought the Six-Day War, turning their beloved state into an occupier of Palestinian territory. This has been a bit detrimental to many Palestinians, to put it mildly.

However, their common point, best expressed by De Swaan, is that trauma isn't (purely) an individual matter. De Swaan was criticised for representing his idea of 'silence and not listening' as too dogmatic. Yes, it's true, the war had (or has) never completely disappeared from the Dutch people's minds, not even in the 'silent' fifties. And yes, newspapers did pay regular attention to the traumas of war victims. And indeed, they did ask patients (clients, guests) to speak out more and more. You could say, therefore, that actually the psychiatrists guided the interest of the Dutch people back to the war. This doesn't alter that 'speech is silver, silence is golden' was the most important proverb until the mid-1960s, and this applied to the newspapers as well. The complaints may indeed have increased around that time, but this was at the very least also the result of a political and societal climate that had changed compared to the 1950s. Complaints were allowed to be expressed, become visible and… increase. But apart from a few actualities – the Breda Three discussion, the hostage-takings, the broadcast of the *Holocaust* series – this new social context played no part in the explanations, neither in those the psychiatrists presented, nor in the given that the newspapers' attention had grown so much from the mid-1960s onwards. On the rare occasion a social context was mentioned, such as the economic malaise of the 1980s, it only led to the warning that this could lead to even more patients because of the resulting increase in violence. Traumas would increase because there would be more triggers for trauma; including traumas that had nothing to do with the new violence, but everything with the old. This didn't affect the individual view of trauma, the individual explanation of trauma, or the individualised method of treatment in any way, at least according to the newspaper articles.

However, in an overview of the development of psychotraumatology in the Netherlands, it's rightly pointed out that this development can't be outlined without taking the social context into consideration.[4] This automatically means that psychological trauma can't be explained detached from the time and place in which the event to which the trauma is attributed occurred. It also means that trauma can't be separated from the political, economic, and social environment in which it arises or is treated. And this then means that an individualised diagnosis and an individualised treatment, fully focused on the individual processing of parenting issues and/or traumatic events, can never be completely successful, regardless of the use of mind-altering drugs like LSD. Those who had remained psychologically imprisoned after the physical liberation of 1945 could never be liberated mentally as well, as long as treatments were based on views focusing on the individual, without paying attention to the societal context of the day.

Post-traumatic stress disorder

The time span of this study ends around the time of Bastiaans' retirement, and more importantly, around the time the new abbreviation PTSD, introduced in the DSM-III in 1980, becomes common knowledge. Despite the general terminology, it can't be separated from the Vietnam War that had ended five years before.[5] Its acceptance in the Netherlands ended a period in which the specific term KZ syndrome transitioned to more general diagnostic terms such as EESS or disaster syndrome; a generalisation that was necessary in order to be able to provide more and more people suffering from similar symptoms with the same and, moreover, appropriate diagnosis, even though the causes of their problems, actual or alleged, often differed widely. In order for the diagnosis to fit the causes, the causes had to be removed from the diagnosis.

The DSM-III was a biologically oriented, much more voluminous revision of the psychoanalytically inspired DSM-II of the 1950s. However, it wasn't just the result of a different focus, diligent scientific thought, and meticulous research work, although this is what was claimed and was generally assumed and what certainly was the initial intention. The psychiatrists responsible for the final editing of the texts didn't escape the influence of the vigorous lobbying of various interest groups. The same, and perhaps above all, was true for the novel diagnosis of PTSD. It was the result of a compromise between, on the one hand, medical insights obtained through research into mental problems, for example in people with burns, and, on the other hand, the influences of widely differing groups like Vietnam veterans who had trouble adjusting after coming home, and feminists. The latter group raised the big issues of matters like assault, rape, and domestic violence and all the problems arising from them. This already led to terms like *Rape Trauma Syndrome*, *Battered Woman Syndrome* or *Abused Child Syndrome* in the 1970s; terminology that focused on causation and that was absorbed into PTSD and was therefore wiped clean socially and causally.

However, it was the veterans in particular who found a willing ear, also because the psychiatrists responsible for the DSM review had often expressed their opposition to the Vietnam War. The psychological problems of returned soldiers both confirmed and reinforced their medical anti-war protest. One of them was Robert Jay Lifton. He subtitled his book *Home from the War*, published in 1973: *Vietnam Veterans – neither victims nor executioners*. Bluntly speaking, in his probably most famous work, *Nazi Doctors. Medical killing and the psychology of genocide* (1986), he reached the same conclusion as Bastiaans did with regard to Hitler, although far more nuanced: Nazi doctors acted the way they did as a result of a troubled childhood, scarred as they were by a nationalistic, authoritarian upbringing and the devastating effects, often personal, always societal, of the First World War. Besides, they studied medicine in a time that fear of degeneration was omnipresent. Highly valued medical professors advocated eugenics as a valuable and practical solution. Racial explanations of medical ailments were commonly accepted, also in circles outside the extreme right. The resemblance between the Nazi doctors of this book and the veterans from *Home from the War*? At the very least, perpetrators weren't just perpetrators. Regardless of the 'neither' in Lifton's subtitle, the Vietnam veterans were also victims, and according to some even completely. It was PTSD that confirmed and recognised their victimhood. This didn't mean, however, that they really got better afterwards, nor that psychological problems were immediately accepted within the various armed forces. In his *The Scars of War* Hugh McManners cites, for example, a military surgeon who called PTSD 'compensationitis' during a training course in 1990.[6]

With diagnostic terminology like shell shock or combat fatigue, war trauma was reserved for the 'perpetrators' until 1945: soldiers who got into psychological trouble because of the violence inflicted by them or their enemies on the fields of battle. Due to the enormous number of civilian dead and injured, because of aerial bombardments but especially as a result of the Shoah, at least in severely stricken Europe the victim perspective largely shifted to the side of those who were solely on the receiving end of all the bloodshed, after the Second World War.[7] The psychological aftermath of the Vietnam War and, in its wake, the wars preceding it, in which, with regard to the Netherlands, Indonesia and Korea have to be considered, caused the perspective to shift back again until a sort of middle ground was reached. It resulted in a name that could be used for both civilians and military personnel, for victims as well as perpetrators, for both camp survivors and hostages (and for the doctors and nurses treating them, who didn't always psychologically survive either).[8] The symptoms became leading, the cause – from having to suffer violence helplessly to (being able to) apply it oneself, either as action or reaction – moved to if not beyond the horizon.

Because of this, it will not come as a surprise that over time publications appeared like Allan Young's *The Harmony of Illusions. Inventing Post-Traumatic Stress Disorder* (1995) or: 'The *invention* of post-traumatic stress disorder and the social usefulness of a psychiatric category,' written by transcultural psychiatrist Derek Summerfield for *The British Medical Journal* in 2001. Certainly this article, in which the author expressed serious criticism of the Western character of PTSD and the influence this had on the treatment method, has led to enough furious reactions. It was a bit like reminiscing the – scarce – Dutch critique on the KZ syndrome. Now it was argued that by stating that PTSD isn't real, but an invention, rather than a scientifically proved fact, trauma and suffering were denied, although, while a lot of research is focused on discovering so called biological markers, the disorder still can't be proved in the sense that it can be seen under a microscope let alone with the naked eye, like so many other illnesses or injuries can. Or, as psychiatrist Berthold Gersons once wrote: "There is no 'blood pressure monitor' for PTSD (yet)." In any case, the critique missed Summerfield's point. What he said was that PTSD is a construct, something that, by the way, is anything but unique to diagnoses, certainly not in the psychiatric world. Therefore, it's riveted to a certain time and place, to certain political, economic, and cultural conditions. It's at least partly the result of choices determined by those circumstances. If they change or disappear, the basis for those choices disappears and the disorder also changes or disappears, at least as a diagnosis. This of course doesn't mean, and the author didn't deny this, that people who have experienced terrible things can't suffer from serious psychological and/or physical complaints.[9]

A handy invention, suited to ideological motives, and embraced by a spoiled audience incapable of dealing with adversity or the result of scientific scrutiny: fact is, few psychiatrists at universities or elsewhere doubted or doubt the truth of the disorder. This belief has become common and, as mentioned, has long since widely exceeded the boundaries of female and veterans' misery. PTSD incorporates and connects groups in their traumatisation that were strictly separated previously and of which critics like Van Heerden wonder whether they should have been connected. After all, psychological problems following a car accident receive the same diagnosis as a long stay in a concentration camp. As a result, the (fairly) normal comes into the same category as the epitome of the abnormal as, vice versa, the abnormal turns normal, or at least becomes more normal. And as a result, the 'normal' is also considered traumatic after which acknowledgement, treatment, and benefits have to follow.[10] Criticism of this equalisation – which can be considered as an unwanted trivialisation of the Shoah – led to the proposal to at least create a separate term for military personnel, the *Combat Reaction Spectrum Disorder,* which referred to the cause of the problems again, as early as the 1980s. This has already become practice, at least in Canada, where the term *Operational Stress Injury* is used. For citizens, the (linguistically speaking horrific) term *Enduring Personality-changes after Catastrophic Experiences* has been proposed, in which a hint of KZ syndrome can be detected. In addition, terms like type-I and -II or complex PTSD indicate that the term itself can't escape diversification. More recent terminology like 'moral injury' become increasingly attractive and will possibly even replace PTSD entirely or in part somewhere in the future.[11]

Jan Bastiaans

As we have seen, the individualised treatment of (war) victims, focused on symptoms and past events and detached from the contemporary context, wasn't without criticism. With this criticism, a link is quickly established to the most important, the most talked-about and the most charismatic person among the Dutch practitioners. Jan Bastiaans, professor of psychiatry in Leiden, has treated hundreds of victims, first in Amsterdam and later in Oegstgeest, from the early 1960s onwards.

That Bastiaans' farewell to the university was rather problematic, to put it mildly, and that he went on and on with his treatment, while questions about his methods and the conclusions he drew from them grew hand over fist, has come to define the perception of the role he played in the preceding decades, just like an acrimonious divorce overshadows previous years of happiness. It became a sad story of someone whose time had come, but who wasn't able to accept this. Perhaps he was indeed blinded by success and admiration, as has been suggested in a broadcast about him and his methods in the already mentioned history programme *Other Times* just a few years after his death,[12] and that's why he carried on with his work longer than medically justified. The death of a patient and a subsequent complaint to the Medical Disciplinary Court brought an unenviable end to a turbulent and overall successful career, although he made at least one applauded comeback, both personally and in terms of public attention, during these years of gradual decline. According to the reporter, he delivered a "magisterial speech" on 15 August 1992, during the commemoration of the end of the Pacific War and referring to the Yugoslav Civil War. It was entitled 'Execution of an Unprocessed Past'.[13]

He died at the age of 80, probably due to Alzheimer's or vascular dementia, five years later. *Trouw,* among others, remembered the man who had become famous for his now called "controversial" treatment of war trauma.

> The big man with the soft voice was a pragmatic scientist. He had a correspondingly broad view of humanity. His clients admired him. To them he was "daddy Bas". He considered it his job to free them from the imprisonment their trauma had brought them, no matter how. There was no acknowledgement by colleagues. They believed that the effect of the Bastiaans' method wasn't so much due to the LSD, but above all to Bastiaans' personality. The criticism aroused his fighting spirit, but in the end, he had to stop the therapeutic use of mind-altering drugs like LSD, a form of treatment that he believed to be more effective than psychoanalysis in case of severe trauma.[14]

in the *NTvG,* the magazine in which the attack on his method was launched at the end of the 1960s, psychiatrist Bas Schreuder, who was the director of Centre '45 then, wrote:

> He has had great significance for the social acknowledgement of the late psychiatric consequences of persecution, resistance, and hostage-taking during the war – a acknowledgement that seems so self-evident today but was anything but in the first 25 years after the Second World War.[15]

But Schreuder didn't stop there. In the last paragraph it wasn't concealed that dealing with Bastiaans wasn't always easy and that he should've stopped practising medicine much earlier than he did.

> He was a striking personality who didn't shy away from conflict and even sought it out. He couldn't live with limitations easily. Leaving was difficult for him, both as a professor in 1985 and at Centre '45 in 1988. When he had to stop working at an advanced age, he could hardly do so.

This, however, didn't alter the fact that first and foremost he remained the "enthusiastic psychiatrist who was always there for his patients" and who would live on in memory "with respect and appreciation".[16]

The man was indeed (and naturally) not without flaws. Even to doctors, including psychiatrists, nothing human is alien. It partly explains the sudden change of opinion about the release of the Breda Three, a change all too clear to everybody, but denied by himself, and inexplicable without looking at the climate of threats. Furthermore, like so many other medical professors in the sixties and seventies,[17] the last few decades of the era in which a professor, and certainly a professor of medicine, was god in *his* department, he was stubborn and always convinced that he was right. Additionally, he didn't shy away from exaggeration if it could serve the – in his eyes – righteous cause. As a result, he played no small part in the emergence of the 'victim culture', the culture of trauma, a necessary step in the by Withuis described wider process that ran from KZ syndrome to the contemporary culture of complaint, and cancel culture for that matter. It's the evolution of psychological trauma from something shameful that had to be hidden, to something that provided identity. The longstanding pension neurosis, detested by most psychiatrists, turned into a distress neurosis they embraced. Suffering became something to hold on to, because without suffering no benefits and without benefits no acknowledgement as a sufferer. Being a victim provided status. *Je suis une victime, donc je le suis.*[18]

In line with this lay that Bastiaans was too gullible when it came to his patients. Like so many at the time (and still today), he took 'victims' at their word.[19] Doubt was the order of the day before the Second World War and also in the decades thereafter – with extensions into the present – and medical and political policy was determined by distrust instead of trust, with all the consequences this entailed for the vast majority of people who didn't simulate and/or merely wanted a justified pension. However, dismissing every doubt as insensitive and inappropriate has its drawbacks just as much if it turns out later that doubt would have been justified. Not only will it question the competence of the doctor then, but also the correctness of the diagnosis in others.

Bastiaans didn't see that treating these 'fake' victims, who throve on his and the general gullibility, wasn't doing his business any good. After it was established that they couldn't have a war trauma, because there were no traumatising events to be found, he stated that they were nonetheless sick. And as a doctor he had to help the sick, even if they didn't suffer from the ailment he initially assumed. In doing so he denied that real or alleged victims have a medical, social and/or financial interest in – consciously or unconsciously – exaggerating or even wholly fabricating a glorious albeit traumatising war past. He also failed to see that the interests could come first and that only thereafter, and because of it, the stories followed, instead of the other way around, and that the supply of a syndrome or disorder can create its own demand.

And yes, his later scientific recording was subpar. And although that is striking on the one hand, because his dissertation was generally lauded for its scientific nature in the 1950s, it's also not surprising at all on the other hand, because his notes were investigated with the view of the democratised and scientific rightly stricter standards of the 1980s, looking back at scientific treatment notes from the 1960s and 1970s. Those reports were written – or better: often not written – by a man in full command of his department, who was trained in psychoanalysis in the 1940s, that then held N=1 to be sacred. For him and for many other physicians, psychiatrists in particular, conclusive evidence for the effectiveness of a method was when it was observed that the individual patient benefited from it, certainly when confirmation by the patient followed. Due to the emergence of evidence-based medicine and the associated randomised trials this completely changed in the 1970s.[20]

Nevertheless, the report raises the question whether constantly treating patients hadn't been at the expense of science, and that raises the second question whether Bastiaans, despite his love for teaching and educating, wasn't more a doctor than a professor, not more a man with a heart for his patients than a man with a heart for the university. That, at his own request, the research was conducted by Van der Ploeg can only mean that he himself was confident in the outcome. This indicates that the change in scientific standards from the time he wrote his dissertation had passed him by.

Bastiaans, and other psychiatrists in his wake, can certainly be blamed of emphasising the unproved inevitability of trauma after shocking events. He has also irresponsibly stretched the numerical limits of the number of traumatised people. It's all true. But what is also true is that, even more than camp survivors such as Cohen, Tas, Kaas or De Wind, it was Bastiaans who made the Dutch population aware that traumatic events (can) leave scars and that these scars can lead to psychological disturbances, even years after the fact. He has played a leading, stimulating, and – indeed, at times a somewhat too – directive role in the necessary debate, both nationally and internationally, about the psychological consequences of the use of violence in general and in war in particular, for three decades. Without him and his zeal for the victims of the horrors of war, of whom a large number in any case *felt* liberated by him eventually, the acceptance of this might not have come at all and would surely have been a lot more problematic. Without him the contemporary medical and social debate about psychological trauma, about making a return pilgrimage to the places of horror, and about possibly starting to use psychedelics in the treatment of trauma once again, would have been completely different, or even practically non-existent, certainly in the Netherlands. This may be seen as his perpetual legacy and great merit, as was noted in the *NTvG* after his death as well.

WORDS OF GRATITUDE

I want to thank all those that contributed to this book on the KZ syndrome and psychiatrist Jan Bastiaans. First of all, Renee Schoffelen and Herman Simissen who were kind enough to have a peak at my English. Secondly, Covid-19, because without the continuous lockdowns this would have been a different book entirely. And thirdly, Eric Vermetten, asking me to write 'something' about his predecessor as a professor in psycho-trauma, and paying for it on top. And last but not last, I want to thank Irma for every once in a while, bringing me a cup of tea and some biscuits during all those hours spent before the computer screen.

Leo van Bergen

Literature

'...in een doolhof', *Leeuwarder Courant*, 22-11-1973

A

'Aanblijven professor Bastiaans bepleit', *Algemeen Dagblad*, 27-2-1985

'Aanbod Endegeest voor opvang patiënten Bastiaans', *NRC Handelsblad*, 11-5-1985

'Aandacht voor vergeten veteranen', *Algemeen Dagblad*, 15-5-1985

'Aanslagen tegen "Holocaust" op Duitse tv', *De Volkskrant*, 20-1-1979

'Aantjes werd voor de wolven gegooid', *Het Vrije Volk*, 9-11-1978

'Aanvallen op onderzoek-Aantjes', *De Waarheid*, 10-11-1978

'Aanvragers oorlogsuitkering vrezen verzwaring bewijslast', *NRC Handelsblad*, 23-3-1987

Aarts, Petra, 'De geschiedenis van het trauma', in: P.G.H. Aarts, R.P.W. Visser, *Trauma: Diagnostiek en behandeling* (Amsterdam: Bohn Stafleu van Loghum, 2007)

'Abba Eban: geen gratie voor "drie"', *Nederlands Dagblad*, 1-3-1972

Abrahams, Frits, 'Discussie ook hier noodzakelijk. Holocaust nuttig ondanks kitsch', *De Volkskrant*, 18-4-1979

'Achteraf bekeken', *Tubantia*, 23-2-1972 / 28-2-1972 / 23-11-1973 / 21-12-1973

Acton, Carol, Jane Potter, *Working in a World of Hurt. Trauma and resilience in the narratives of medical personnel in warzones* (Manchester: Manchester UP, 2015)

'"Afdoen schade duurt te lang"', *Het Parool*, 24-10-1981

'Afgrijselijke jeugdervaring bracht geobsedeerde vrouw tot kindermoord', *Het Vrije Volk*, 12-9-1962

'Afwijzende reacties op pleidooi om Drie van Breda weg te zenden', *Trouw*, 17-3-1976

Aker, H., 'Prof. Bastiaans', *De Telegraaf*, 28-1-1986

Alink, Lize, 'Recht & slecht. Schreeuw om hulp', *Het Vrije Volk*, 21-7-1979

- 'Gevolgen van de oorlog zijn nog lang niet opgevangen', *Het Vrije Volk*, 10-5-1980

Alons, W., 'Prof. Bastiaans', *De Telegraaf*, 13-3-1985

'"Als Bastiaans gelijk heeft stopt de LSP"', *Het Vrije Volk*, 27-3-1981

'Alsnog gedenkteken voor slachtoffers Englandspiel', *Leeuwarder Courant*, 15-5-1979

Amesz, Hans, 'Er staan nu bloemen voor de ramen van de commandant…', *Het Nieuws van het Noorden,* 26-6-1980

Amsterdam, Herman van, 'LSD: onberekenbaar medicijn', *Algemeen Dagblad*, 8-2-1986

'Amsterdamse actie na "Wijster" gepland', *Trouw*, 22-12-1975

Andere Tijden, 'Bastiaans en de LSD therapie. Controverse rond een psychiatrisch experiment in Nederland', Anderetijden.nl/aflevering/657/Bastiaans (seen: 8-5-2021)

'Artsen beticht van ingreep in hersenen', *De Volkskrant*, 7-9-1979

'Artsen roepen op tot aanpassing abortuswet', *De Volkskrant*, 5-6-1976

'"Artsenij" ontrafelt het "rampensyndroom"', *Het Nieuws van het Noorden,* 10-4-1980

'Auschwitz Comité niet gekend in voorlichting over Holocaust', *NIW*, 16-2-1979

'Auschwitz Comité vindt Holocaust goede film', *Leeuwarder Courant*, 8-2-1979

B

Baan, P.A.H., 'J. Bastiaans, Psychosomatische gevolgen van onderdrukking en verzet', *NTvG*, 28-3-1959, 676

Baarda, Frits, 'Vrede met Vietnam', *Het Vrije Volk*, 28-3-1987

'Baarnse activist de Booy voor bedreiging in kort geding', *Het Parool*, 18-12-1975

Babington, Antony, *Shell-Shock. A history of the changing attitudes towards war-neurosis* (London: Leo Cooper, 1997)

Bagijn, Karel, 'Gijzelaars hebben nog lang angst', *Algemeen Dagblad*, 29-9-1981

Bank, Jan, 'KZ-slachtoffers "herontdekt" op televisie', *De Volkskrant*, 26-2-1972

Bastiaans, J., *Psychosomatische Gevolgen van Onderdrukking en Verzet* (Amsterdam: Noord-Hollandsche Uitgevers Maatschappij, 1957)

- 'Begrijpt u nu waarom ik huil', *NTvG*, 21-1-1970, 302-303
- 'Vom Menschen im KZ und vom KZ im Menschen. Ein Beitrag zur Behandlung des KZ-syndroms und dessen Spätfolgen', in: B.A. Sijes, S. Wiesenthal (red.), *Essays über Naziverbrechen. Simon Wiesenthal gewidmet* (Amsterdam: Wiesenthal Fonds, 1973) 177-202
- 'Het KZ-syndroom en de menselijke vrijheid', *NTvG*, 11-3-1974, 1173-1178

- ‘De behandeling van oorlogsslachtoffers’, *Arts & Wereld*, 17, 1 (januari 1984) 8-18
- ‘Hollands dagboek’, *NRC Handelsblad*, 6-4-1985
- *Isolement en Bevrijding* (Amsterdam: Balans, 1986)
- ‘Executie van een onverwerkt verleden’. Lezing Stichting Herdenk 15 augustus, archief KITLV Leiden, collectie Frits Jan Suyderhoud, nr. 23

Bastiaans, J., et al., *Leven na een Oorlog* (Amsterdam: Nationaal Centrum Geestelijke Volksgezondheid, 1972)

Bastiaans, J., S. Mulder, W.K. van Dijk, H.M. van der Ploeg, *Mensen bij Gijzelingen* (Alphen aan de Rijn: A.W. Sijthoff, 1981)

‘Bastiaans (bijna 70) werkt drie opvolgers in’, *Trouw*, 21-8-1987

‘Bastiaans bij afscheid: onzekerheid leidt tot isolement’, *Algemeen Dagblad*, 29-6-1985

‘Bastiaans blijft bij Jelgersmakliniek’, *De Waarheid*, 8-2-1983

‘Bastiaans kan oorlogsslachtoffers blijven behandelen’, *Het Nieuws van het Noorden*, 9-5-1985

‘Bastiaans komt tegemoet aan eisen inspecteur’, *De Volkskrant*, 24-1-1986

‘Bastiaans krijgt half jaar voor regelen opvolger’, *De Volkskrant*, 18-6-1987

‘Bastiaans laat een onzekere toekomst achter’, *Trouw*, 3-12-1987

‘Bastiaans mag LSD blijven toepassen’, *De Volkskrant*, 6-2-1986

‘Bastiaans mag LSD gebruiken’, *NRC Handelsblad*, 6-2-1986

‘Bastiaans mag LSD methode blijven toepassen’, *Algemeen Dagblad*, 6-2-1986

‘Bastiaans mag met LSD blijven werken’, *Het Vrije Volk*, 6-2-1986

‘Bastiaans mag slachtoffers oorlog blijven behandelen’, *Trouw*, 27-2-1985

‘Bastiaans mag tot in 1985 behandelen’, *Trouw*, 5-2-1983

‘Bastiaans neemt afscheid van universiteit’, *De Waarheid*, 29-6-1985

‘Bastiaans opgevolgd door drie man bij Centrum 45’, *De Volkskrant*, 21-11-1987

‘Bastiaans tegen Stuyt over filmvertoning’, *NRC Handelsblad*, 19-4-1972

‘Bastiaans wil niet verhuizen’, *Het Vrije Volk*, 21-9-1982

‘Bastiaans wint kort geding tegen De Booy’, *NRC Handelsblad*, 27-12-1975

‘Bastiaans zoekt tijdelijk onderdak’, *De Waarheid*, 14-4-1987

‘Bastiaans: bestraffen oorlogsmisdadiger “dwaas”’, *Het Parool*, 16-11-1987

‘Bastiaans’, *De Volkskrant*, 29-10-1982

‘Bastiaans’, *De Waarheid*, 23-5-1985

‘Bastiaans’, *De Waarheid*, 16-4-1987

‘Bastiaans’, *De Waarheid*, 18-6-1987

‘Beeldspraak’, *De Waarheid*, 8-6-1977

Benders, H., ‘Een gijzeling en de nazorg’, *Het Nieuws van het Noorden,* 7-2-1981
‘Begrijpt u nu waarom ik huil’, *Trouw*, 16-5-1969
‘“Begrijpt u nu waarom ik huil…”’, *Tubantia*, 14-5-1969
‘“Begrijpt u nu waarom ik huil?” op VARA-tv’, *Leeuwarder Courant*, 25-2-1972
‘“Begrijpt u nu waarom ik huil?” vandaag voor tv’, *Trouw*, 26-2-1972
‘“Behandeling nieuwe patiënten met LSD voorlopig verbieden”’, *Nederlands Dagblad*, 5-2-1986
‘Behandeling patiënten met oorlogstrauma in gevaar. Opvolging Bastiaans nog niet geregeld’, *Algemeen Dagblad*, 28-2-1987
‘Behandelploeg Bastiaans rond’, *Het Nieuws van het Noorden,* 23-1-1986
Bekkering, P.G., M. Bekkering-Mertens, ‘De Japanse kampen; nog geen verleden tijd’, *NTvG*, 28-1-1980, 467-473
‘Beoordeling van daders “neutraal”’, *Het Nieuws van het Noorden,* 22-6-1979
Berg, Harm van den, ‘Slachtoffers van oorlog bepleiten bij Kamer voortzetting therapie-Bastiaans’, *Het Parool*, 27-2-1985
- ‘Prof. Bastiaans moet nu echt stoppen’, *Het Parool*, 31-10-1987
- ‘Bastiaans tuimelt van voetstuk’, *Het Parool*, 14-11-1987
‘Behandelaar van oorlogstrauma’s Bastiaans overleden’, *De Volkskrant*, 1-11-1997
Berg, Harm van den, Wera de Lange, ‘De zaak-Rost past in beeld van affaire “Drie van Breda”’, *Het Parool*, 24-11-1986
Bergen, Leo van, *De Zwaargewonden Eerst? Het Nederlandsche Roode Kruis en het vraagstuk van oorlog en vrede* (Rotterdam: Erasmus, 1994)
- *Van Genezen in Geloof tot Geloof in Genezen. De medische faculteit van de Vrije Universiteit 1880-2000* (Amsterdam: Veen, 2005)
- *Zacht en Eervol. Lijden en sterven in de Grote Oorlog* (Antwerpen: Manteau, 2014)
- *Pro Patria et Patienti. De Nederlandse militaire geneeskunde 1795-1950* (Nijmegen: Van Tilt/NIMH, 2019)
‘Beroep op begrip’, *Leeuwarder Courant*, 28-2-1972
‘Beroering bij universiteiten over bouwstop. Leidse hoogleraren dringen aan op protest’, *De Waarheid*, 6-1-1965
Bertina, B.J., ‘Van Gasteren maakte geen objectief drama’, *De Volkskrant*, 16-5-1969
- ‘Begrijpt u nu waarom ik huil’, *De Volkskrant*, 30-5-1969
‘Beslissing’, *NRC Handelsblad*, 6-2-1979

'Bewindsman bemoeit zich niet met opvolging dr. J. Bastiaans', *Nederlands Dagblad*, 13-2-1986

'Bewindsman beziet of opvolger Bastiaans met LSD mag werken', *De Volkskrant*, 12-9-1984

'Bewindsman steunt Bastiaans in voortzetten hulp oorlogsvervolgden', *De Volkskrant*, 28-3-1985

'Bewindsman streeft ernaar werk Bastiaans te redden. Mogelijk in een aparte stichting', *De Volkskrant*, 28-2-1985

'Bewindsman wil Bastiaans behouden, dat wel', *De Waarheid*, 1-3-1985

'Bij bijna alle slachtoffers van gijzelingen nadelige gevolgen', *Leeuwarder Courant*, 22-6-1979

'Bij het slaan van een eerste paal. Autoriteiten ontdekken een nieuw syndroom', *De Waarheid*, 22-4-1972

'Bij Kamerleden meer twijfels over de "Drie"', *Het Parool*, 24-2-1972

'Bij nazorg gijzelaars huisarts betrekken', *Algemeen Dagblad*, 20-12-1975

'Binnenland', *NRC Handelsblad*, 17-5-1973

Binneveld, Hans, *Om de Geest van Jan Soldaat. Beknopte geschiedenis van de militaire psychiatrie* (Rotterdam: Erasmus Publishing, 1995)

Blijham, H., 'Het dilemma van het existentieel getraumatiseerd zijn', Psychotraumanet.org/nl/het-dilemma-van-het-existentieel-getraumatiseerd-zijn (seen: 16-3-2021)

Bloch, M.B., 'Het post-concentratiekampsyndroom', *Nederlands Militair Geneeskundig Tijdschrift*, 1971, 165-166

'Bloemen voor de ramen van de kommandatur', *Leeuwarder Courant*, 28-6-1980

Blok, Gemma, *Baas in eigen Brein. 'Antipsychiatrie' in Nederland, 1965-1985* (Amsterdam: Uitgeverij Nieuwezijds, 2004)

Blokker, Jan, 'Loch Ness', *De Volkskrant*, 26-3-1983

Boas, Henriette, 'Een afwijkende mening over de "Drie van Breda"', *Het Parool*, 24-2-1972

- 'Drie van Breda (4)', *Trouw*, 4-2-1976

Bodewes, Johan, 'Emoties uit het verleden', *Het Nieuws van het Noorden,* 9-3-1972

'Boek over de gevolgen van gijzelingen', *NRC Handelsblad*, 29-9-1981

'Boek over kampsyndroom in voorbereiding', *Het Parool*, 17-3-1972

'Boek over KZ-syndroom', *Het Vrije Volk*, 20-3-1972

'Boek over leed NSB-kinderen', *Het Nieuws van het Noorden,* 13-1-1981

Boer, E.J., 'Centrum '45: liever controverses begraven', *NRC Handelsblad*, 18-5-1973

- 'De echte kater komt nog', *NRC Handelsblad*, 18-6-1977

- 'Stress. Risicofactor achter de schermen', *NRC Handelsblad*, 17-3-1983
- 'Bestaat er een bepaalde kankerpersoonlijkheid?', *NRC Handelsblad*, 2-2-1984
- 'Slechts weinig onderzoek gedaan', *NRC Handelsblad*, 7-2-1986
- 'Oorlogsslachtoffers en literatuuronderzoek', *NRC Handelsblad*, 9-4-1987

'Boete als dr. Tom de Booy dr. Bastiaans zal beledigen', *Het Nieuws van het Noorden,* 24-12-1975

Bogers, Hans, Stephen Snelders, Hans Plomp, *De Psychedelische (R)evolutie. Geschiedenis en recente ontwikkelingen in het onderzoek naar veranderde bewustzijnsstaten* (Amsterdam: Bres, z.j. [1994])

Bolle, Lex, 'Bastiaans', *Het Parool*, 3-12-1987

Boltendal, Rudi, 'Keilsons proefschrift tevens kroniek van menselijk leven en lijden', *Leeuwarder Courant*, 20-7-1979
- 'Mensen bij Gijzelingen', *Leeuwarder Courant*, 21-8-1982

Bolwijn, Lennart, 'Reemst, Theo van' (Spanjestrijders.nl/bio/reemst-theo-van (seen: 16-3-2021))

'Bomalarm in VARA-studio', *Het Vrije Volk*, 28-2-1972

'Bommeldingen na eerste uitzending Holocaust', *Het Nieuws van het Noorden,* 24-4-1979

Booij, J., 'Farmacotherapie en psychotherapie. LSD als adjuvans bij de psychotherapie', *NTvG*, 6-1-1968, 2-7
- 'Vraagstukken rondom de psychotherapie', *NTvG*, 14-9-1968, 1621-1624

Bossenbroek, Martin, *De Meelstreep. Terugkeer en opvang na de Tweede Wereldoorlog* (Amsterdam: Bert Bakker, 2001)

Bossum, Bernard van, 'Ons recht, de slachtoffers en de drie', *De Tijd*, 28-2-1972

Braber, Ben, 'Ontsnapt aan deportatie. Verzet van Joden in Westerbork', *De Waarheid*, 26-4-1983

Brabers, Jan, *Hippocrates op Heyendaal. Ontstaan en ontplooiing van de faculteit der Medische Wetenschappen van de Radboud Universiteit Nijmegen 1951-2001* (Nijmegen: Valkhof Pers, 2009)

Bramsen, I., J.E. Dirkzwager, H.M. van der Ploeg, *Deelname aan Vredesmissies: gevolgen, opvang en nazorg* (Amsterdam: Vrije Universiteit, 1997)

'Brieven', *NRC Handelsblad*, 14-2-1983 / 16-4-1987

'Brits leger tussen twee vuren', *Het Parool*, 18-5-1974

'Brochure over KZ-syndroom. Vriend kan ook helpen bij naweeën van oorlog', *De Volkskrant*, 4-3-1972

Bröcker, F.J., 'De LSD controverse', *NTvG*, 28-5-1966, 999-1004
- 'Farmacotherapie en psychotherapie', *NTvG*, 2-3-1968, 420-421 (incl. reactie. Joh. Booij)

Brugmans, I.J., *Nederlands-Indië onder Japanse bezetting* (Franeker: Wever, 1960)

Bruinsma, Jet, '"Buitenwereld maakt van Bastiaans soort goeroe"', *De Volkskrant*, 12-12-1987
- '"Sluiten wetten slachtoffers oorlog aantasting ereschuld"', *De Volkskrant*, 3-9-1985
- 'Inspectie kritiseert therapie Bastiaans', *De Volkskrant*, 23-1-1986
- 'Pionierswerk Centrum '40-'45 zeker zinvol', *De Volkskrant*, 24-1-1984

'Bundel opstellen van Milikowski', *De Volkskrant*, 1-12-1973

Bueren, Peter van, 'Begrijpt u nu waarom ik huil… Slachtoffers van de Tweede Wereldoorlog leven nog', *De Tijd*, 16-5-1969

Buijze, Roy, 'Vergeten kampslachtoffers', *Het Parool*, 9-8-1980
- 'De patiënt is altijd gestoord', *Het Parool*, 31-10-1981
- 'Niet alleen verzet Meertens roept vragen op', *Het Parool*, 23-2-1984
- '"Je moet opnieuw door de hel, maar ik wil het nu afmaken"', *Het Parool*, 17-3-1984
- 'Bastiaans verliest', *Het Parool*, 28-2-1985

'Bundel informatie over oorlogsleed', *Algemeen Dagblad*, 8-3-1972

'Bundel informatie over oorlogsleed', *Limburgsch Dagblad*, 8-3-1972

Busby, Mattha, 'Will the magic of psychedelics transform psychiatry?', *The Observer*, 7-11-2021

C

'Centrum '45 accepteert de methode-Bastiaans', *Trouw*, 18-6-1987

'Centrum '45 door koningin geopend', *Nederlands Dagblad*, 17-5-1973

'Centrum '45 geopend door Koningin', *Het Parool*, 16-5-1973

'Centrum '45 geopend', *De Waarheid*, 16-5-1973

'Centrum '45 is geopend', *Algemeen Dagblad*, 17-5-1973

'Centrum '45 neemt hulp oorlogsslachtoffers van prof. Bastiaans over', *NRC Handelsblad*, 20-6-1985

'Centrum '45 start zonder staf', *NRC Handelsblad*, 2-3-1973

'Centrum '45 voor verzetsslachtoffers nu gereed', *De Waarheid*, 2-3-1973

'Centrum '45 zet werk van prof. J. Bastiaans voort', *De Volkskrant*, 20-6-1985

'Centrum '45: "TROS moet Holocaust uitstellen"', *Trouw*, 7-2-1979

'Centrum '45 over samenwerking met prof. Bastiaans', *NRC Handelsblad*, 6-6-1973

'Centrum voor behandeling KZ-syndroom officieel geopend', *Tubantia*, 16-5-1973
'Centrum voor behandeling van KZ-syndroom officieel geopend', *Tubantia*, 16-5-1973
'Centrum', *NIW*, 1-6-1973
Chatenier, Hilde Maria du, 'Leemte', *Algemeen Dagblad*, 9-3-1985
Citroen, Michal, *U wordt door Niemand Verwacht. Nederlandse joden na kampen en onderduik* (Utrecht: Het Spectrum, 1999)
Cohen, E.A., *Het Duitse Concentratiekamp. Een medische en psychologische studie* (Amsterdam: H.J. Paris, 1952)
- 'Kampgevolgen', *NIW*, 29-1-1965
- 'Het post-concentratiekampsyndroom', *NTvG*, 15-11-1969, 2049-2054
- 'Vechten om ziek te mogen zijn', *NRC Handelsblad*, 13-3-1971
- 'Het post-concentratiekampsyndroom: een "disaster"-syndroom', *NTvG*, 7-4-1972, 1680-1685
'Commissie schadevergoeding Nazi-slachtoffers', *NIW*, 6-11-1959
'Commissie ziet kansen voor continueren werk Bastiaans', *De Volkskrant*, 22-5-1985
'Concentratiekamp II', *De Volkskrant*, 20-5-1969
'Concentratiekampen eisen nog steeds slachtoffers', *De Tijd*, 2-3-1967
'Concentratiekampziekte tast de hersenen aan', *Algemeen Dagblad*, 30-10-1954
'Conclusie informatiebundel: over oorlogservaringen kan worden gepraat', *Leeuwarder Courant*, 4-3-1972
'Conclusies psychiaters zouden kabinet goed uitkomen. Afbraak zorg oorlogsgetroffenen dreigt', *De Volkskrant*, 7-4-1987
'Conflict ontsiert opening "Centrum '45"', *De Telegraaf*, 16-5-1973
'Conflict opgelost: Bastiaans kan nog oorlogsslachtoffers behandelen', *Algemeen Dagblad*, 7-2-1983
'Conflict rondom prof. Bastiaans. Minister Vorrink passeert prof. Baan', *Het Nieuws van het Noorden,* 26-5-1973
'Controverse nasleep affaire-Dennendal. Prof. Speijer vervroegd met pensioen', *Het Parool*, 1-6-1972
Croes-de Groot, A.H., 'Prof. Bastiaans', *De Telegraaf*, 22-8-1987

D

Dam, G.G. van, 'Zelf doen', *Het Vrije Volk*, 27-12-1975
Damme, Leon van, 'Veertig jaar geleden: de Drie van Breda' (montesquieu-instituut.nl) (seen: 10-12-2020))
'De "Drie" stuk voor stuk vrij', *De Telegraaf*, 28-2-1972
'De aangrijpende LSD film van prof. Bastiaans', *Het Vrije Volk*, 8-11-1966

'De Booy moet zich matigen tegenover prof. Bastiaans', *Het Parool*, 27-12-1975

'De drie voelen zich veilig in Breda. Toenemend aantal protesten tegen vrijlating', *Algemeen Dagblad*, 24-2-1972

'De echo van dertien bange en barre dagen', *Het Nieuws van het Noorden*, 30-11-1985

'De mens van nu wordt steeds egocentrischer', *De Telegraaf*, 9-12-1969

'De methode-Bastiaans', *Trouw*, 8-2-1986

'De prijs van overleven', *Trouw*, 2-5-2005

'De strijd, die niet ophield. Dr. H. Milikowski over het omgekeerde KZ-syndroom', *De Waarheid*, 9-2-1974

'De verstokte', *Leeuwarder Courant*, 16-2-1981

Dean jr., Eric T., *Shook over Hell. Post-Traumatic Stress, Vietnam, and the Civil War* (Cambridge, Mass./London: Harvard UP, 1997)

'Debat over Bredase "3" direct op televisie', *Limburgsch Dagblad*, 26-2-1972

Dehue, Trudy, *De Depressie-epIbidemie. Over de plicht het lot in eigen hand te nemen* (Amsterdam/Antwerpen: Augustus, 2008)

'Den Uyl onder de indruk van woorden van prof. Bastiaans. "Nazorg voor vrijgelatenen organiseren"', *Trouw*, 15-12-1975

'Den Uyl over gesprek met Zuidmolukkers: Proberen herhalingen kapingen en gijzelingen te voorkomen', *Leeuwarder Courant*, 20-12-1975

Derksen, Leo, 'Zes miljoen doden op de toonbank', *De Telegraaf*, 31-3-1979

- 'Op zicht. Het grote zwijgen (1)', *De Telegraaf*, 1-12-1982

'Deze maand begint bouw KZ-paviljoen', *De Volkskrant*, 1-4-1972

Diepstraten, Johan, 'Nuttige discussie over oorlogsjaren', *De Volkskrant*, 9-4-1980

Dijk, A.J. van, 'Signalement van een onmogelijkheid', *NRC Handelsblad*, 14-12-1978

Dijk, Ale van, 'Aart C. Gisolf en 't "rampen-syndroom". "Telefoonnummers lossen niets op"', *Het Vrije Volk*, 9-4-1980

Dijk, Rob van, 'LSD: Van alles gaan de helften uiteen', *Het Parool*, 8-2-1986

Dikkers, Irene, 'Echte dromen van Annemie McGillary', *De Telegraaf*, 23-5-1980

- 'Uitkering aan Indische ex-kampmensen een afvalrace', *De Telegraaf*, 15-8-1981

'Directeur kliniek aangeklaagd voor LSD behandeling', *Algemeen Dagblad*, 7-9-1979

'Dossier-Wijster is nog niet afgesloten', *Algemeen Dagblad*, 16-12-1978

'Dr. A. Sunier, Joodse Geestelijke Gezondheidszorg: Hulpverlening kan leren van onze kennis', *NIW*, 6-4-1979
'Dr. Bastiaans hoogleraar psychiatrie', *Het Parool*, 11-11-1963
'Dr. Bastiaans hoogleraar te Leiden', *Algemeen Handelsblad*, 12 -11-1963
'Dr. Tom de Booy verliest kort geding', *Leeuwarder Courant*, 24-12-1975
Drayer, Elma, 'Hoe het kamp het bestaan vergiftigde', *Trouw*, 3-4-2010
'"Drie" niet vrij bij verzet Kamer', *NRC Handelsblad*, 24-2-1972
'Drie artsen "leren" methode Bastiaans', *Nederlands Dagblad*, 22-8-1987
'Drie artsen opvolgers van psychiater Bastiaans', *NRC Handelsblad*, 20-11-1987
'Drie niet gelijktijdig vrij', *Algemeen Dagblad*, 17-3-1972
Driever, Jan, *De Onderlinge Belofte. Zeventig jaar Stichting 1940-1945* (Amsterdam: Boom, 2015)
Duijn, Roel van, 'Moffenhoer? Nee, een verzetsheldin!', *Trouw*, 16-4-2016
Dunning, A.J., 'Altijd wat', *NRC Handelsblad*, 21-4-1983
Duynstee, F., 'Tweede Kamer heeft ernstig gefaald…', *De Telegraaf*, 29-2-1972

E

'Een medisch document van de eerste orde', *Tubantia*, 14-5-1969
Eeraerts, Mark, 'LSD', *Trouw*, 30-5-1985
'Eerste paal van centrum lijders aan KZ-syndroom', *Limburgsch Dagblad*, 18-4-1972
'Eerste paal voor KZ-syndroomkliniek', *NRC Handelsblad*, 18-4-1972
'Eibert Meester om gezondheidsredenen uit Eerste Kamer', *NRC Handelsblad*, 2-8-1976
'Eibert Meester treedt terug', *Het Vrije Volk*, 2-8-1976
'Eibert Meester uit Eerste Kamer', *Leeuwarder Courant*, 2-8-1976
'Eibert Meester uit Senaat', *Het Parool*, 2-8-1976
'Eibert Meester vraagt minister over beleid rond Centrum '45', *Het Vrije Volk*, 18-5-1973
'Eibert Meester', *De Volkskrant*, 2-8-1976
'Einde van oorlog herdacht. Geïsoleerde positie Indische Nederlanders centraal', *Trouw*, 16-8-1980
Eiselin, Ferry, 'Levenslang is discriminatie', *Het Parool*, 24-2-1972
- 'Centrum '45 start met conflict', *Het Parool*, 17-5-1973
Eiselin-Hoon, F., 'Kliniek', *Trouw*, 3-3-1972
Emde Boas, C. van, 'Van Gasteren filmt het KZ-syndroom en velen moeten het zien', *Algemeen Handelsblad*, 17-5-1969
'Emoties maken veel indruk op Van Agt', *De Volkskrant*, 24-2-1972
'Emoties op de hoorzitting niet in bedwang te houden', *Tubantia*, 25-2-1972

Ende, Hannah van den, '*Vergeet niet dat je arts bent'. Joodse artsen in Nederland 1940-1945* (Amsterdam: Boom, 2015)

Engelbrecht, Corina, 'Het Indische kampsyndroom', *NRC Handelsblad*, 30-5-1980 (naschrift: Rudy Kousbroek)

- 'Gevangenen van de vrede', *NRC Handelsblad*, 23-7-1980

Engelsman, A. (red.), *Oorlogstrauma's na 45 jaar? Politiek en psychiatrisch ongeduld* (Amsterdam: Van Gennep, 1989)

Enning, Bram, *De Oorlog van Bastiaans* (Amsterdam: Augustus, 2009)

'Er komt geen anti-terreurgroep onder ministerie van defensie', *Nederlands Dagblad*, 21-10-1977

'Ernstige kritiek van ex-gijzelaars op nazorg', *Nederlands Dagblad*, 13-2-1976

'Ernstige moeilijkheden rond nieuwe kliniek van prof. Bastiaans. Prins steunt compromispoging', *Het Parool*, 19-5-1973

'Ernstige moeilijkheden rond nieuwe kliniek van prof. Bastiaans', *Het Parool*, 19-5-1973

'Ervaringen geleerden in boek gepubliceerd', *De Waarheid*, 30-9-1981

'Examens', *De Tijd*, 2-2-1957

'"Executie van een onverwerkt verleden". Indrukwekkende rede prof. J. Bastiaans tijdens 15 augustus-herdenking' (bron onbekend. Kopie in bezit auteur)

'"Experts twijfelen aan methode Bastiaans"', *Het Parool*, 19-5-1973

'Ex-gegijzelden hebben kritiek op autoriteiten', *Het Nieuws van het Noorden,* 22-6-1979

'Ex-gevangenen verzetten zich tegen vrijlating Drie van Breda', *NRC Handelsblad*, 17-3-1976

'Ex-gijzelaar vindt begeleiding "te ambtelijk"', *NRC Handelsblad*, 12-2-1976

'Expogé biedt Tros hulp bij nazorg', *NIW*, 16-2-1979

'Expogé-voorzitter C. (sic) Aalders overleden', *Het Vrije Volk*, 28-2-1972

F

Fahrenfort, Jacques, 'Van Agt's aftreden ondanks geestelijke terreur nog net voorkomen', *De Telegraaf*, 4-3-1972

'Film KZ-syndroom roept veel positieve reacties op', *Tubantia*, 28-2-1972

'Film KZ-syndroom: veel reacties', *De Volkskrant*, 28-2-1972

'Film over behandeling kamp-syndroom vanavond uitgezonden', *De Volkskrant*, 26-2-1972

'Film over KZ-syndroom vanavond op tv', *Tubantia*, 26-2-1972

'Film', *Trouw*, 28-2-1972

'Foresterprijs uitgereikt aan prof. Bastiaans', *NRC Handelsblad*, 27-2-1973

Fortuin, Johanna, '"Wat worden wij daar nou wijzer van, papa Bas?"', *Het Parool*, 31-10-1987
- 'De deskundigheid van prof. J. Bastiaans lijkt grenzeloos', *Het Parool*, 26-11-1987

Frequin, Louis, *Ga Maar Rustig Slapen* (Maasbree: Corrie Zeelen, 1980)

G

'Gardeniers is voor monument in Westerbork', *Het Parool*, 29-1-1981

Garschagen, Agaath, 'Therapeut: Bastiaans is nooit helemaal te vervangen', *NRC Handelsblad*, 31-12-1987

Gasteren, Louis van, 'Begrijpt U?...', *De Telegraaf*, 16-5-1984

'Gebruik van LSD in psychiatrie blijft uiterst discutabel', *De Waarheid*, 15-11-1975

'Gedenkteken slachtoffers Englandspiel', *Het Vrije Volk*, 12-5-1979

'"Geen korting geld oorlogsslachtoffers"', *Het Parool*, 28-3-1985

'Geen nieuwe patiënten voor artsen met opiumverlof', *Algemeen Dagblad*, 4-2-1986

'Geen vervolging van vrouw die kinderen doodde', *Het Parool*, 25-9-1962

'Geen voortzetting van LSD therapie', *Het Parool*, 21-12-1987

'Geestelijk gestoorde PTT-beambte verduisterde twintig mille', *De Maasbode*, 17-2-1954

'Geestelijke stoornissen bij ex-concentratiekampgevangenen', *De Waarheid*, 16-12-1961

'Gegevens ontbreken voor onderzoek Bastiaans', *Het Parool*, 6-11-1987

'Gegijzelden houden nog lang klachten', *Het Vrije Volk*, 22-6-1979

'Gegijzelden zijn soms te diep in de put gedrukt', *Het Nieuws van het Noorden*, 31-7-1979

Gersons, Berthold, 'Traumaspectrumstoornissen: van enkelvoudig trauma tot complexe PTSS', in: Eric Vermetten, Rolf Kleber, Onno van der Hart (red.), *Handboek Posttraumatische Stressstoornis* (Amsterdam: Boom, 2012) 65-81

'Gesprekken Hendriks-Bastiaans', *De Waarheid*, 20-12-1975

'Gestoord gevoelsleven ook zaak voor de huisarts. Te veel beheersing door opvoeding oudere generatie', *De Volkskrant*, 9-10-1965

Geurtsen, A., 'Waarom ik "om" ging', *Het Nieuws van het Noorden,* 29-2-1972
- 'Waarom ik "om" ging', *Limburgsch Dagblad*, 29-2-1972

'Gevoelens. NIW Commentaar', *NIW*, 9-2-1979

'Gevolgen van de hongerwinter en de kampen', *Het Vrije Volk*, 4-3-1955

'Gijzelaars kregen hersenspoeling', *Het Vrije Volk*, 20-12-1975

'Gijzelaars krijgen ook op lange termijn begeleiding', *NRC Handelsblad*, 15-12-1975
'Gijzelaars willen spontane hulp', *De Volkskrant*, 22-6-1979
'Gijzeling heeft soms ook positief gevolg', *NRC Handelsblad*, 22-6-1979
'Gijzeling laat doorgaans lange tijd sporen na', *Trouw*, 22-6-1979
'Gijzelingen werkten positief uit op slachtoffers', *Het Parool*, 22-6-1979
Gisolf, Aart, 'Na de oorlog geboren, soms toch "oorlogservaring"', *Algemeen Dagblad*, 4-5-1976
- 'Er gebeurde iets vreemds met de ex-mariniers', *Algemeen Dagblad*, 4-5-1977
- 'Het kampsyndroom: Vergeten kan niet maar praten is goed', *Algemeen Dagblad*, 4-5-1977
- 'Kind uit het verzet', *Algemeen Dagblad*, 4-5-1977
- 'Oorlog is weer actueel', *Algemeen Dagblad*, 3-5-1978
- 'De behandeling', *Algemeen Dagblad*, 3-5-1978
- 'Twee levens', *Algemeen Dagblad*, 3-5-1978
- 'Bastiaans: bewonderd en gehaat', *Algemeen Dagblad*, 14-2-1983
Glimmerveen, Henk, 'Psychiatrie van de mollegang. Het Mulder-syndroom', *De Waarheid*, 6-10-1981
Gnirrep, Yvonne, 'Holocaust – de niet te bevatten werkelijkheid', *De Waarheid*, 5-5-1979
Godschalk, J.J., 'Het Blow-up effect van de televisie informatie', *NRC Handelsblad*, 11-3-1972
Gonggrijp, Frits, 'Prof. Speyer is uitgekeken op de universiteit', *De Telegraaf*, 9-6-1972
- 'Incident bij opening van "Centrum '45"', *De Telegraaf*, 17-5-1973
- 'Sciëntologen krijgen ongelijk van het Medisch Tuchtcollege', *De Telegraaf*, 8-10-1980
Goudriaan, Huib, 'Noodzaak van K.Z.-kliniek laat ingezien', *Trouw*, 22-4-1972
- 'Koningin opent kliniek voor oorlogsslachtoffers, *Trouw*, 5-5-1973
- 'Dertig jaar na "Korea". Het ergste komt later', *Trouw*, 8-10-1983
- 'Oud Indonesiëgangers: We willen steun en eerherstel', *Trouw*, 24-4-1985
Goulooze, Henk, 'Lijdensweg voor politieke gevangenen in Sowjet-Unie', *Algemeen Dagblad*, 18-11-1975
'Gratiebesluit staat vast. Steun kabinet voor Van Agt', *De Volkskrant*, 26-2-1972
'Gratiedebat onzeker', *De Telegraaf*, 25-2-1972
Grijpma, Paul, 'Na 35 jaar weerzien met Auschwitz', *Het Parool*, 25-6-1980

'Groeiende nood onder oorlogsslachtoffers', *Het Parool*, 29-1-1981
Groen-Prakken, J., 'Trauma en ontwikkelingsinterferentie: Een diagnostisch onderscheid bij de behandeling van getraumatiseerden en hun kinderen uit een psychoanalytisch referentiekader' (psychotraumanet.org/nl/trauma-en-ontwikkelingsinterferentie-een-diagnostisch-onderscheid-bij-de-behandeling-van)
Groenendijk, Bas, 'Vaak klap na voor verkeersslachtoffers. Interview met prof. J. Bastiaans', *Algemeen Dagblad*, 29-12-1983
Groot, Jan Hein de, 'Gijzelingenrapport: verplichte studie voor elke hulpverlener', *Het Vrije Volk*, 22-6-1979
- 'Bevrijding… spreekkamers zullen volstromen', *Het Vrije Volk*, 1-4-1985
- 'Patiënt van prof. Bastiaans: "Het hoofd van die dode man zit in m'n kop"', *Het Vrije Volk*, 2-4-1985
- 'De mensen voor wie de oorlog telkens weer begint', *Het Vrije Volk*, 4-4-1985
'Groot aantal meldingen voor hearing', *Het Parool*, 22-2-1972
Grüter, Regina, *Een Fantast schrijft Geschiedenis. De affaires rond Friedrich Weinreb* (Amsterdam: Balans, 1997)
- *Kwesties van Leven en Dood. Het Nederlandse Rode Kruis in de Tweede Wereldoorlog* (Amsterdam: Boom, 2017)

H
Hafkenscheid, Anton, 'Het (on)gewone in de diagnostiek en de behandeling van oorlogsslachtoffers', *Tijdschrift voor Psychotherapie*, 31 (3), (Juni 2005) 185-204
Hagers, Jos, 'Spanningen tussen medewerkers. Directeur Centrum '45 ontslagen', *De Telegraaf*, 31-7-1981
- 'Oorlogssyndroom neemt toe', *De Telegraaf*, 4-5-1984
- '"Joegoslavië roept oorlogsherinneringen op". Prof. dr. J. Bastiaans bij herdenking Japanse capitulatie', *De Telegraaf*, 15-8-1992
Haijtema, Arno 'Overlevingskunst', *De Volkskrant*, 9-4-2021
Hart, Maarten 't, 'De overijlde resignatie', *NRC Handelsblad*, 9-6-1983
Hart, Onno van der, Annemarie Broeze, 'Posttraumatische stress en de posttraumatische stressstoornis: een historisch overzicht', in: Vermetten, Kleber,Van der Hart, *Handboek Posttraumatische Stressstoornis*, 25-44
Hart, Onno van der, Frank Hermans, Rolf Kleber, Eric Vermetten, 'Psychotraumatologie in Nederland: historische ontwikkelingen', in: Vermetten, Kleber, Van der Hart, *Handboek Posttraumatische Stressstoornis*, 45-64

Hartmans, Rob, 'Schimmige herinneringen', *De Groene Amsterdammer*, 8-4-2009

Haveman, Ben, 'Ze kunnen De Waarheid nooit vertellen, nooit', *De Volkskrant*, 21-4-1979

- 'En dan ga je naar de beul', *De Volkskrant*, 16-3-1985
- 'De eeuw van het oorlogstrauma', *De Volkskrant*, 24-4-1999

Heerden, Jaap van, 'Het onduidelijke KZ-syndroom', *NRC Handelsblad*, 3-2-1983

Heertje, [Arnold], 'Een rapport dat maar geheim moet blijven', *Het Parool*, 21-3-1987

Heijermans, H.L., 'Lijvig verhaal over LSD', *Het Vrije Volk*, 28-2-1967

Heijmans, Jan, 'Dit was een Jappenkamp. Het gruwelijk verleden leeft nog steeds', *Algemeen Dagblad*, 14-1982

Heil, Piet, 'Drugs wekken emotie in Zürich', *Het Vrije Volk*, 16-1-1970

- 'De betrokkene', *Het Vrije Volk*, 10-7-1979

'Helft slachtoffers positief over eigen rol', *Het Nieuws van het Noorden,* 22-6-1979

'Helpers Ex-Gijzelaars. Betere nazorg slachtoffers geweld bepleit', *De Volkskrant*, 15-1-1976

Helversteijn, Wim, 'Kliniek voor slachtoffers van syndroom', *De Tijd*, 5-5-1973

'Henk Leliefeld, algemeen medicus: "Coördinatie, dat is het wat wij al jaren missen"', *NIW*, 6-4-1979

Herbergs, Ben, 'Terug naar Oegstgeest', *Het Vrije Volk*, 23-6-1973

- 'De hulpverleners belagen de gegijzelden', *Het Vrije Volk*, 4-6-1977
- 'Een half jaar nazorg aan ex-gegijzelden: "Hadden de psychiaters er zich maar niet mee bemoeit"', *Het Vrije Volk*, 31-12-1977

'Herdenking eind Tweede Wereldoorlog', *De Waarheid*, 14-7-1980

'Herdenking einde van oorlog 1945', *NRC Handelsblad*, 10-7-1980

Hers, J.F.Ph., J.L. Terpstra (eds.), *Stress. Medical and legal analysis of late effects of World War II suffering in the Netherlands* (Leiden: Kooyker, 1988)

Herzberg, Abel J., 'Laat, om onzentwil, de Drie van Breda vrij', *Trouw*, 27-1-1976

- *Kroniek der Jodenvervolging 1950-1945* (Amsterdam: Meulenhoff) 1978 [30)
- 'Holocaust verzwakt de werkelijkheid', *Het Nieuws van het Noorden,* 30-4-1979

'Het post-concentratiekampsyndroom', *NIW*, 25-9-1970

'Het syndroom van "maatschappelijke begeleiders"', *De Waarheid*, 23-8-1978

Hieselaar, Loek, 'Na 26 jaar kliniek voor slachtoffers concentratiekampen. Mensen die na de oorlog geestelijk wrak zijn gebleven', *De Tijd*, 29-5-1971
- 'Psychiater Bastiaans: Velen zijn gevangene van zichzelf', *De Tijd*, 3-3-1973

Hilfman, M.M., 'Bestrijding van Narcotica', *NTvG*, 20-9-1969, 1663
Historianet.nl/oorlog/tweede-wereldoorlog/hitler/had-hitler-maar-een-testikel seen: 30-3-2021)
Hoeden, J.A. van der, 'Farmacotherapie en psychotherapie', *NTvG*, 13-4-1968, 707
Hoek, Sietze van der, 'Prof. Bastiaans over "Teheran": "Gijzelaars ernstig ontwricht"', *De Volkskrant*, 20-1-1981
- 'Mensen bij gijzelingen', *De Volkskrant*, 1-10-1981
- 'Hebt u onder de bom gezeten dan?', *De Volkskrant*, 3-3-1986

Hofhuizen, Herman, 'Gezien', *De Tijd*, 23-2-1972
- 'Gezien. Huiveringwekkend', *De Tijd*, 28-2-1972

Hofstede, B.P., 'Tros brengt Holocaust: Het toevallige geweten der natie', *NRC Handelsblad*, 6-2-1979
Hofstede, Peter, 'De media en Aantjes', *NRC Handelsblad*, 18-11-1987
'Holocaust begeleid door radioserie', *De Volkskrant*, 8-2-1979
'Holocaust op Nederlandse tv', *Het Nieuws van het Noorden,* 7-4-1979
'Holocaust toch in Duitse versie', *Algemeen Dagblad*, 8-2-1979
'Holocaust vertoond voor Friese hulpverleners', *Leeuwarder Courant*, 4-4-1979
'Holocaust, huiveringwekkend stuk geschiedenis, op tv', *Leeuwarder Courant*, 2-4-1979
'Holocaust: nog niet erg veel heftige emoties', *Het Parool*, 24-4-1979
'Holocaust: weer vele reacties', *De Volkskrant*, 30-4-1979
'Holocaust-hallucinaties tijdens Leidse LSD kuur te boek gesteld', *NRC Handelsblad*, 29-5-1987
'Honderden reacties op omstreden film', *Limburgsch Dagblad*, 28-2-1972
Hondius, Dienke, *Terugkeer. Antisemitisme in Nederland rond de bevrijding* (The Hague: SDU, 1998)
Hoof, Jan van, 'Prof. dr. J. Bastiaans: "Drie van Breda" roept opnieuw angsten op bij slachtoffers', *De Tijd*, 19-2-1972
Hooff, Joost van der, 'Ik heb de gijzeling positief uitgebuit…', *Het Vrije Volk*, 10-10-1979
- 'Jan Bastiaans en het contactisolement. "Ook een rotjeugd kan leiden tot een soort KZ-situatie"', *Het Vrije Volk*, 10-6-1985 / 13-6-1985
- 'De barre lijdensweg van kandidaten voor een uitkering voor oorlogsslachtoffers', *Het Vrije Volk*, 10-7-1986

'Hoogleraar in psychiatrie: Beleid van regering bij uitbreiding universiteiten is politieke waanzin', *Algemeen Dagblad*, 10-12-1964
'Hoogleraar psychiatrie prof. J. Bastiaans: in 70 procent van gevalleen van kanker stress oorzaak', *Nederlands Dagblad*, 26-3-1983
'Hoogleraar weigert verhuizing patiënten', *De Volkskrant*, 21-9-1982
'Hoogleraar wijst op onderzoeken. Langdurige stress kan kanker bevorderen', *De Volkskrant*, 25-3-1983
'Hoogleraren pleiten voor andere abortuswetgeving', *De Waarheid*, 5-6-1976
'Hoogleraren voor en tegen gratie. "Niet alle slachtoffers tegen"', *De Telegraaf*, 23-2-1972
Hoorn, W. van, 'De vergelijking tussen de methodes van Bastiaans en Freud is misplaatst', *NRC Handelsblad*, 20-2-1986
'Hoorzitting over "Drie" begint in gespannen sfeer', *Het Vrije Volk*, 24-2-1972
Houten, Annelies van den, 'Landelijk centrum geeft informatie aan oorlogsgetroffenen', *NIW*, 23-2-1979
- 'Belevingsboeken over oorlog meer dan naakt feitenmateriaal', *NIW*, 2-5-1980
Hovens, J.E., G.J. van der Ploeg, 'Hoe het trauma het gewone leven binnendrong. De geschiedenis van de PTSS sinds de negentiende eeuw', *Tijdschrift voor Psychiatrie*, 44 (2002), 12, 803-811
'HP deze week', *Het Parool*, 22-12-1976
Huijskens, Charles, 'Degradatie prof. Bastiaans wekt alom bevreemding', *De Telegraaf*, 23-1-1986
- 'Professor Bastiaans mag LSD therapie blijven toepassen', *De Telegraaf*, 6-2-1986
- 'Weer aan het werk en nog subsidie ook', *De Telegraaf*, 8-2-1986
'Huisarts moet ex-gegijzelde direct helpen', *Algemeen Dagblad*, 22-6-1979
'Hulp blijft voor oorlogsslachtoffers', *Het Vrije Volk*, 18-6-1987
'Hulp slachtoffers oorlog uitgebreid', *Trouw*, 21-6-1985
'Hulpdienst verwerkte 500 reacties na Holocaust', *NIW*, 27-4-1979
'Hulpverlening oorlogsgetroffenen is veel te laat', *NIW*, 6-4-1979
Hulsman, L.H.C., 'Gratie van de Drie van Breda minste van twee kwaden', *De Tijd*, 28-2-1972
Hulst, Wiecher, 'Indisch oorlogsleed en Nederlands onbegrip: "Nooit zullen ze er wat van snappen"', *NRC Handelsblad*, 25-8-1979
Huygen, Maarten, 'Prof Bastiaans kijkt terug bij emeritaat: Verdringing minder sterk', *NRC Handelsblad*, 3-7-1985
Hydra, Ton, 'Vreemde dag', *Trouw*, 15-12-1975
- 'Natuurlijk', *Trouw*, 17-3-1976

- 'Ondergang en late bevrijding', *Trouw*, 14-7-1978
- 'Er knaagt iets aan de helden zonder glorie', *Trouw*, 1-2-1979

I

'Ik zie het zo', *De Waarheid*, 25-9-1971

Immateriële Hulpverlening aan Oorlogsgetroffenen. Eindrapport van het Werk- en Adviescollege (The Hague: Staatsuitgeverij, 1978)

'In centrum KZ-syndroom staat openheid voorop', *Het Vrije Volk*, 18-4-1972

'Informatiebundel over verwerken van oorlogsleed', *Leeuwarder Courant*, 29-2-1972

'Installatie van commissie voor kamp-syndroom', *De Volkskrant*, 16-1-1971

'Installatie van projectgroep nazorg van ex-gijzelaars', *Trouw*, 14-1-1976

'Installatie werkgroep kampsyndroom', *Het Parool*, 15-1-1971

'Intensieve begeleiding "Holocaust" in Nederland', *Limburgsch Dagblad*, 8-2-1979

'Ir. G.S. Vrijburg: "Echt bevrijd zijn wij niet"', *Het Vrije Volk*, 9-8-1980

'Ir. Manusama acht nieuwe harde acties niet uitgesloten', *Leeuwarder Courant*, 15-12-1975

'Israël: laat drie niet vrij', *De Tijd*, 29-2-1972

J

Jacobus, Simone, 'Stichting opgericht voor slachtoffers van geweld', *NIW*, 28-6-1985

Jansen, Han J.A., 'Gesprek met goede vriend leert: Prins vindt het vervelend om ouder te worden', *De Volkskrant*, 26-6-1971
- 'Speciale kliniek opgezet. Slachtoffers van nazi's krijgen extra zorg', *De Volkskrant*, 23-2-1972

Jansma, Klaas, 'Bovensmilde ultimatum', *Het Parool*, 25-5-1977
- 'Opvang al optimaal geregeld', *Het Parool*, 25-5-1977

'Japanse overgave herdacht', *Algemeen Dagblad*, 16-8-1980

'Jodenvervolging als TV spel. Voor of tegen Holocaust?', *Trouw*, 17-4-1979

Jones, Edgar, Simon Wessely, *Shell Shock to PTSD. Military psychiatry from 1900 to the Gulf War* (Hove/New York: Psychology Press, 2005)

'Jom-Kipoer-oorlog eiste erg veel psychische slachtoffers', *Tubantia*, 21-2-1974

Jong, Joop de, 'Impressies uit Japanse hel goed onderbouwd', *De Volkskrant*, 15-6-1983

Jong, Wim de, 'Meer kans op kanker bij rustige mensen', *Het Vrije Volk*, 25-3-1983
'Joop Wolff verwijt justitie gebrek aan wil. Plicht tot actieve opsporing oorlogsmisdadigers', *De Waarheid*, 31-7-1978
Jungman, [Wim], 'Zwaar geschut en polarisatie', *Het Parool*, 28-2-1972
- 'Een oorlog en zijn nasleep', *Het Parool*, 23-11-1973
- 'Pratend over Colditz', *Het Parool*, 21-4-1975
- 'Van Klinkklaar naar Beilen', *Het Parool*, 15-12-1975
- 'De kijk van Jungman', *Het Parool*, 22-1-1979

K

Kaas, A.J.W., 'Over de psychologie der politieke gevangenen in het concentratiekamp', *De Nieuwe Stem*, 1946, 409-422
- 'De Duitse concentratiekampen', in: J. Bolhuis et al. (red.), *Onderdrukking en Verzet. Nederland in oorlogstijd*, deel 1 (Nijmegen: G.J. Thieme, z.j. [1949]) 609-664
- *Buchenwald. Conclusie na twintig jaar* (Arnhem: Van Loghum Slaterus, 1968)
Ka-Tzetnik 135633, *Shivitti. A vision* (San Franscio: Harper and Row, 1989)
'Kabinet beslist misschien zelf', *Limburgsch Dagblad*, 25-2-1972
'Kabinet wil toch gratie', *De Telegraaf*, 26-2-1972
Kalk, Dick, 'Het verzet "loont" niet', *Het Vrije Volk*, 1-4-1972
'Kamer steunt zuinig kabinet in kwestie oorlogsslachtoffers', *De Waarheid*, 29-3-1985
'Kamer wankelt onder protest tegen gratie', *Het Nieuws van het Noorden,* 23-2-1972
'Kamer wil snel opvolger Bastiaans', *Algemeen Dagblad*, 18-6-1987
'Kamer wil therapie Bastiaans behouden', *Nederlands Dagblad*, 1-3-1985
'Kamer: werk prof. Bastiaans moet voortgezet', *Trouw*, 29-3-1985
'Kamer: werk van Bastiaans moet doorgaan', *De Telegraaf*, 29-3-1985
'Kamerleden bezorgd over vertrek van prof. Bastiaans', *De Telegraaf*, 5-7-1984
'Kamerleden herzien mening over gratie', *De Volkskrant*, 23-2-1972
'Kamerleden zien film over kamp-syndroom', *De Tijd*, 24-2-1972
'Kamerlid Geurtsen ging "om" door losgeslagen emoties', *Tubantia*, 29-2-1972
'Kamerlid in opspraak', *Het Vrije Volk*, 1-4-1976
'Kamerlid wil onderzoek naar conflicten rond Centrum '45', *De Tijd*, 18-5-1973
'Kamermeerderheid is tegen collectieve vrijlating', *Leeuwarder Courant*, 29-2-1972

Kamphuis, Herma, 'De negentien treinen naar Sobibor', *Het Nieuws van het Noorden,* 21-4-1979
Kat, P.J., 'Vrijlating van de "Drie van Breda" zou een aanval in de rug van voormalig verzet zijn', *NRC Handelsblad*, 23-2-1972
- 'De schaduwen van het kamp zullen blijven', *NRC Handelsblad*, 13-3-1972
Kater, J., 'Concentratiekamp-syndroom', *Algemeen Dagblad*, 30-5-1964
Katz, Renate, 'Kliniek "Het Centrum" voor oorlogsslachtoffers geopend', *NIW*, 18-5-1973
'Kenmerk besteedt aandacht aan werk prof. Bastiaans', *De Volkskrant*, 21-7-1987
Kessel, Anne van, 'De wetenschap tript weer', *Trouw*, 21-5-2016
'Kijk niet', *NIW*, 20-4-1979
'Kijken naar Holocaust afgeraden', *NRC Handelsblad*, 23-4-1979
'Kind van NSB'er klaagt zijn nood', *Algemeen Dagblad*, 13-1-1983
'Kinderen uit hongerwinter nu nog gestoord. Nazi-slachtoffers doorleefden weer folteringen', *De Volkskrant*, 5-11-1966
'Kinderen van NSB'ers komen nu in de problemen', *De Waarheid*, 14-1-1983
'Klacht na toediening LSD door hoogleraar', *NRC Handelsblad*, 7-9-1979
'Klacht over psychiater afgewezen', *NRC Handelsblad*, 8-10-1980
'Klacht tegen Bastiaans na behandeling', *Trouw*, 7-9-1979
'Klacht tegen professor Bastiaans', *Het Vrije Volk*, 7-9-1979
Kleijer, Pauline, 'Geen jager, maar prooi', *De Volkskrant*, 11-2-2021
Klein, Annemieke, *Verlangen naar Verbetering. 375 Jaar academische geneeskunde in Utrecht* (Amsterdam: Boom, 2010)
Kleisen, A.D., 'Openbare diagnoses?', *Het Vrije Volk*, 11-1-1977
Kleyn, Leo, 'Verzetsverleden steeds moeilijker na te gaan', *Trouw*, 14-8-1976
- 'Elke dag krijg je wel een flits van het concentratiekamp', *Trouw*, 11-1-1986
'Kliniek Bastiaans tijdelijk dakloos', *Het Parool*, 14-4-1987
'Kliniek voor oorlogsslachtoffers', *Algemeen Dagblad*, 2-3-1973
Klinkenberg, Wim, 'Hannie Schafts ideologie is in film verdoezeld', *De Volkskrant*, 1-10-1981
Knoop, Hans, 'Nieuwe kans voor historie', *NIW*, 2-6-1978
Kolk, Bessel van der, *The Body Keeps the Score. Brain, mind, and body in the healing of trauma* (New York: Penguin, 2014)
'Komt 25 februari naar de Dokwerker!', *De Waarheid*, 1-2-1964
Komrij, Gerrit, 'Een en ander', *NRC Handelsblad*, 2-2-1983
'Koningin opende Centrum '45', *Limburgsch Dagblad*, 17-5-1973

'Koningin opent Centrum '45', *Het Nieuws van het Noorden,* 16-5-1973
'Koningin opent vandaag kliniek Centrum '45', *Algemeen Dagblad*, 16-5-1973
Koolbergen, Michiel, 'Kernwapens en pudding. Uit de weekbladen', *Trouw*, 8-10-1981
Koopman, Theo, 'Belangstelling voor Tweede Wereldoorlog leeft in 1978 plotseling weer fel op', *Het Nieuws van het Noorden,* 2-12-1978
Koopmans, G., 'Prof. Bastiaans', *Het Parool*, 24-5-1973
Kopuit, M., 'Jom Kippoeroorlog vergt nog jaren slachtoffers', *NIW*, 18-1-1974
'Kort', *De Waarheid*, 28-2-1985
Kousbroek, Rudy, 'Terug naar Negri Panerkomst 20 (slot): De grote vedwijntruc', *NRC Handelsblad*, 11-4-1980
- 'Terug naar Negri Panerkomst 21. Een nabetrachting: Het kampsyndroom', *NRC Handelsblad*, 2-5-1980
- *Het Oostindisch Kampsyndroom* (Amsterdam: Meulenhoff, 1992)
Kreutzer, Ruud, 'Lange tijd is leed in Jappenkampen verdrongen', *Het Nieuws van het Noorden,* 29-8-1983
Kuin, Riëtte, 'Prof. J. Bastiaans "tendeert naar vrijlating". Dilemma: óf de klap ineens óf steeds maar weer wonden openrijten', *Trouw*, 24-2-1972
- '"Voor slachtoffers is tot nu toe erg weinig gedaan"', *Trouw*, 11-3-1972
Kuipers, Henk, 'Ex-gegijzelde mevrouw Giessen: "Ik geniet intenser"', *Het Nieuws van het Noorden,* 29-11-1980
- 'Ex-gegijzelde Ger Vaders: "Hulp en nazorg kwamen te laat"', *Het Nieuws van het Noorden,* 29-11-1980
- 'Nederlandse psychiaters adviseren bij hulp aan Amerikaanse gijzelaars', *Het Nieuws van het Noorden,* 20-1-1981
- 'Groninger drukker vraagt helderziende om adviezen', *Het Nieuws van het Noorden,* 20-5-1981
Kuipers-de Haan, W.J., 'Kampsyndroom', *NRC Handelsblad*, 30-5-1980
'KZ-syndroom kliniek wordt enige ter wereld', *Het Vrije Volk*, 2-3-1972
'KZ-syndroom: "Iedereen kan helpen"', *De Tijd*, 4-3-1972

L

'Laat men bezwaren brengen waar ze horen', *Het Parool*, 6-8-1977
'Laat optredende gevolgen van oorlogsschade', *NIW*, 18-6-1965
'Laatste deel Englandspiel vanavond op het TV scherm', *Limburgsch Dagblad*, 1-2-1979

'Lages, Aus der Fünten en Kotälla mogen niet vrij!', *De Waarheid*, 23-12-1959

Lange, Wera de, 'Ben Polak vreest voor oorlogsgetroffenen', *De Waarheid*, 2-9-1985

Langerak, Henk, 'Wisselende reacties op Holocaust', *Algemeen Dagblad*, 25-4-1979

Lardenoye, Fred, 'Indiëveteraan was ook actief in het oorlogsverzet. Interview met Willem Wilbrink (94)', *De Kareoler*, 2021, 3, 6-8

'Late gevolgen van concentratiekamp', *Algemeen Dagblad*, 4-3-1955

Laudy, Yvonne, 'Bevrijder uit het innerlijke kamp. Prof. Bastiaans (76) helpt wanhopige patiënten zo lang hij kan', *De Telegraaf*, 8-1-1994

'Leed in Jappenkampen lange tijd verdrongen', *Limburgsch Dagblad*, 27-8-1983

'Leed van kampleven duurt nog voort. Congres over dwangneurose besloten', *De Volkskrant*, 31-7-1965

'"Leed van kinderen van NSB'ers vaak onderschat"', *Nederlands Dagblad*, 14-1-1983

Leeuw, Kees de, 'Oud-verzetsman in kliniek terug naar oorlogsjaren', *Trouw*, 7-4-1975

\- 'Reacties op Holocaust zijn nauwelijks te voorspellen', *Trouw*, 21-4-1979

'Leidse professor gaf oorlogsveteraan zijn geheugen terug', *Leeuwarder Courant*, 23-9-1974

'Leidse psychiatrie blijkt ernstig ziek', *De Telegraaf*, 20-10-1972

Lerner, Paul, *Hysterical Men* (Ithaca/London: Cornell UP, 2003)

'Leven na een oorlog: praten is mogelijk', *NRC Handelsblad*, 4-3-1972

'"Leven in een doolhof": het oorlogs-syndroom', *Limburgsch Dagblad*, 22-11-1973

'"Leven na een oorlog" gebundeld', *Het Parool*, 7-3-1972

Lifton, Robert Jay, *Home from the War. Vietnam Veterans: neither victims nor executioners* (New York: Basic Books, 1973

\- *Nazi-doctors. Medical killing and the psychology of genocide* (New York: Basic books, 1986

Loggem, M. van, 'Ex-illegalen lijden vaak aan psychische zieketen', *Het Vrije Volk*, 2-2-1957

Look, H.P.Th., 'De Drie van Breda', *NRC Handelsblad*, 29-2-1972

Loon, H.F. van, '800 Vergeten oorlogshelden wachten op een gebaar van Den Haag', *De Telegraaf*, 22-7-1977

\- 'Vier geleerden schreven boek over gijzelingen', *De Telegraaf*, 29-9-1981

Loonstein, Marja, 'Joods Nederland bekeek Holocaustserie nauwelijks', *NIW*, 27-4-1979
Los, P.L., 'Leven na een oorlog', *Nederlands Dagblad*, 6-4-1972
- 'Prof. Bastiaans helpt vernielde mensen', *Nederlands Dagblad*, 6-2-1987
Loth, Julia, *Militaire Psychiatrie in de Krijgsmacht: innovatie en discontinuïteit* (ongep. man.)
Luirink, Bart, 'Methode Bastiaans dreigt te verdwijnen', *De Waarheid*, 12-5-1987
'Louis van Gasteren: "Dat Europa, dat is toch iets"', *Het Nieuws van het Noorden,* 29-6-1972
'LSD beschadigt de chromosomen', *NTvG*, 3-4-1971, 628
'LSD en chromosomen', *NTvG*, 6-6-1970, 978
'LSD hulp voor KZ-patiënten', *Het Vrije Volk*, 21-3-1975
'LSD therapie voortgezet', *Het Parool*, 6-2-1986
Lu, Donna, '"Psychedelics renaissance": new wave of research puts hallucinogenics forward to treat mental health', *The Guardian*, 25-9-2021
Lulofs, B., 'Zootje', *De Telegraaf*, 21-8-1976
- 'Taboe', *De Telegraaf*, 5-2-1983
- 'Ontslag', *De Telegraaf*, 9-3-1985

M

'Maar meneer', *Het Parool*, 12-11-1987
'Malik: "Acties tegen Indonesië hard aanpakken"', *NRC Handelsblad*, 22-12-1975
'"Man in gezin vaak op tweede plaats". Dr. Bastiaans over geboorteregeling', *Het Parool*, 14-5-1960
Mari, Henk de, 'Oude oorlogshelden bestoken elkaar met grof geschut', *De Telegraaf*, 24-2-1979
- 'Verwoest naar Oegstgeest', *De Telegraaf*, 11-3-1981
Matussek, Paul, *Die Konzentrationslagerhaft und ihre Folgen* (Berlin/Heidelberg/New York: Springer Verlag, 1971)
McManners, Hugh, *The Scars of War* (London: HarperCollins, 1993)
'Meedogenloze machtsstrijd schakelt prof. Bastiaans uit', *Tubantia*, 17-5-1973
'Meerderheid laat belang slachtoffers prevaleren', *Trouw*, 1-3-1972
Meerloo, A.M., *Total War and the Human Mind. A psychologist's experiences in occupied Holland* (London: Allen & Unwin, 1944)
- *Homo Militans. De psychologie van oorlog en vrede in de mens* (The Hague: Servire, 1964 (1e druk 1939)

'Meester stapt op', *De Telegraaf*, 2-8-1976
'Meester uit Kamer', *Algemeen Dagblad*, 2-8-1976
Meijer, Ischa, *Brief aan mijn Moeder* (Amsterdam: Bert Bakker, 1975)
Melkman, J., 'Psychische invloed van vervolging op symposium', *NIW*, 11-11-1977
Memelink, O.W., 'Toen voelde ik dat mijn bevrijding voltooid was', *NRC Handelsblad*, 14-11-1987
'Mensen', *Algemeen Dagblad*, 10-2-1973
'"Methode Bastiaans handhaven"', *Het Parool*, 28-2-1985
'Methode Belinfante-Dekker', *Het Parool*, 3-8-1960
Metz, Tracy, 'Bastiaans: verdachte consul is volledig ontoerekeningsvatbaar', *NRC Handelsblad*, 5-12-1986
- 'Ton boete, geen cel geëist tegen oud-consul', *NRC Handelsblad*, 7-2-1987
Meulenberg, Frans, 'Het experiment met LSD therapie', *Trouw*, 2-8-2000
Meurs, A.J. van, *Over de Gevechtsuitputting* (Rotterdam: W.L. & J. Brusse, 1955)
'Mevrouw Donker: zaak tegen Menten is nooit geseponeerd', *Leeuwarder Courant*, 6-12-1978
Milikowski, Herman, 'Het KZ-syndroom en de psychiatrische mythen', in: Ibidem, *Sociologie als Verzet. Over KZ-syndroom, gezinsproblemen, sociale en seksuele relaties en agressie* (Amsterdam: Van Gennep, 1975 [2e druk])
'Minister en Kamerleden zagen kampsyndroomfilm', *De Telegraaf*, 24-2-1972
'Minister Engels was tegen uitzending', *Het Parool*, 28-2-1972
'Minister heeft vertoning film niet verboden', *Leeuwarder Courant*, 28-2-1972
'Minister stelt richtlijnen voor. "TV uitzendingen over de oorlog goed begeleiden"', *Het Parool*, 3-2-1979
'Minister van Agt: Geen programma voor vrijlating Drie van Breda', *Limburgsch Dagblad*, 17-3-1972
'Minister ziet film over syndroom', *NRC Handelsblad*, 24-2-1972
'Misbruik psychiatrie op grote schaal in Rusland', *Het Nieuws van het Noorden,* 14-10-1978
Mitchell, Jennifer M., Michael Bogenschutz, Rick Doblin, 'MDMA-assisted therapy for severe PTSD: a randomized, double-blind, placebo-controlled phase 3 study', *Nature Medicine*, 27 (2021) 1025-1033
'Moeder vergaste haar zoontjes (4 en 7 jaar). Triest drama voor rechtbank', *Nieuwe Tilburgsche Courant*, 12-9-1962

'Moeten we 4 en 5 mei nog altijd vieren?', *De Tijd*, 3-5-1969

Montgomery, Adam, *The Invisible Injured. Psychological trauma in the Canadian military from the First World War to Afghanistan* (Montreal: McGill Queen's UP, 2017)

Mooij, Annet, 'De langste schaduw. Het denken over psychische oorlogsgevolgen', in: Conny Kristel (red.), *Binnenskamers. Terugkeer en opvang na de Tweede Wereldoorlog, Besluitvorming* (Amsterdam: Bert Bakker, 2002) 261-291

- 'Bastiaans, Jan', *Biografisch woordenboek van Nederland* (Resources.huygens.knaw.nl/bwn1880-2000/lemmata/ bwn6/bastiaans)

'Monument Ravensbrück', *NIW*, 29-5-1959

Moulin, D. de, 'Kankerpersoonlijkheid (2)', *NRC Handelsblad*, 23-3-1984

'Mr. Aalders van Expogé overleden', *Leeuwarder Courant*, 28-2-1972

Müller-Bauseneik, Jens, 'Die US-Fernsehserie "Holocaust" im Spiegel der deutschen Presse (Januar-März 12979): eine Dokumentation', *Historical Social Research*, 30 (2005), 4, 128-140

Musaph, H., 'Late reacties op oorlogsleed. Gevolgen van onderdrukking en verzet', *NIW*, 29-3-1957

- 'LSD wordt steeds minder gebruikt', *NRC Handelsblad*, 7-2-1986

N

Nanninga, Wilma, 'Oud-consul moet boeten voor fraude: eis 1 ton', *De Telegraaf*, 7-2-1987

'Na dertig jaar eigen "thuis" voor oorlogsslachtoffers', *Het Vrije Volk*, 2-3-1973

'Na Holocaust 400 tot 500 telefoontjes', *Leeuwarder Courant*, 24-4-1979

'Na kabinetsbesluit over Drie van Breda. PvdA-fractie denkt aan interpellatie', *Leeuwarder Courant*, 6-3-1972

'Na vertrek van Bastiaans toepassing LSD niet toegestaan', *NRC Handelsblad*, 12-9-1984

'Nationaal centrum volksgezondheid geeft boekje uit. Antwoord op vragen over het KZ-syndroom', *Trouw*, 3-3-1972

'Nazorg voor àlle slachtoffers van geweld en rampen', *Het Vrije Volk*, 31-12-1977

'Nazorg, ja, maar zó mag het nooit meer', *Het Vrije Volk*, 10-10-1979

'Nazorg-groep ex-gijzelaars samengesteld', *De Volkskrant*, 14-1-1976

'Nederland ontvangt Holocaust beheerst', *Het Vrije Volk*, 24-4-1979

'Nederlanders over hun "rampen"-syndroom', *De Telegraaf*, 9-4-1980

'Nederlands Auschwitz Comité vindt Holocaust "goede" film', *Het Nieuws van het Noorden*, 10-2-1979

'Neo-nazi's van aanslag op TV masten verdacht', *De Telegraaf*, 20-1-1979
'Neo-nazi's willen meer acties tegen TV serie Holocaust', *Trouw*, 22-1-1979
Neyenhuys, Leo, 'Oorlogsslachtoffers nog geen uitstervende groep', *De Volkskrant*, 18-12-1976
Nieboer, W., 'Terrorisme niet los te zien van publieke norm-ondergraving', *Nederlands Dagblad*, 14-6-1982
'Niet vrijlaten', *Friese Koerier*, 29-12-1959
Nietsch, Hetty, 'Bastiaans: de sterken en de stillen komen het laatst', *Trouw*, 5-2-1983
- 'Niets mogen doen: dan ligt stress op de loer', *Trouw*, 25-3-1983
'Nieuw conflict over methode Bastiaans', *Het Parool*, 1-2-1986
'Nieuwe behandelingen met LSD verboden', *NRC Handelsblad*, 4-2-1986
'Nieuwe instelling voor oorlogsslachtoffers', *Het Nieuws van het Noorden*, 21-2-1979
'Nieuwe medicijnen beïnvloeden chemische hersenwerking', *Nederlands Dagblad*, 6-2-1978
'Nieuwe poging van Agt. "Bredase Drie" weer in kabinet', *Het Vrije Volk*, 17-3-1976
'Nieuws. Prijs', *NRC Handelsblad*, 27-2-1973
Nijkamp-van Doornik, P., '"Onvoltooid verleden" – NS-documentaire over rampen-syndroom', *Nederlands Dagblad*, 10-4-1980
'Nog duizenden lijden aan naweeën oorlog. Aparte kliniek wordt opgericht', *De Tijd*, 21-4-1971
'Nog eens "de Drie van Breda"', *Trouw*, 3-6-1972
'NOS-radio met documentaires over zelfmoord', *Leeuwarder Courant*, 28-2-1974
'NSB-kinderen: "Niet de schuld, wel de straf"', *Het Vrije Volk*, 13-1-1983
'NSB-kinderen: niet de schuld, wel de straf', *Trouw*, 14-1-1983

O

'Officier eist plaatsing in een inrichting. Vrouw vergaste twee kinderen', *Leeuwarder Courant*, 12-9-1962
'Oktober-oorlog eiste veel psychische slachtoffers onder militairen Israël', *Leeuwarder Courant*, 22-2-1974
'Onderscheiding aan ziekbed', *De Telegraaf*, 28-4-1973
'Onderzoek gevraagd naar Centrum '45', *NRC Handelsblad*, 18-5-1973
'Onderzoek gevraagd naar de gang van zaken rond Centrum '45 in Oegstgeest', *Leeuwarder Courant*, 18-5-1973
'Onderzoek gevraagd naar passeren prof. Bastiaans', *Tubantia*, 18-5-1973
'Onderzoek methode-Bastiaans mislukt', *Nederlands Dagblad*, 7-11-1987

'Onderzoek methode-Bastiaans mislukt', *Het Nieuws van het Noorden,* 6-11-1987
'Onderzoek naar Centrum '45', *De Tijd*, 25-5-1973
'Onderzoek naar Centrum '45', *Het Vrije Volk*, 4-6-1973
'Onderzoek naar conflict bij Centrum '45 gevraagd', *Trouw*, 18-5-1973
'Onderzoek naar conflict over Centrum '40-'45', *Het Vrije Volk*, 25-5-1973
'Onderzoek naar gebruik LSD in therapie Bastiaans', *Het Parool*, 23-1-1986
'Onderzoek naar gevolg LSD-behandeling Bastiaans mislukt', *De Volkskrant*, 6-11-1987
'Onderzoek naar langdurige begeleiding van gegijzelden', *Algemeen Dagblad*, 15-12-1975
'Onderzoek naar methode Bastiaans is mislukking', *Trouw*, 6-11-1987
'Onderzoek naar methode Bastiaans', *Trouw*, 24-1-1986
'Onderzoek naar resultaten therapie is mislukt', *De Telegraaf*, 6-11-1987
'Onderzoek naar werkmethoden van professor J. Bastiaans', *Nederlands Dagblad*, 24-1-1986
'Onderzoek zegt: Stress kan oorzaak zijn van kanker', *Het Nieuws van het Noorden,* 25-3-1983
'Ontsnapping KZ-syndroom met LSD kuur', *De Telegraaf*, 21-3-1975
'Onvoltooid verleden', *De Waarheid*, 10-4-1980
'Oorlogsgetroffenen vragen Brinkman duidelijkheid', *De Waarheid*, 13-5-1987
'"Oorlogsslachtoffers hebben vooral behoefte aan rust"', *De Volkskrant*, 23-3-1987
'Oorlogsslachtoffers klagen arts van Centrum '45 aan', *De Volkskrant*, 30-11-1987
'Oorlogsslachtoffers krijgen meer hulp. Hoogleraar maakt inhaalprogramma', *De Volkskrant*, 7-3-1972
'Oorlogsslachtoffers moeten tijdelijk ondergebracht. Professor Bastiaans en patiënten worden enkele maanden dakloos', *De Volkskrant*, 14-4-1987
'Oorlogsslachtoffers nog steeds in het verdomhoekje', *Het Vrije Volk*, 3-12-1979
Oosten, Ad van, 'Het verzet en het onbegrip van twee psychiaters', *De Waarheid*, 4-5-1987
'Oplossing nabij voor patiënten van Bastiaans', *Trouw*, 22-5-1985
'Oplossing voor patiënten prof. Bastiaans in zicht', *Nederlands Dagblad*, 23-5-1985
'Oplossing voor werk Bastiaans', *Het Parool*, 22-5-1985
'Oproep voor onthulling museum in Ravensbrück', *De Waarheid*, 19-5-1959

‘Opvang en begeleiding tijdens Holocaust-serie’, *Algemeen Dagblad*, 8-2-1979
‘Opvolger Bastiaans vraagt toestemming voor gebruik LSD’, *De Volkskrant*, 22-12-1987
Os, Pieter van, *Liever dier dan mens. Een overlevingsverhaal* (Amsterdam: Prometheus, 2021 [11])
‘Oud-verzetslieden in beroep tegen beslissing van officier’, *Trouw*, 11-1-1978
Overeem, Emmy van, ‘Oorlog duurt voort in Centrum ’45’, *NRC Handelsblad*, 14-5-1973
- ‘Nietes-welles: realiteit van Beilen heeft twee kanten’, *NRC Handelsblad*, 18-12-1975
- ‘Hulpverleners, bemoei je er niet mee’, *NRC Handelsblad*, 28-5-1977
- ‘Ervaring voor Joodse wezen les voor alle traumata’, *NRC Handelsblad*, 22-2-1979
- ‘De druppel die de emmer doet overlopen’, *NRC Handelsblad*, 29-10-1979

‘Overleg opgeschort over Centrum ’45’, *Het Nieuws van het Noorden,* 18-12-1985
‘Overleg over positie van prof. Bastiaans’, *Tubantia*, 6-6-1973
‘Overval consulaat “spontaan” plan’, *De Volkskrant*, 22-12-1975
‘Overval op consulaat was niet gepland’, *De Waarheid*, 22-12-1975

P

Pam, Max, ‘Ordinaire smartlap’, *Het Vrije Volk*, 28-2-1973
Panhuysen, L.H.H.M., ‘De ongewenste werkingen na het innemen van LSD’, *NTvG*, 25-4-1970, 723-727
Pannekoek, Yvo, *Memoires* (Amsterdam: Van Oorschot, 1983)
‘Patiënten Bastiaans tijdelijk dakloos’, *NRC Handelsblad*, 14-4-1987
‘Patiënten bezorgd over toekomst methode-Bastiaans’, *De Volkskrant*, 3-12-1987
‘Patiënten bezorgd over voortbestaan methode-Bastiaans’, *De Waarheid*, 3-12-1987
‘Patiënten dringen aan op aanblijven prof. Bastiaans bij centrum’, *NRC Handelsblad*, 3-12-1987
‘Patiënten op de bres voor “hun” Bastiaans’, *Het Vrije Volk*, 26-1-1983
‘Patiënten prof. Bastiaans mogen college niet meer in’, *Trouw*, 26-4-1983
‘Patiëntenactie voor aanblijven Bastiaans’, *Het Parool*, 2-12-1987
Peereboom, Klaas, ‘Begrijpt u nu waarom ik huil…’, *Het Parool*, 17-5-1969
- ‘De protesterende jongeren stemmen psychiater Bastiaans niet optimistisch’, *Het Parool*, 12-9-1970

- 'Pensioen zou helpen bij behandeling KZ-syndroom', *Het Parool*, 18-3-1972
- 'De straf voor verzetswerk', *Het Parool*, 31-3-1972
- 'Waardevol boek over KZ-syndroom', *Het Parool*, 3-5-1975
- 'Kapers en gijzelaars als één groep', *Het Parool*, 17-12-1975
- '"Van oorlogsslachtoffer werd problematiek niet begrepen". Interview met prof. Bastiaans', *Het Parool*, 26-3-1977
- 'De oorlog werkt bij velen nog diep na', *Het Parool*, 4-5-1977
- 'Littekens gijzeling blijven', *Het Parool*, 5-1-1980
- 'Het trauma van de gegijzelde mens', *Het Parool*, 17-10-1981

Pennewaard, Wiebe, 'Na veertig jaar', *Leeuwarder Courant*, 4-5-1987

'Pensioenrechten voor slachtoffers van concentratie-kampen bepleit', *Nederlands Dagblad*, 22-2-1968

'Pentothal-behandeling Bastiaans onderzocht', *NRC Handelsblad*, 23-1-1986

'Personalia', *Trouw*, 10-2-1973

Piersma, Hinke, *De Drie van Breda. Duitse oorlogsmisdadigers in Nederlandse gevangenschap 1945-1989* (Amsterdam: Balans, 2005)
- *Jaap le Poole, verzetsman voor het leven* (Boom: Amsterdam, 2006)

Piët, Susanne, 'In een geur van braadvlees. Uit de weekbladen', *NRC Handelsblad*, 9-9-1976
- 'Uit de weekbladen', *NRC Handelsblad*, 23-12-1976

Pijper, Jan, 'Meertens bemiddelde bij prins voor schimmige sjeik', *Het Vrije Volk*, 23-2-1984

'Pleidooi heropenen van kliniek Bastiaans', *NRC Handelsblad*, 21-5-1985

Ploeg, Hans van der, 'Stress en psychotrauma's. Voer voor psychologen en psychiaters', in: M.W. Hengeveld et al. (red.), *Nuchtere Psychiatrie. Liber amicorum bij het afscheid van prof. dr. H.G.M. Rooijmans* (Houten/Diegem: Bohn Stafleu Van Loghum, 1999) 1-11
- 'LSD in de psychiatrie', *NRC Handelsblad*, 16-6-2000
- 'Preludium: "Dit was Brandpunt. Goedenavond"', in: Vermetten, Kleber, Van der Hart, *Handboek Posttraumatische Stressstoornis*, 23-24

Ploeg, H.M. van der, J.W. Reerds, W.Chr. Kleijn, J. Mook, P.P. Moorman, *Onderzoek naar de Behandeling van Oorlogsslachtoffers met LSD psychotherapie: een verslag van een vooronderzoek* (Rijksuniversiteit Leiden, vakgroep psychiatrie, september 1987)

Ploeg, H.M. van der, J.M.P. Weerts (red.), *Veteranen in Nederland. Onderzoek naar de gevolgen van oorlogservaringen – Tweede Wereldoorlog – Politionele acties – Korea* (Lisse: Swets&Zeitlinger, 1995)

Poel, Cor van de, 'Zo mag ik 't zien', *Leeuwarder Courant*, 24-4-1979 / 11-4-1980 / 27-3-1981
Polak, Nico, 'Verzetsgroepen in actie tegen Stichting '40-'45', *Het Vrije Volk*, 23-2-1984
- 'Van Meekren, waarom?', *Het Vrije Volk*, 29-11-1986
'Politici menen na 85 stemmen tegen: "De Drie" blijven nog in Breda', *Het Vrije Volk*, 1-3-1972
Pons, Cornelis, 'Mei geen jubelmaand voor ex-verzetsmensen: "Van deze dagen wordt je bloed dunner"', *Het Vrije Volk*, 4-4-1985 / 11-4-1985
'Post-Abortussyndroom onderwerp bijeenkomst Nederl. Artsenverbond', *Nederlands Dagblad*, 25-10-1979
Praag, H.M. van, 'Hallucinogenen, het paard van Troje?', *NTvG*, 2-11-1968, 1985-1989
'Premier Van Agt ontvangt boek "Mensen bij gijzelingen". "Overheid moet aanleiding tot gijzelingen voorkomen"', *Het Nieuws van het Noorden*, 29-9-1981
'Prijs prof. Bastiaans', *Het Parool*, 27-2-1973
'Prijs voor prof. Bastiaans', *Het Parool*, 9-2-1973
'Prijs', *NRC Handelsblad*, 30-10-1982
'Prins bij begin bouw kliniek. Bouw KZ-centrum "ere-verplichting"', *De Volkskrant*, 18-4-1972
'Prins sloeg paal voor z'n vrinden', *De Telegraaf*, 18-4-1972
'Problemen Centrum '45 worden uitgepraat', *Het Parool*, 6-6-1973
'Problemen oorlogsslachtoffers worden nog steeds onderschat', *Trouw*, 17-2-1979
'Problemen rond Centrum '45 lijken opgelost', *De Volkskrant*, 6-6-1973
'Prof Bastiaans mag therapie voortzetten', *Trouw*, 6-2-1986
'Prof Bastiaans op symposium: spanningen zijn vaak de oorzaak van kanker', *De Waarheid*, 26-3-1983
'Prof Bastiaans op symposium: Stress zou oorzaak van kanker kunnen zijn', *Leeuwarder Courant*, 25-3-1983
'Prof Bastiaans verduidelijkt kritiek op Centrum '45', *NRC Handelsblad*, 25-5-1973
'Prof Bastiaans vindt uitlating minister Stuyt "onbegrijpelijk"', *Het Parool*, 19-4-1972
'Prof Bastiaans voorziet weinig problemen na verbod gebruik LSD', *Leeuwarder Courant*, 3-2-1986
'Prof Bastiaans: "Behandeling van Aantjes onmenselijk"', *De Telegraaf*, 10-11-1978
'Prof Bastiaans: Aantjes publiekelijk gegijzeld met zijn gezin', *Nederlands Dagblad*, 10-11-1978

'Prof Bastiaans mag bij nieuwe patiënten geen LSD gebruiken', *De Telegraaf*, 3-2-1986
'Prof. Bastiaans bij presentatie boek van Cohen: "Massamoord op Joden nog steeds ontkend"', *Het Nieuws van het Noorden,* 24-4-1979
'Prof. Bastiaans blijft nog tot 1985 werken', *Het Nieuws van het Noorden,* 7-2-1983
'Prof. Bastiaans blijft werken onder oorlogsslachtoffers', *Nederlands Dagblad*, 8-2-1983
'Prof. Bastiaans contra Stuyt', *Het Vrije Volk*, 19-4-1972
'Prof. Bastiaans dreigt dakloos te worden', *De Telegraaf*, 14-4-1987
'Prof. Bastiaans heeft genoeg van belediging', *Het Vrije Volk*, 18-12-1975
'Prof. Bastiaans in brief aan prof. Muntendam: "Leidse universiteit moet zaak regelen"', *Trouw*, 25-5-1973
'Prof. Bastiaans in Leiden: als medicus vind ik dit onmenselijk. "Mr. Aantjes wordt publiekelijk met zijn gezin gegijzeld"', *Leeuwarder Courant*, 9-11-1978
'Prof. Bastiaans kan doorgaan met behandeling', *Leeuwarder Courant*, 9-5-1985
'Prof. Bastiaans kan doorgaan', *Het Vrije Volk*, 7-2-1983
'Prof. Bastiaans kan oorlogsslachtoffers blijven behandelen', *De Volkskrant*, 8-2-1983
'Prof. Bastiaans krijgt ruimte op Endegeest', *Het Parool*, 11-5-1985
'Prof. Bastiaans mag behandeling oorlogssyndroom voortzetten', *De Telegraaf*, 7-2-1983
'Prof. Bastiaans mag patiënten niet toelaten tot collegezaal', *NRC Handelsblad*, 26-4-1983
'Prof. Bastiaans mag van Kamer behandeling nog even voortzetten', *NRC Handelsblad*, 27-2-1985
'Prof. Bastiaans moet stoppen met kliniek', *Het Nieuws van het Noorden,* 13-4-1987
'Prof. Bastiaans neemt afscheid als hoogleraar', *Het Parool*, 29-6-1985
'Prof. Bastiaans ontkent verklaring in kort geding. "Bewering over LSP in de mond gelegd"', *De Telegraaf*, 15-4-1981
'Prof. Bastiaans over conflict Centrum '45: "Er zijn in deze zaak nare dingen gebeurd"', *Het Parool*, 19-05-1973
'Prof. Bastiaans over drama bij Wijster: "Aantal gijzelaars onderging duidelijk hersenspoeling"', *Het Vrije Volk*, 20-12-1975
'Prof. Bastiaans over gegijzelden in Teheran. "Aan 'bekentenissen' Amerikanen ging vast hersenspoeling vooraf"', *Leeuwarder Courant*, 11-4-1980

'Prof. Bastiaans over gijzelaars in Teheran. Naweeën duren nog jaren', *Het Nieuws van het Noorden,* 14-4-1980
'Prof. Bastiaans over voorspellende waarde kankerpersoonlijkheid', *NRC Handelsblad*, 25-3-1983
'Prof. Bastiaans pleit voor een centraal behandelingsapparaat oorlogsslachtoffers', *Het Parool*, 8-3-1972
'Prof. Bastiaans teleurgesteld over centrum lijders KZ-syndroom', *De Tijd*, 17-5-1973
'Prof. Bastiaans vindt uitlating minister Stuyt onbegrijpelijk', *Het Nieuws van het Noorden,* 19-4-1972
'Prof. Bastiaans waarschuwt voor acute ziekteverergering. Steeds meer twijfel over gratie in parlement', *Het Vrije Volk*, 23-2-1972
'Prof. Bastiaans werkt mee aan rapport', *Het Parool*, 28-7-1973
'Prof. Bastiaans werkt opvolgers in', *Het Parool*, 11-7-1987
'Prof. Bastiaans werkt zelf zijn drie opvolgers in', *Trouw*, 11-7-1987
'Prof. Bastiaans wil functie niet neerleggen', *Trouw*, 20-1-1983
'Prof. Bastiaans wint kort geding', *Het Vrije Volk*, 27-12-1975
'Prof. Bastiaans zet werk voort', *NRC Handelsblad*, 7-2-1983
'Prof. Bastiaans: geen sprake van ruzie', *Nederlands Dagblad*, 26-5-1973
'Prof. Bastiaans: goede samenwerking met staf van Centrum '45', *Leeuwarder Courant*, 25-5-1973
'Prof. Bastiaans: LSD kan het slot openen', *Leeuwarder Courant*, 14-12-1987
'Prof. Bastiaans: Samenwerking goed met staf Centrum '45', *De Volkskrant*, 25-5-1973
'Prof. Bastiaans: samenwerking met staf Centrum '45 goed', *Tubantia*, 25-5-1973
'Prof. Bastiaans: Voldoende hulp voor gijzelaars', *De Telegraaf*, 21-1-1981
'Prof. Bastiaans', *Het Nieuws van het Noorden,* 6-2-1986
'Prof. dr. J. Bastiaans heeft liever meer hulp voor hun slachtoffers dan een actief opsporingsbeleid naar oorlogsmisdadigers', *De Volkskrant*, 12-8-1978
'Prof. dr. J. Bastiaans over affaire-Aantjes: Presentatie rapport "soort volkstribunaal"', *Trouw*, 10-11-1978
'Prof. dr. J. Bastiaans over toestand gegijzelden in Teheran. "Grootste klap komt als mensen vrij zijn"', *Limburgsch Dagblad*, 16-4-1980
'Prof. dr. J. Bastiaans: 14% gegijzelden komen om volgens statistieken', *Het Vrije Volk*, 16-6-1977
'Prof. J. Bastiaans op symposium: Stress zou oorzaak van kanker kunnen zijn', *Leeuwarder Courant*, 25-3-1983

'Prof. J. Bastiaans, "Bemanning Centrum '45 onvoldoende"', *De Volkskrant*, 17-5-1973
'Prof. Jan Bastiaans (1917-1997)', *Trouw*, 3-11-1997
'Prof. Weijel hekelt "bot beleid" regering', *De Volkskrant*, 28-2-1972
'Professor Bastiaans over oorlogsslachtoffers. "Grote ontevredenheid over bureaucratie"', *De Waarheid*, 17-7-1981
'Professor Bastiaans slachtoffer van de universitaire machtsstrijd', *Het Nieuws van het Noorden,* 16-5-1973
'Professor Bastiaans: "Behandeling van oorlogsslachtoffers naar dieptepunt"', *De Telegraaf*, 16-7-1981
'Projectgroep gijzelaars begint', *Het Vrije Volk*, 14-1-1976
'Projectgroep nazorg gijzelaars ingesteld', *Nederlands Dagblad*, 15-1-1976
'Projectgroep nazorg van ex-gijzelaars kan aan het werk', *NRC Handelsblad*, 14-1-1976
'Protest van vele honderden in Amersfoort', *Het Parool*, 24-2-1972
'Protesten tegen vrijlating "Drie"', *Trouw*, 23-2-1972
'PSP-Kamerlid: Eibert M. moet toch vervolgd voor pensioenfraude', *Leeuwarder Courant*, 11-1-1978
'Psychiater D. Mulder in boek "Mensen bij gijzelingen": "Terrorisme zal zich sterk uitbreiden; voor vrouw grotere rol"', *Leeuwarder Courant*, 29-9-1981
'Psychiater D. Mulder in boek "Mensen bij gijzelingen": Terrorisme zal zich sterk uitbreiden', *Limburgsch Dagblad*, 29-9-1981
'Psychiater door Tuchtcollege vrijgesproken', *Het Parool*, 8-10-1980
'Psychiater verwacht sterke uitbreiding terrorisme', *Het Parool*, 28-9-1981
'Psychiatrie met politieke bijsmaak in Sowjet-Unie', *Leeuwarder Courant*, 25-8-1978
'Psychiatrisch centrum wil doorgaan met opvang van oorlogsslachtoffers', *Trouw*, 11-5-1985
'Psychisch leed – twintig jaar na de oorlog', *Het Parool*, 29-7-1965
'Psychische factor belangrijk bij behandeling van astma', *Het Parool*, 30-12-1958
'"Psychische gevolgen van oorlogservaringen veel te laat ontdekt"', *NRC Handelsblad*, 8-5-1985
Psychotraumanet.org/nl/de-thematiek-van-trauma-en-oorlog-analystische-kring (seen: 16-3-2021)
'Psycho-analyse van regeringsbeleid', *De Volkskrant*, 10-12-1964
Put, Paul van der, 'Maar deze mug blijft doorgaan', *Het Vrije Volk*, 6-1-1979
- 'Wim des Celles al jarenlang ondergedoken in zijn "vaderland"', *Het Vrije Volk*, 9-8-1980

R

'"Rampen-syndroom" in Artsenij', *Leeuwarder Courant*, 10-4-1980
'Rapport haalt basis van recht oorlogsslachtoffer op een uitkering weg. "Geen verband oorlog en leed"', *Het Parool*, 19-3-1987
'Rapport Leidse onderzoekers: Nazorg gijzeling niet voldoende na "Bovensmilde"', *Het Nieuws van het Noorden,* 22-6-1979
'Rapport roept op tot actieve hulpverlening: "Slachtoffers gijzelingen te vaak verwaarloosd"', *De Telegraaf*, 22-6-1979
'Reacties verdeeld', *Limburgsch Dagblad*, 6-3-1972
Ree, Hans, 'Arts en Auto', *NRC Handelsblad*, 7-2-1984
Ree, F. van, 'Gewoontevorming, verslaving en gewenning bij gebruik van alcohol, marihuana en LSD', *NTvG*, 13-4-1968, 707-709
- 'Een behandeling van een suïcidale patiënt met LSD 25', *NTvG*, 23-8-1969, 1470-1472
Reemst, Th.E. van, 'Arts schreef proefschrift over ziekten uit verzet '40-'45', *De Waarheid*, 7-2-1957
'Regering houdt nog vast aan gratie. Kamerleden bedreigd', *De Volkskrant*, 25-2-1972
'Regering zou willen afzien van Kamerdebat', *Leeuwarder Courant*, 25-2-1972
'Regeringsbesluit over de Drie verdeeld ontvangen', *Tubantia*, 6-3-1972
Rep, Jelte, 'Trix Terwindt: tot het einde toe een strijdbare vrouw', *Trouw*, 9-4-1987
'Richtlijnen van CRM voor uitzendingen over oorlog', *NIW*, 9-2-1979
Ridder, Tom de, Jolande Withuis, '"Scheldend op mezelf voel ik dat ik een wrak ben". Het gebroken leven van A.J.W. Kaas, psychiater in Buchenwald (1908-1976), *De Gids*, 168 (2005) 378-396
Ris, Ernst, 'Gat in Avenue-stijl', *Het Vrije Volk*, 21-12-1973
Romme, Erik, 'Van Bastiaans tot nu. Een kwart eeuw traumabehandeling in Stichting Centrum '45', *Cogiscope*, 2012, 3, 2-5
Rondagh, Ferd., 'LSD gesprekken met verzetsman. Het oorlogsleed van Willem van Salland', *De Volkskrant*, 28-3-1975
- 'Vermoeden psycholoog: Gegijzelden voelden zich als kinderen. KZ-syndroom valt niet te verwachten', *De Volkskrant*, 15-12-1975
Rooijmans, H.G.M., 'Bastiaans', *De Volkskrant*, 6-4-1985
- *99 Jaar tussen Wal en Schip. Geschiedenis van de Leidse Universitaire Psychiatrie (1899-1998)* (Houten: Bohn Stafleu Van Loghum, 1998)
Rosen, Gerald M., Scott O. Lilienfeld, 'Posttraumatic stress disorder: an empirical evaluation of core assumptions', *Clinical Psychological Review*, 28, 5 (June 2008) 837-868

Rosenthal, Eddo, 'Psychiater Mulder in Israël: plan anti-gijzelgroep onder Defensie', *De Volkskrant*, 19-10-1977
'Ruime meerderheid is tegen vrijlating', *De Tijd*, 29-2-1972
'Ruimte voor oorlogspatiënten aangeboden', *Algemeen Dagblad*, 11-5-1985
'Rust voor vrijgelaten gegijzelden het belangrijkst', *Leeuwarder Courant*, 9-12-1975
Ruyter, Martin, '"We horen vaak: Je moet niet zeuren". Milikowski: andere kijk op Van Gasterens film', *De Volkskrant*, 22-5-1969
- 'Mr van de Poel: Voor mijn gevoel geen nederlaag. Anders wordt 't afwegen van leed', *De Volkskrant*, 30-3-1971
- 'De verlate belangstelling voor de kampslachtoffers', *De Volkskrant*, 12-5-1973
'Ruzie bij opening van nieuwe oorlogsslachtoffers-kliniek', *Het Vrije Volk*, 17-5-1973

S
Sant, Roelfien, 'Holocaust wordt nú al begeleid door de TROS', *Het Parool*, 26-3-1979
Scagliola, S.I., *Last van de Oorlog. De Nederlandse oorlogsmisdaden in Indonesië en hun verwerking* (Amsterdam: Balans, 2002)
Scheepmaker, Nico, 'Collin Welland: de Pinter van het moderne TV spel', *Leeuwarder Courant*, 23-2-1972
Scheepmaker, Nico, 'Standbeeld voor gefolterde mens van twintigste eeuw', *Leeuwarder Courant*, 28-2-1972
- 'Kastje kijken', *Het Nieuws van het Noorden,* 28-2-1972 / 23-11-1973 / 21-12-1973
- '"En wij, wij leven voort in een doolhof…"', *Leeuwarder Courant*, 23-11-1973
- '"Wij leven voort" was in vreemde vorm gegoten', *Leeuwarder Courant*, 21-12-1973
- 'Trijfel', *Het Nieuws van het Noorden,* 21-2-1983
Schie, Joop van, 'Hoe ziek zijn zij die om vervolging roepen?', *De Volkskrant*, 12-8-1978
Schreuder, B.J.N., 'In memoriam prof. dr. J. Bastiaans', *NTvG*, 13-12-1997, 2479-2480
Schumacher, Peter, 'De oorlog duurt voort…', *NRC Handelsblad*, 10-7-1976
Schütz, Mathias, 'Memory Unbound, Unfounded Memory? On Medicine, the Holocaust, and Bioethical Reflection', *European Journal for the History of Medicine and Health*, 78 (2021), 74-95

Schuurman, C.J., 'Farmacotherapie en psychotherapie: LSD als adjuvans bij de psychotherapie', *NTvG*, 8-6-1968, 1095-1096

'Scientology-sekte klaagt LSD kuur in psychiatrie aan', *Leeuwarder Courant*, 19-2-1980

'Senator wil onderzoek bij Centrum '45', *Het Parool*, 18-5-1973

Sereny, Gitta, *De Duisternis Tegemoet* (Brussels/The Hague: Manteau, 1975)

'Sfeervolle herdenking van Japanse capitulatie in 1945', *Nederlands Dagblad*, 16-8-1980

Shepard, Ben, *A War of Nerves. Soldiers and psychiatrists 1914-1994* (London: Jonathan Cape, 2000)

Shorter, Edward, *A History of Psychiatry. From the era of the asylum to the age of Prozac* (New York: John Wiley & Sons, 1997)

Sinner, Louis, 'Na concentratiekamp sterker dan gemiddelde Nederlander', Algemeen Dagblad, 8-1-1977

'Slachtoffers concentratiekampen beleven gruwel weer op Duitse tv', *De Telegraaf*, 5-11-1966

'Slachtoffers geweld in de kou. Centrum '45 sluit deuren voor grote groep patiënten', *Het Parool*, 18-9-1987

'Slachtoffers in Ned.-Indië herdacht', *Het Parool*, 15-8-1980

'Slachtoffers van KZ-syndroom komen nu los. Vara en prof. dr. Bastiaans tevreden na uitzending', *Het Vrije Volk*, 28-2-1972

'"Slechte opvang van militairen uit Indonesië leidt nu tot trauma's"', *NRC Handelsblad*, 22-5-1987

'Sluiting dreigt voor kliniek van Bastiaans', *Leeuwarder Courant*, 13-4-1987

'Snel intensieve hulp voor ex-gijzelaars', *Het Nieuws van het Noorden*, 28-9-1981

Snelders, Stephen, 'The LSD Therapy Career of Jan Bastiaans, M.D.', *Newsletter of the Multidisciplinary Association for Psychedelic Studies*, 8, 1 (Spring 1998) 18-20

\- *LSD en de Psychiatrie in Nederland* (proefschrift UvA 1999)

Snelders, S., T. Pieters, 'De opkomst, val en mogelijke opkomst van LSD', *Tijdschrift voor Psychiatrie*, 62 (2020) 8, 707-711

'Snelle publikatie over KZ-syndroom', *De Tijd*, 8-3-1972

'Sociologisch onderzoek reacties op KZ-syndroom', *Tubantia*, 17-3-1972

Soetendorp, Awraham, 'Blijf kinderen van slachtoffers oorlog helpen!', *Het Parool*, 1-4-1986

Spaan, Henk, 'Goede raad is duur', *Het Parool*, 21-1-1981

Spanjer, Marjanke, 'Bastiaans: "Na abortus geen KZ-syndroom"', *NRC Handelsblad*, 31-10-1979

'Spanning en emotie tijdens hoorzitting', *De Tijd*, 25-2-1972
'Speciaal opvangteam', *Algemeen Dagblad*, 22-12-1975
'Speciaal vandaag', *De Telegraaf*, 7-6-1977
'Specialisten uren bezig met psycho-somatische ziekten', *Het Vrije Volk*, 30-7-1965
'Spoedig uitslag over pensioen E. Meester', *NRC Handelsblad*, 3-4-1976
Sprenger, W.H., 'Drie van Breda: verleden dat brandend actueel is', *De Volkskrant*, 27-3-1976
'Staalkaart van opvattingen over astma', *Trouw*, 2-6-1978
'Staatssecretaris installeert projectgroep. Nazorg gijzelaars gestart', *Algemeen Dagblad*, 15-1-1976
'Staatssecretaris reikt Centrum '45 helpende hand', *Nederlands Dagblad*, 21-6-1985
'Staatssecretaris Van der Reijden weigert toezegging. Behandelingsmethode niet verloren bij vertrek Bastiaans', *Trouw*, 28-2-1985
'Steeds meer aandacht voor Nazi-slachtoffers', *De Volkskrant*, 23-2-1972
Steen, Paul van der, 'Uithuilen aan de borst van papa Bas', *Trouw*, 4-4-2009
Steijns, M.J.E., 'Oud-Natzweilers', *Trouw*, 25-6-1966
Stein-Olman, Wilma, 'Isolement en bevrijding voor de medische boekenkast', *NIW*, 27-3-1987
'Stichting '40-'45 "is nog lang niet klaar met werk"', *Het Parool*, 11-5-1985
'Stichting '40-'45 blij met laat begrip voor oorlogsslachtoffers', *Trouw*, 6-10-1972
'Stichting voor slachtoffers van oorlog en geweld', *Algemeen Dagblad*, 20-6-1985
Stout, Gerrie, 'Kampsyndroom', *NRC Handelsblad*, 30-5-1980
'Stress kan oorzaak kanker zijn', *Het Parool*, 25-3-1983
'Stress kan oorzaak van kanker zijn', *Limburgsch Dagblad*, 26-3-1983
'"Stress oorzaak kanker"', *Algemeen Dagblad*, 25-3-1983
'Studenten', *Algemeen Dagblad*, 20-2-1965
'Studie methode-Bastiaans mislukt', *NRC Handelsblad*, 6-11-1987
'Stuyt twijfelt aan medische ethiek bij film KZ-syndroom', *Het Parool*, 12-4-1972
'Stuyt veroordeelt vertoning film over KZ-syndroom', *De Volkskrant*, 12-4-1972
'Stuyt: "Begrijpt u nu…" op televisie was onjuist', *Het Vrije Volk*, 12-4-1972
Summerfield, Derek, 'The invention of post-traumatic stress disorder and the social usefulness of a psychiatric category', *British Medical Journal*, 2001, 322

Swaan, A. de, 'Het onvermogen om te luisteren. Individuele kampervaringen en collectief onbegrip', *NRC Handelsblad*, 3-5-1980
'Syndroom', *De Telegraaf*, 22-11-1986
'Syndroom', *De Volkskrant*, 3-11-1979
'Syndroomfilm: 800 reacties', *NRC Handelsblad*, 28-2-1972

T

Tas, J., 'Psychotherapie en pharmaca', *NTvG*, 17-2-1968, 325-326
'Te weinig gegevens voor onderzoek van resultaten methode prof. Bastiaans', *Leeuwarder Courant*, 6-11-1987
'Tehuis voorlijders aan KZ-syndroom', *Nederlands Dagblad*, 18-4-1972
'Telefoon al tijdens uitzending Holocaust roodgloeiend', *Algemeen Dagblad*, 4-5-1979
'Telefoon roodgloeiend na derde deel Holocaust', *Algemeen Dagblad*, 30-4-1979
'Televisienieuws', *NRC Handelsblad*, 23-2-1972
'Televizier Magazine', *Het Nieuws van het Noorden,* 26-3-1983
'Televizier', *NRC Handelsblad*, 24-10-1980
'Televizier-Magazine over jaar gijzelaars in Iran', *Leeuwarder Courant*, 24-10-1980
'Terroristen zoeken naar nieuwe vormen van actie', *Trouw*, 28-9-1981
'Terug naar Alfaques om afstand te kunnen nemen', *De Telegraaf*, 14-7-1979
Terwindt, Trix, 'Bastiaans', *Het Parool*, 25-5-1973
- 'Syndroom', *De Telegraaf*, 9-5-1984
- 'Bastiaans', *De Telegraaf*, 15-3-1985
Thomas, Gregory M., *Treating the Trauma of the Great War. Soldiers, civilians, and psychiatry in France, 1914-1940* (Baton Rouge: Louisiana State UP, 2009)
Thomassen, Michel, 'Universiteit van Leiden ontslaat directeur kliniek', *Algemeen Dagblad*, 19-1-1983
'Tien jaar na Wijster', *Leeuwarder Courant*, 30-11-1985
Tijn, M. van, 'Leven na een oorlog', *NIW*, 24-3-1972
Tijn, Philip van, 'Film terecht uitgezonden', *Het Vrije Volk*, 28-2-1972
Timmers, S., 'Vraagtekens bij de film "Begrijpt u nu waarom ik huil"', *NTvG*, 7-1-1970, 73
- 'Begrijpt u nu waarom ik huil?', *NTvG*, 18-2-1970, 779-780
'Toediening LSD bij behandelen patiënten voorlopig verboden', *De Volkskrant*, 4-2-1986
'Toezegging van gesprek maakt eind aan gijzeling', *Het Parool*, 20-12-1975

Toonen, Hans, 'In dienst van uitstervend oorlogsleed. ABP-directeur drs. F. Gudde aan het hoofd van uitkering slachtoffers 1940-'45', *Limburgsch Dagblad*, 28-11-1987
'Trieste gang van gefolterd leven', *Algemeen Dagblad*, 12-9-1962
'TROS bereidt zich voor op reacties TV serie Holocaust', *De Telegraaf*, 30-1-1979
'Tros brengt "Holocaust"', *Leeuwarder Courant*, 20-1-1979
'TROS dringt terecht aan op begeleiding van "Holocaust"', *Nederlands Dagblad*, 7-3-1979
'TROS zal de serie Holocaust niet uitstellen', *Trouw*, 8-2-1979
'Tros' informatie gaat aan te veel voorbij', *De Waarheid*, 21-4-1979
'Tuchtcollege pleit psychiater vrij', *De Volkskrant*, 8-10-1980
'Twee psychiaters moeten Bastiaans opvolgen', *De Telegraaf*, 13-2-1986
'Twee verzetslieden eisen vervolging van oud-kamerlid', *Algemeen Dagblad*, 11-1-1978
'Tweede kliniek Centrum '45', *Het Parool*, 20-6-1985
'Twijfel wint terrein', *Limburgsch Dagblad*, 24-2-1972
'Twijfels over film', *Het Nieuws van het Noorden,* 12-4-1972

U

Udink, Betsy, 'Verpleegster in de vleesfabriek Vietnam', *De Volkskrant*, 27-4-1985
'Uit de Gooise lucht gegrepen', *De Telegraaf*, 23-2-1972 / 28-2-1972
'Uit de weekbladen', *Trouw*, 1-2-1979
'"Uitkering burgeroorlogsslachtoffers een lijdensweg"', *Het Vrije Volk*, 25-10-1986
'Uitvlucht', *De Waarheid*, 18-8-1975
'Universiteit wil na 1 juni van hoogleraar af. Toekomst werk Bastiaans onzeker', *De Volkskrant*, 29-3-1985

V

Vaal, O.M. de, 'LSD als helper van de psychiater', *Het Parool*, 17-5-1969
Vaders, Ger, 'Moet dat nou, Holocaust', *Het Nieuws van het Noorden,* 6-4-1979
- 'Einde van een illusie', *Het Nieuws van het Noorden,* 29-9-1981
- 'Prof. Bastiaans. Vaders' visie', *Het Nieuws van het Noorden,* 12-2-1986

'Van der Reijden (WVC): "Behoud van methode-Bastiaans nog onzeker"', *Het Nieuws van het Noorden,* 28-3-1985
'Van der Reijden bereid Centrum '45 uit te breiden', *De Waarheid*, 21-6-1985

'Van der Reijden regelt opvolgen Bastiaans niet', *Algemeen Dagblad*, 13-2-1986
'Van der Reijden voor methode van Bastiaans', *NRC Handelsblad*, 28-2-1985
'Van der Reijden weigert garantie aanblijven prof. Bastiaans', *Leeuwarder Courant*, 28-2-1985
'Van der Reijden: voortzetting werk Bastiaans onzeker', *Algemeen Dagblad*, 28-2-1985
'Van Gasteren filmde medische verkenning met LSD', *De Telegraaf*, 16-5-1969
'Vara blijft erbij: LSP-groep slecht', *Algemeen Dagblad*, 15-4-1981
'Veel emoties op hoorzitting "drie" Breda', *NRC Handelsblad*, 25-2-1972
'Veel extra leed oorlogsslachtoffers', *Het Vrije Volk*, 1-6-1977
'Veel kritiek op procedure Aantjes', *Limburgsch Dagblad*, 10-11-1978
'Veel slachtoffers verkeren nu in uitputtingsfase', *Limburgsch Dagblad*, 13-12-1978
Veen, Evelien van, 'Het trauma zit in het hele lichaam', *De Volkskrant*, 16-10-2021
Veld, N.K.C.A. in 't Veld, *De Zuivering van Artsen en Advocaten. Een bijdrage tot de geschiedschrijving van de zuivering van het vrije beroep* (The Hague: SDU, 1983)
Velden, D. van, *De Japanse burgerkampen* (Franeker: Wever, 1977)
Veltkamp, J.J., 'Kan prof. Bastiaans echt niet weg?', *De Volkskrant*, 27-3-1985
'"Verbijsterend wat kinderen van NSB'ers na de oorlog is aangedaan"', *Het Parool*, 13-1-1983
'Verbod op kuren met hallucinerende middelen', *Trouw*, 4-2-1986
Verburgh, H.S., 'Prof Bastiaans in conflict met Leidse universiteit. "Ik heb een symbolische functie…"', *NRC Handelsblad*, 27-1-1983
Verhoog, Gertjan, 'Kinderen uit Jappenkamp worstelen met vergeten jeugd', *Leeuwarder Courant*, 7-6-1986
'Verhouding stemmen in kamer nog onduidelijk', *Trouw*, 25-2-1972
'Verleden kamerlid onder de loep', *Algemeen Dagblad*, 2-4-1976
'Verontrusting over lot van psychiaters in de Sovjet-Unie', *Het Parool*, 18-4-1978
'Vertoont het post-abortus-syndroom overeenkomst met het KZ-syndroom?', *Nederlands Dagblad*, 1-11-79
'Verzet bepleit voortzetting van therapie Bastiaans', *De Volkskrant*, 27-2-1985
'Verzet is ongerust over trage behandeling werk van professor Bastiaans', *De Telegraaf*, 13-12-1985

'Verzet tegen gratie voor de laatste Duitse oorlogsmisdadigers', *Algemeen Handelsblad*, 14-11-1963
'Verzetsgroepen in actie tegen Stichting '40-'45', *Het Vrije Volk*, 18-2-1984
'Verzoek van Centrum '45 aan TROS: "Stel uitzending Holocaust uit"', *De Waarheid*, 8-2-1979
Voituron, Gerard, 'Gijzelaars bedreigd door kampsyndroom', *Algemeen Dagblad*, 29-10-1980
Vonderen, J.P. van, 'Brief van oud-vrijwilliger basis voor documentaire', *De Telegraaf*, 22-11-1973
Voolen, Edward van, 'Wiesenthals jubileum herdacht met bundel essays', *NIW*, 7-6-1974
'Voor milieu gevaarlijke produkten belast', *Leeuwarder Courant*, 12-4-1972
'Voor opvolging prof. Bastiaans 2 kandidaten', *Het Parool*, 13-2-1986
'Voormalig verzetsstrijdster Trix Terwindt overleden', *De Volkskrant*, 10-4-1987
'Voorstanders door anonymi bestookt. Zware dreigementen tegen kamerleden', *De Telegraaf*, 25-2-1972
'Voorstanders vrijlating door luid geschreeuw onderbroken', *Leeuwarder Courant*, 25-2-1972
'Voorstel Bastiaans over Centrum '45: "Via universiteit samenwerking kliniek regelen"', *Het Parool*, 25-5-1973
'Voortzetting van therapie Bastiaans is nog onzeker', *Het Nieuws van het Noorden,* 28-2-1985
'Voorwaarden aan LSD therapie. Kamer bezorgd over voortzetting werk Bastiaans', *Het Nieuws van het Noorden,* 6-2-1986
'Vragen over Centrum '45', *Algemeen Dagblad*, 18-5-1973
'Vragen over film KZ-syndroom', *Tubantia*, 12-4-1972
Vreede, Mathijs de, 'Echtpaar uit syndroomfilm zat gespannen te kijken', *Het Parool*, 29-2-1972
- 'Na dertig jaar nog niet vrij', *Het Parool*, 3-5-1975
Vries, H.R. de, 'Bijsmaak', *De Volkskrant*, 30-5-1969
'*Vrij Nederland*: zwarte handel', *Trouw*, 9-9-1976
'Vrijlaten "drie" nog steeds onhaalbaar', *De Volkskrant*, 17-3-1976
Vroom, M.G., *Schrik, Angst en Vrees: Een psychiatrische en phenomenologische studie naar aanleiding van vliegtuigbombardementen* (Den Helder: C. de Boer, 1942)
Vroon, Piet, 'Binnenvetters', *De Volkskrant*, 2-4-1983
- 'Luchtje', *De Volkskrant*, 5-11-1983
- 'Geurtjes', *De Volkskrant*, 4-5-1985
- 'LSD', *De Volkskrant*, 1-2-1986

'Vrouw die twee kinderen ombracht voor rechtbank', *Het Parool*, 12-9-1962
'Vrouwen van de Drie zijn verdwenen', *Het Vrije Volk*, 29-2-1972

W
'"Waanzin", zegt Leidse prof', *De Telegraaf*, 10-12-1964
Wallagh, Constant, 'Indrukwekkend verslag van Van Gasteren', *Algemeen Dagblad*, 15-5-1969
Waltmans, Astrid, 'Overeem, Emmy van (1931-2012)' (Resources.huygens.knaw.nl/vrouwenlexicon/lemmata/data/Overeem (seen: 16-3-2021))
'Was moeder niet toerekenbaar voor moord op zoontjes?', *Limburgsch Dagblad*, 12-9-1962
'Wat hebben jullie met onze meisjes gedaan', *Limburgsch Dagblad*, 14-7-1978
'"Wat hebben jullie met onze meisjes gedaan?" Over Max Bueno de Mesquita', *Leeuwarder Courant*, 13-7-1978
'We hebben 't juist uitstekend gedaan', *Het Vrije Volk*, 31-12-1977
'Weduwe Donker ontkent handeltje met Menten', *De Waarheid*, 7-12-1978
'Weekbladen', *De Volkskrant*, 27-3-1975 / 22-12-1976 / 11-4-1985 / 16-7-1987
'Weekbladen van week tot week', *Leeuwarder Courant*, 27-3-1975 / 2-5-1975 / 23-12-1976
'Weekbladeren', *Leeuwarder Courant*, 12-4-1979 / 2-8-1984 / 4-9-1987
Welgraven, Co, 'Wat 25 jaar na zijn dood vooral beklijft: Ischa Meijer schond de norm dat je oorlogsslachtoffers ontziet', *Trouw*, 29-1-2020
Wennekes, Wim, *Allemaal rottigheid allemaal ellende. Het KZ-syndroom van Willem van Salland* (Amsterdam: Wetenschappelijke uitgeverij, 1975)
'Werk Bastiaans zal worden voortgezet', *NIW*, 5-4-1985
'Werkgroep onderzoekt concentratiekampsyndroom', *Trouw*, 16-1-1971
'Werkgroep onderzoekt post-concentratiekampsyndroom', *Trouw*, 23-12-1970
'Werkgroep voor behandeling concentratiekampslachtoffers', *De Waarheid*, 15-1-1971
'Werkgroep wil voortzetting van therapie prof. Bastiaans', *Trouw*, 30-1-1984
Westerman Holstijn, A.J., 'Ziekte en verzet', *Het Parool*, 23-3-1957
'Wetenschap die problemen van hele mensheid raakt. Geslaagd psycho-analytisch congres', *Algemeen Dagblad*, 31-7-1965

Wibaut, F., 'Psychische zieken probleem voor sociale zorg', *Het Parool*, 6-8-1955
Wiese, Kees, 'Te veel publiciteit?', *Het Nieuws van het Noorden,* 29-11-1980
Wigbold, Herman, 'De hoofd- en bijzaken in de affaire-Aantjes', *Het Vrije Volk*, 10-11-1978
Wild, Kees van der, 'Kamerlid H.J.L. Vonhoff: "Categorie verzetsmensen schandalig achtergesteld"', *De Telegraaf*, 9-12-1970
Wilke, Jürgen, 'Die Fernsehserie "Holocaust" als Medienereignis', *Historical Social Research*, 30 (2005), 4, 9-17
Willems, Menzo, 'Libanon-syndroom na gewelddadige ervaringen. Veel Unifillers in geestelijke nood', *De Telegraaf*, 25-10-1986
- 'Prof. Bastiaans (70) staakt met tegenzin zijn controversiële werkwijze', *De Telegraaf*, 31-10-1987
Wilschut, Johannes, *Tussen Psychiatrie en Filosofie. De dynamische psychiatrie van Eugène A.D.E. Carp (1895-1983)* (Amsterdam: proefschrift Vrije Universiteit, 1998)
Wind, Eddy de, *Eindstation… Auschwitz* (Amsterdam: Republiek der Letteren, 1946)
- 'Confrontatie met de Dood', *Folia Psychiatrica, Neurologica et Neurochirurgica Neerlandica*, 52 (1949), December, 459-466
- 'Overleven – veertig jaar later', *NRC Handelsblad*, 14-2-1981
- 'De onvoorspelbaarheid van het late optreden van oorlogstrauma's. De halve waarheden van Schudel', *NRC Handelsblad*, 22-4-1987
Witsen, E. van, *Krijgsgevangenen in de Pacific-oorlog* (Franeker: Wever, 1971)
Withuis, Jolande, *Erkenning. Van oorlogstrauma naar klaagcultuur* (Amsterdam: De Bezige Bij, 2002)
- *Weest manlijk, zijt sterk* (Amsterdam: De Bezige Bij, 2009)
- 'De opmars van het slachtoffer', *Trouw*, 28-11-2009
- 'Opkomst en neergang van PTSS. Een sociologische duiding van het succes van de posttraumatische stressstoornis', *Directieve Therapie*, 30 (2010) 149-159
Withuis, Jolande, Annet Mooij, 'From Totalitarianism to Trauma', in: Jolande Withuis, Annet Mooij (eds.), *The Politics of War Trauma. The aftermath of World War II in eleven European countries* (Amsterdam: Aksant, 2010), pp. 193-239
- 'Conclusion', in: Withuis, Mooij (eds.), *The Politics of War Trauma*, 323-331
Wolff, F., 'Bastiaans', *Het Parool*, 3-12-1987

Woltz, W., 'Buitenlandse deskundigen: bewondering voor snelle besluitvorming', *NRC Handelsblad*, 18-6-1977
Woltz, W., 'Trip naar "42"', *Algemeen Handelsblad*, 7-6-1969
'Wrok maar ook begrip', *Limburgsch Dagblad*, 7-12-1985

Y
Young, Allan, *The Harmony of Illusions. Inventing Post-Traumatic Stress Disorder* (Princeton: Princeton UP, 1995)

Z
'Zes verslagen LSD therapieën', *NRC Handelsblad*, 21-3-1975
'"Zij zijn erg eenzaam"', *Algemeen Dagblad*, 14-8-1982
'Zware keus vanavond', *Het Parool*, 22-11-1973
Zweden, G.C. van, 'Dodenkamp Sobibor aan de vergetelheid ontrukt', *Trouw*, 24-4-1979

ABBREVIATIONS

ADHD	Attention Deficit Hyperactivity Disorder
ARP	Anti-Revolutionary Party
BNMO	Association of Dutch Military War Victims
CBOG	Central Policy and Support Group for the Aftercare of Former Hostages / Committee on Guidance and Reception of Hostages
CDA	Christian Democratic Appeal
CIA	Central Intelligence Agency
COVID	Corona Virus Disease
COVVS	Central Body Former Resistance and Victims
CPN	Communist Party Netherlands
CRM	Culture, Recreation and Social Work
DS'70	Democratic Socialists 1970
DSM	Diagnostic and Statistical Manual of Mental Disorders
EESS	Existential Emotional Stress Syndrome
EO	Evangelical Broadcasting
ICODO	Information and Coordination Body for War Victims for Service and Relief to War Victims
ISOG	International Foundation for the Victims of War and Violence
JMW	Jewish Social Work
KGB	Committee for State Security)
KL	KonzentrationsLager (concentration camp)
KRO	Catholic Radio Broadcasting
KVP	Catholic People's Party
KZ	KonZentrationslager (concentration camp)
LSD	Lyserg-Säure-Diathylamid
NAV	Dutch Doctors Association
NCRV	Dutch Christian Radio Association
NIOD	Netherlands Institute for War Documentation
NIPG	Netherlands Institute for Preventive Medicine
NIW	New Israeli Weekly
NRC	New Rotterdam Daily
NSB	National Socialist Movement
NTvG	Dutch Journal of Medicine

NVO	Dutch Association of War Victims
PAI	Psycho-Analytical Institute
PSP	Pacifist Socialist Party
PTSD	Post-Traumatic Stress Disorder
PTT	Post, Telegraph and Telephone
PvdA	Labour Party
RMS	Republik Maluku Selatan (Republic of South Maluku)
SS	Schutzstaffel
TROS	Television & Radio Broadcasting Foundation
USSR	Union of Soviet Socialist Republics (Soviet Union)
UvA	University of Amsterdam
VARA	United Workers Radio Amateurs
UN	United Nations
VVD	People's Party for Freedom and Democracy
WAC	Tutorial and Advisory Board for intangible assistance to war victims
WBP	Extraordinary Pension Act
WPA	World Psychiatric Association
WUV	Benefits Act for Persecution Victims
WVF	World Veterans Federation

ENDNOTES

Epigraph

1: Drayer, 'Hoe het kamp het bestaan vergiftigde', 3-4-2010
2: Haijtema, 'Overlevingskunst', 9-4-2021
3: Van Veen, 'Het trauma zit in het hele lichaam'
4: Bastiaans, 'Het KZ-syndroom en de menselijke vrijheid', 1173

Introduction

1: Kater, 'Concentratiekamp-syndroom', 30-5-1964
2: 'Centrum voor behandeling van KZ-syndroom officieel geopend', 16-5-1973; Renate Katz, 'Kliniek "Het Centrum" voor oorlogsslachtoffers geopend', 18-5-1973; Groen-Prakken, 'Trauma en ontwikkelingsinterferentie'; Crocq, Crocq, 'From shell shock', 52-53
3: Kater, 'Concentratiekamp-syndroom', 30-5-1964; Van den Ende, '*Vergeet niet dat je arts bent*', 161; Aarts, De geschiedenis', 26-27
4: Bastiaans, 'Het KZ-syndroom en de menselijke vrijheid'
5: Snelders, 'The LSD Therapy Career of Jan Bastiaans, M.D.', 18-20
6: Enning, *De Oorlog van Bastiaans*, 97
7: Withuis, *Erkenning*, 91-92, 106-107; Cohen, *Het Duitse Concentratiekamp*, 107
8: Kater, 'Concentratiekamp-syndroom', 30-5-1964; Van den Ende, *'Vergeet niet dat je arts bent'*, 272
9: Quoted from: Van der Hart, Broeze, 'Posttraumatische stress', 25
10: Lerner, *Hysterical Men*, 74-79
11: Van Bergen, *Pro Patria et Patienti*, 277-279; Loth, *De Militaire Psychiatrie in de Krijgsmacht*
12: Cohen, *Het Duitse Concentratiekamp*, IX
13: Snelders, Pieters, 'De opkomst, val en mogelijke opkomst vanLSD', 709; Withuis, *Erkenning*, 93, 102, 120, 138, 239-240; Withuis, 'De opmars van het slachtoffer'; Mooij, 'De langste schaduw', 263, 268; Van der Hart et al., 'Psychotraumatologie', 46-47
14: Withuis, *Erkenning*, 29

15: Bastiaans, *Psychosomatische Gevolgen*, 461-466; Withuis, *Erkenning*, 33-34; Mooij, 'De langste schaduw', 272; Van der Hart et al., 'Psychotraumatologie', 48
16: Kater, 'Concentratiekamp-syndroom', 30-5-1964
17: Hij was de opvolger van Eugéne Carp. Wilschut, *Tussen Psychiatrie en Filosofie*; Rooijmans, *99 Jaar tussen Wal en Schip*, 49-94
18: Snelders, *LSD en de Psychiatrie in Nederland*, 198-199
19: Van Voolen, 'Wiesenthals jubileum herdacht', 7-6-1974; Bastiaans, 'Vom Menschen'; Mooij, 'Bastiaans, Jan'
20: In the Auschwitz guest book an entry of June 1980 reads: 'From people in concentration camps to the concentration camp in people', signed: J. Bastiaans. Amesz, 'Er staan nu bloemen voor de ramen van de commandant…', 26-6-1980; 'Bloemen voor de ramen van de kommandatur', 28-6-1980
21: 'Leidse professor gaf oorlogsveteraan zijn geheugen terug', 23-9-1974
22: Grijpma, 'Na 35 jaar weerzien met Auschwitz', 25-6-1980; Amesz, 'Er staan nu bloemen voor de ramen van de commandant…', 26-6-1980; 'Bloemen voor de ramen van de kommandatur', 28-6-1980
23: Lardenoye, 'Indiëveteraan', 6, 8
24: Enning, *De Oorlog van Bastiaans*, 29-30
25: Andere Tijden, 'Bastiaans'
26: De Wind, *Eindstation... Auschwitz*, 171; Withuis, Mooij, 'From totalitarianism to trauma', 200-1
27: Verburgh, 'Prof Bastiaans in conflict met Leidse universiteit', 27-1-1983; Kaas, *Buchenwald*, 118-119; Piersma, *De Drie van Breda*, 106
28: Andere Tijden, 'Bastiaans'
29: 'Moeder vergaste haar zoontjes', 12-9-1962; 'Trieste gang van gefolterd leven', 12-9-1962; 'Vrouw die twee kinderen ombracht voor rechtbank', 12-9-1962; 'Afgrijselijke jeugdervaring bracht geobsedeerde vrouw tot kindermoord', 12-9-1962; 'Officier eist plaatsing in een inrichting', 12-9-1962; 'Was moeder niet toerekenbaar voor moord op zoontjes?', 12-9-1962; 'Geen vervolging van vrouw die kinderen doodde', 25-9-1962
30: 'Gestoord gevoelsleven ook zaak voor de huisarts', 9-10-1965
31: 'NOS-radio met documentaires over zelfmoord', 28-2-1974
32: 'Staalkaart van opvattingen over astma', 2-6-1978
33: '"Afdoen schade duurt te lang"', 24-10-1981; Buijze, 'De patiënt is altijd gestoord', 31-10-1981; Groenendijk, 'Vaak klap na voor verkeersslachtoffers', 29-12-1983
34: Van der Hooff, 'Jan Bastiaans en het contactisolement', 10-6-1985/13-6-1985. Also: Bastiaans, *Isolement en bevrijding*, 68-86

35: 'Prof. Bastiaans over voorspellende waarde kankerpersoonlijkheid', 25-3-1983; Boer, 'Stress', 17-3-1983; '"Stress oorzaak kanker"', 25-3-1983; 'Hoogleraar wijst op onderzoeken', 25-3-1983; 'Stress kan oorzaak kanker zijn', 25-3-1983; De Jong, 'Meer kans op kanker bij rustige mensen', 25-3-1983; 'Prof. J. Bastiaans op symposium: Stress', 25-3-1983; 'Onderzoek zegt: Stress', 25-3-1983; Nietsch, 'Niets mogen doen', 25-3-1983; 'Prof Bastiaans op symposium: spanningen', 26-3-1983; 'Hoogleraar psychiatrie prof. J. Bastiaans: in 70 procent', 26-3-1983; 'Televizier Magazine', 26-3-1983; 'Stress kan oorzaak van kanker zijn', 26-3-1983; Blokker, 'Loch Ness', 26-3-1983; Vroon, 'Binnenvetters', 2-4-1983; Dunning, 'Altijd wat', 21-4-1983; 't Hart, 'De overijlde resignatie', 9-6-1983; Vroon, 'Luchtje', 5-11-1983; Boer, 'Bestaat er een bepaalde kankerpersoonlijkheid?', 2-2-1984; Ree, 'Arts en Auto', 7-2-1984; De Moulin, 'Kankerpersoonlijkheid (2)', 23-3-1984

36: '"Man in gezin vaak op tweede plaats"', 14-5-1960

37: 'De mens van nu wordt steeds egocentrischer', 9-12-1969

38: Peereboom, 'De protesterende jongeren stemmen psychiater Bastiaans niet optimistisch', 12-9-1970

39: '"Als Bastiaans gelijk heeft stopt de LSP"', 27-3-1981; Van de Poel, 'Zo mag ik 't zien', 27-3-1981; 'Vara blijft erbij: LSP-groep slecht', 15-4-1981; 'Prof. Bastiaans ontkent verklaring in kort geding', 15-4-1981

40: F.i.: 'Klacht tegen Bastiaans na behandeling', 7-9-1979; '"Als Bastiaans gelijk heeft stopt de LSP"', 27-3-1981; 'Bastiaans mag tot in 1985 behandelen', 5-2-1983; Nietsch, 'Bastiaans', 5-2-1983; 'Bastiaans blijft bij Jelgersmakliniek', 8-2-1983

41: Van Kessel, 'De wetenschap tript weer', 21-5-2016; Mitchell et al., 'MDMA-assisted therapy for severe PTSD'; Lu, '"Psychedelics renaissance"'; Busby, 'Will the magic of psychedelics'

42: Van der Kolk, *The Body Keeps the Score*, 225-226; Van Veen, 'Het trauma zit in het hele lichaam'

43: Shorter, *A History of Psychiatry*, 264

44: Wilschut, *Tussen Psychiatrie en Filosofie*, 200 (incl. noot 187)

45: Snelders, Pieters, 'De opkomst, val en mogelijke opkomst vanLSD', 707; Mooij, 'De langste schaduw', 273; Piersma, *De Drie van Breda*, 107

46: Enning, *De Oorlog van Bastiaans*, 127

47: Laudy, 'Bevrijder uit het innerlijke kamp'; Bossenbroek, *De Meelstreep*, 573. For Bastiaans and his usage of LSD, see: Snelders, *LSD en de Psychiatrie in Nederland*, 98-124

48: Shorter, *A History of Psychiatry*, 264-265; Mooij, 'Bastiaans, Jan'

49: 'LSD beschadigt de chromosomen'; 'LSD en chromosomen'

50: Snelders, *LSD en de Psychiatrie in Nederland*, 8-9, 197-202 (Handelseditie: *LSD therapie in Nederland*)
51: Snelders, *LSD en de Psychiatrie in Nederland*
52: Kleijer, 'Geen jager, maar prooi', 11-2-2021
53: Meulenberg, 'Het experiment met LSD therapie, 2-8-2000
54: Snelders, Pieters, 'De opkomst, val en mogelijke opkomst vanLSD', 708-710; Snelders, *LSD Therapie In Nederland*; Bogers, Snelders, Plomp, *De Psychedelische (R)evolutie*
55: See f.i. also the book *U wordt door Niemand Verwacht* of Michal Citroen who will have been one of the last persons to interview Bastiaans.
56: Romme, 'Van Bastiaans tot nu', 4; Interview Allart Bastiaans, 5-10-2020
57: Enning, *De Oorlog van Bastiaans*
58: F.i.: Kaas, *Buchenwald*, 21
59: F.i.: Citroen, *U wordt door Niemand Verwacht*, 151-152
60: Braber, 'Ontsnapt aan deportatie', 26-4-1983
61: Withuis, *Erkenning*, 109-116, 136, 189; Hondius, *Terugkeer*.
62: Withuis, *Erkenning*, 121-123. On the Breda Three discussion, see: Piersma, *De Drie van Breda*
63: Withuis, Mooij, 'From totalitarianism to trauma'; Withuis, Mooij, 'Conclusion', 325
64: Withuis, *Erkenning*, 31; Withuis, Mooij, 'From Totalitarianism to trauma', 198-9, 203-4
65: Enning, *De Oorlog van Bastiaans*, 105; Withuis, *Erkenning*, 235; Withuis, Mooij, 'From totalitarianism to trauma', 211
66: Gersons, 'Traumaspectrumstoornissen', 76-77
67: Milikowski, 'Het KZ-syndroom', 108-109; Withuis, *Erkenning*, 55-56
68: Withuis, *Erkenning*, 170-171
69: Binneveld, *Om de Geest van Jan Soldaat*, 239
70: Gersons, 'Traumaspectrumstoornissen', 74-76
71: Udink, 'Verpleegster in de vleesfabriek Vietnam', 27-4-1985; Baarda, 'Vrede met Vietnam', 28-3-1987; Van der Hart, Broeze, 'Posttraumatische stress', 34; Van der Hart et al., 'Psychotraumatologie', 49; Gersons, 'Traumaspectrumstoornissen', 69, 72-73
72: Van der Hart, Broeze, 'Posttraumatische stress', 26; Withuis, 'Opkomst en neergang van PTSS'
73: Gersons, 'Traumaspectrumstoornissen', 69
74: Van Overeem, 'Oorlog duurt voort in Centrum '45', 14-5-1973; Van Overeem, 'De druppel die de emmer doet overlopen', 29-10-1979; Blijham, 'Het dilemma van het existentieel getraumatiseerd zijn'; Withuis, *Erkenning*, 52, 55, 213

75: Hovens, Van der Ploeg, 'Hoe het trauma het gewone leven binnendrong', 809
76: Jones, Wessely, *Shell Shock to PTSD*, 193, 208; Montgomery, *The Invisible Injured*, 215; Young, *The Harmony of Illusions*; Thomas, *Treating the Trauma of the Great War*
77: Van Bergen, *Zacht en Eervol*, 257-290
78: Cohen, *Het Duitse Concentratiekamp*, 39-40
79: Kousbroek,'Terug naar Negri Panerkomst 21'; Kousbroek, *Het Oostindisch Kampsyndroom*, 366; De Jong, 'Impressies uit Japanse hel goed onderbouwd', 15-6-1983
80: Kousbroek, *Het Oostindisch Kampsyndroom*, 370; Scagliola, *Last van de Oorlog*, 13, 112-113
81: Withuis, *Erkenning*, 123
82: Kousbroek, *Het Oostindisch Kampsyndroom*, 369-370; Komrij, 'Een en ander', 2-2-1983
83: Komrij, 'Een en ander', 2-2-1983. Also: Van der Steen, 'Uithuilen aan de borst van papa Bas', 4-4-2009; Hartmans, 'Schimmige herinneringen'
84: Kuipers, 'Groninger drukker vraagt helderziende om adviezen', 20-5-1981
85: Haveman, 'De eeuw van het oorlogstrauma', 24-4-1999
86: Enning, *De Oorlog van Bastiaans*, 179-181
87: Withuis, *Erkenning*, 88
88: For this see: Dehue, *De Depressie-epIbidemie*
89: Hovens, Van der Ploeg, 'Hoe het trauma het gewone leven binnendrong', 804
90: Withuis, *Erkenning*, 57-58; Mooij, 'De langste schaduw', 288.

1. The first reports about the KZ syndrome and Bastiaans' thesis

1: Kater, 'Concentratiekamp-syndroom', 30-5-1964; '"Psychologische gevolgen van oorlogservaringen veel te laat ontdekt"', 8-5-1985; psychotraumanet.org/nl/de-thematiek-van-trauma-en-oorlog-analystische-kring; Mooij, 'De langste schaduw', 263; Hondius, *Terugkeer*, 170, Van der Hart et al, 'Psychotraumatologie', 48; Withuis, Mooij, 'From totalitarianism to trauma', 199-200
2: Vroom, *Schrik, Angst en Vrees*; Van der Hart et al., 'Psychotraumatologie', 47
3: F.i.: Meerloo, *Homo Militans*, 5; Meerloo, *Total War*; Withuis, *Erkenning*, 20; Mooij, 'De langste schaduw', 261-262; Enning, *De oorlog*

van Bastiaans, 97; Van der Hart et al., 'Psychotraumatologie', 47; Hondius, *Terugkeer*, 86; Withuis, Mooij, 'From totalitarianism to trauma', 201
4: Cohen, *Het Duitse Concentratiekamp*, IX, 231-232; Van der Hart et al., 'Psychotraumatologie', 48
5: Cohen, *Het Duitse Concentratiekamp*, XI
6: Cohen, 'Het post-concentratiekampsyndroom', 1969/1972
7: Kleyn, 'Elke dag krijg je wel een flits van het concentratiekamp', 11-1-1986
8: Kaas, 'De Duitse concentratiekampen'
9: Kaas, *Buchenwald*, 11, 18, 121-123; Kaas, 'Over de psychologie'; De Ridder, Withuis, '"Scheldend op mezelf"'
10: De Wind, *Eindstation... Auschwitz*, 172
11: De Wind, 'Confrontatie met de Dood'
12: De Wind, 'Overleven – veertig jaar later', 14-2-1981; Withuis, *Erkenning*, 7, 37-40, 44; Mooij, 'De langste schaduw', 279; Van der Hart et al., 'Psychotraumatologie', 48
13: Cohen, 'Kampgevolgen', 29-1-1965
14: Mooij, 'De langste schaduw', 268-270; Withuis, Mooij, 'From totalitarianism to trauma', 201-2; Enning, *De Oorlog van Bastiaans*, 93; Van der Hart et al., 'Psychotraumatologie', 48-49
15: 'Geestelijk gestoorde PTT-beambte verduisterde twintig mille', 17-2-1954
16: Matussek, *Die Konzentrationslagerhaft*, 267
17: 'Concentratiekampziekte tast de hersenen aan', 30-10-1954; Milikowski, 'Het KZ-syndroom', 87
18: Andere Tijden, 'Bastiaans'
19: In 't Veld, *De Zuivering van Artsen*, 20-21; Van den Ende, '*Vergeet niet dat je arts bent*', 274
20: 'Gevolgen van de hongerwinter en de kampen', 4-3-1955; 'Late gevolgen van concentratiekamp', 4-3-1955
21: Wibaut, 'Psychische zieken probleem voor sociale zorg', 6-8-1955
22: F.i.: 'Examens', 2-2-1957
23: Bastiaans, *Psychosomatische Gevolgen van Onderdrukking en Verzet*
24: Rooijmans, *99 Jaar tussen Wal en Schip*, 88, 101
25: Matussek, *Die Konzentrationslagerhaft*
26: Westerman Holstijn, 'Ziekte en verzet', 23-3-1957; Aarts, 'De geschiedenis', 27
27: Enning, *De Oorlog van Bastiaans*, 38
28: Musaph, 'Late reacties op oorlogsleed', 29-3-1957
29: Westerman Holstijn, 'Ziekte en verzet', 23-3-1957

30: Also: 'Psychische factor belangrijk bij behandeling van astma', 30-12-1958
31: Van Loggem, 'Ex-illegalen lijden vaak aan psychische ziekten', 2-2-1957; Westerman Holstijn, 'Ziekte en verzet', 23-3-1957
32: Van Reemst, 'Arts schreef proefschrift over ziekten uit verzet '40-'45', 7-2-1957; Bolwijn, 'Reemst'
33: Enning, *De Oorlog van Bastiaans*, 201
34: Van Reemst, 'Arts schreef proefschrift over ziekten uit verzet '40-'45', 7-2-1957
35: Ibidem
36: 'Commissie schadevergoeding Nazi-slachtoffers', 6-11-1959; 'Niet vrijlaten', 29-12-1959
37: 'Oproep voor onthulling museum in Ravensbrück', 19-5-1959; 'Monument Ravensbrück', 29-5-1959
38: 'Lages, Aus der Fünten en Kotälla mogen niet vrij!', 23-12-1959
39: 'Verzet tegen gratie voor de laatste Duitse oorlogsmisdadigers', 14-11-1963

2. Attention is increasing

1: 'Geestelijke stoornissen bij ex-concentratiekampgevangenen', 16-12-1961; Mooij, 'De langste schaduw', 271
2: 'Geestelijke stoornissen bij ex-concentratiekampgevangenen', 16-12-1961
3: Ibidem
4: 'Dr. Bastiaans hoogleraar psychiatrie', 11-11-1963; 'Dr. Bastiaans hoogleraar te Leiden', 12 -11-1963; For Heringa f.i. also; In 't Veld, *De Zuivering van Artsen*, 34-49
5: 'Komt 25 februari naar de Dokwerker!', 1-2-1964
6: Kater, 'Concentratiekamp-syndroom', 30-5-1964; Aarts, 'De geschiedenis', 23
7: Cohen, 'Kampgevolgen', 29-1-1965
8: Ibidem
9: 'Het post-concentratiekampsyndroom', 25-9-1970. Also: Van Os, *Liever dier dan mens*, 315-317, 337-339
10: Cohen, *Het Duitse Concentratiekamp*, 124-125
11: 'Psycho-analyse van regeringsbeleid', 10-12-1964; 'Beroering bij universiteiten over bouwstop. Leidse hoogleraren dringen aan op protest', 6-1-1965; 'Hoogleraar in psychiatrie: Beleid', 10-12-1964; '"Waanzin", zegt Leidse prof', 10-12-1964; 'Studenten', 20-2-1965

3. The psychoanalytic conference in Amsterdam in July 1965

1: 'Laat optredende gevolgen van oorlogsschade', 18-6-1965
2: 'Wetenschap die problemen van hele mensheid raakt', 31-7-1965
3: 'Leed van kampleven duurt nog voort', 31-7-1965; Withuis, *Erkenning*, 32-33
4: 'Wetenschap die problemen van hele mensheid raakt', 31-7-1965
5: 'Specialisten uren bezig met psycho-somatische ziekten', 30-7-1965
6: 'Wetenschap die problemen van hele mensheid raakt', 31-7-1965
7: 'Specialisten uren bezig met psycho-somatische ziekten', 30-7-1965
8: Interview Allart Bastiaans, 20-10-2020
9: 'Leed van kampleven duurt nog voort', 31-7-1965
10: 'Specialisten uren bezig met psycho-somatische ziekten', 30-7-1965
11: 'Psychisch leed – twintig jaar na de oorlog', 29-7-1965
12: Kaas, *Buchenwald*, 9; De Ridder, Withuis, '"Scheldend op mezelf"'; Enning, *De oorlog van Bastiaans*, 143
13: 'Psychisch leed – twintig jaar na de oorlog', 29-7-1965; 'Leed van kampleven duurt nog voort', 31-7-1965
14: 'Psychisch leed – twintig jaar na de oorlog', 29-7-1965
15: 'Slachtoffers concentratiekampen beleven gruwel weer op Duitse tv', 5-11-1966; 'De aangrijpende LSD film van prof. Bastiaans', 8-11-1966; 'Concentratiekampen eisen nog steeds slachtoffers', 2-3-1967; Milikowski, 'Het KZ-syndroom', 89; Enning, *De Oorlog van Bastiaans*, 116
16: 'Psychisch leed – twintig jaar na de oorlog', 29-7-1965
17: Ibidem
18: Ibidem
19: Ibidem
20: Steijns, 'Oud-Natzweilers', 25-6-1966; Withuis, *Weest manlijk, zijt sterk*, 360-361 (noot 63)

4. About LSD and the reverse burden of proof

1: Snelders, *LSD therapie in Nederland*
2: 'Slachtoffers concentratiekampen beleven gruwel weer op Duitse tv', 5-11-1966; 'De aangrijpende LSD film van prof. Bastiaans', 8-11-1966; 'Concentratiekampen eisen nog steeds slachtoffers', 2-3-1967
3: 'Slachtoffers concentratiekampen beleven gruwel weer op Duitse tv', 5-11-1966
4: 'Kinderen uit hongerwinter nu nog gestoord', 5-11-1966
5: 'De aangrijpende LSD film van prof. Bastiaans', 8-11-1966

6: Ibidem
7: Ibidem
8: 'LSD hulp voor KZ-patiënten', 21-3-1975
9: 'De aangrijpende LSD film van prof. Bastiaans', 8-11-1966
10: Heijermans, 'Lijvig verhaal over LSD', 28-2-1967
11: 'Concentratiekampen eisen nog steeds slachtoffers', 2-3-1967
12: Ibidem
13: Ibidem
14: Ibidem
15: Enning, *De oorlog van Bastiaans*, 38-39, 149, 178, 296; Withuis, Mooij, 'From totalitarianism to trauma', 195-196, 208-9
16: Enning, *De oorlog van Bastiaans*, 180, 216
17: Withuis, *Erkenning*, 113
18: 'Pensioenrechten voor slachtoffers van concentratie-kampen bepleit', 22-2-1968; Aarts, 'De geschiedenis', 23

5. The movie *Do you now understand why I cry…*

1: youtube.com/watch?v=Fq4RuGLMIb4; Enning, *De Oorlog van Bastiaans*, 116-127
2: Peereboom, 'Begrijpt u nu waarom ik huil…', 17-5-1969
3: '"Begrijpt u nu waarom ik huil…"', 14-5-1969; 'Van Gasteren filmde medische verkenning met LSD', 16-5-1969
4: Van Emde Boas, 'Van Gasteren filmt het KZ-syndroom en velen moeten het zien', 17-5-1969
5: Peereboom, 'Begrijpt u nu waarom ik huil…', 17-5-1969; 'Slachtoffers van KZ-syndroom komen nu los', 28-2-1972; Enning, *De Oorlog van Bastiaans*, 123
6: Van Emde Boas, 'Van Gasteren filmt het KZ-syndroom en velen moeten het zien', 17-5-1969; 'Van Gasteren filmde medische verkenning met LSD', 16-5-1969
7: Van Emde Boas, 'Van Gasteren filmt het KZ-syndroom en velen moeten het zien', 17-5-1969; 'Van Gasteren filmde medische verkenning met LSD', 16-5-1969
8: Van Emde Boas, 'Van Gasteren filmt het KZ-syndroom en velen moeten het zien', 17-5-1969; 'Van Gasteren filmde medische verkenning met LSD', 16-5-1969
9: '"Begrijpt u nu waarom ik huil…"', 14-5-1969; Wallagh, 'Indrukwekkend verslag van Van Gasteren', 15-5-1969; 'Begrijpt u nu waarom ik huil', 16-5-1969
10: '"Begrijpt u nu waarom ik huil…"', 14-5-1969

11: '"Begrijpt u nu waarom ik huil…"', 14-5-1969; Wallagh, 'Indrukwekkend verslag van Van Gasteren', 15-5-1969
12: '"Begrijpt u nu waarom ik huil…"', 14-5-1969
13: Van Emde Boas, 'Van Gasteren filmt het KZ-syndroom en velen moeten het zien', 17-5-1969; Peereboom, 'Begrijpt u nu waarom ik huil…', 17-5-1969
14: 'De prijs van overleven', 2-5-2005; Van der Hart et al., 'Psychotraumatologie', 51
15: 'Een medisch document van de eerste orde', 14-5-1969; Sinner, 'Na concentratiekamp', 8-1-1977
16: Bröcker, 'De LSD controverse', 999; Snelders, *LSD en de Psychiatrie in Nederland*, 172-176
17: Booij, 'Farmacotherapie en psychotherapie'; Booij, 'Vraagstukken rondom de psychotherapie'; Snelders, *LSD en de Psychiatrie in Nederland*, 60-62, 178-191; Enning, *De Oorlog van Bastiaans*, 66, 86-87; Bossenbroek, *De Meelstreep*, 496-497
18: Bröcker, 'De LSD controverse'
19: Bröcker, 'Farmacotherapie en psychotherapie'; Van Ree, 'Gewoontevorming, verslaving en gewenning bij gebruik van alcohol, marihuana en LSD'; Van Ree, 'Een behandeling van een suïcidale patiënt met LSD 25'; Schuurman, 'Farmacotherapie en psychotherapie'; Van Praag, 'Hallucinogenen, het paard van Troje?'; Panhuysen, 'De ongewenste werkingen na het innemen van LSD'
20: Tas, 'Psychotherapie en pharmaca'; Van der Hoeden, 'Farmacotherapie en psychotherapie'
21: Timmers, 'Vraagtekens bij de film "Begrijpt u nu waarom ik huil"'; Bastiaans, 'Begrijpt u nu waarom ik huil?'; Timmers, 'Begrijpt u nu waarom ik huil?'
22: Van Bergen, *Van Genezen in Geloof*, 359-360, 381-386, 473-481, 589-590
23: Peereboom, 'Begrijpt u nu waarom ik huil…', 17-5-1969
24: Van Bueren, 'Begrijpt u nu waarom ik huil…', 16-5-1969
25: 'Moeten we 4 en 5 mei nog altijd vieren?', 3-5-1969
26: Van Bueren, 'Begrijpt u nu waarom ik huil…', 16-5-1969
27: 'Begrijpt u nu waarom ik huil', 16-5-1969
28: Wallagh, 'Indrukwekkend verslag van Van Gasteren', 15-5-1969
29: Ibidem
30: Bertina, 'Van Gasteren maakte geen objectief drama', 16-5-1969
31: Ibidem; Enning, *De Oorlog van Bastiaans*, 122
32: 'Concentratiekamp II', 20-5-1969

33: De Vaal, 'LSD als helper van de psychiater', 17-5-1969; Enning, *De Oorlog van Bastiaans*, 123
34: De Vries, 'Bijsmaak', 30-5-1969
35: Enning, *De Oorlog van Bastiaans*, 125
36: Ruyter, '"We horen vaak: Je moet niet zeuren"', 22-5-1969; Milikowski, 'Het KZ-syndroom', 197; Enning, *De Oorlog van Bastiaans*, 123
37: Ruyter, '"We horen vaak: Je moet niet zeuren"', 22-5-1969; For a much more critical review, written some years later, of as well Bastiaans as Van Gasteren's picture, see: Milikowski, 'Het KZ-syndroom'; Enning, *De Oorlog van Bastiaans*, 123
38: Bertina, 'Begrijpt u nu waarom ik huil', 30-5-1969
39: Ibidem
40: Ibidem
41: Ibidem
42: Woltz, 'Trip naar "42"', 7-6-1969.
43: Enning, *De Oorlog van Bastiaans*, 128
44: Kaas, *Buchenwald*, 43, 46, 49-50, 87-88, 100-105, 125, 138; De Ridder, Withuis, '"Scheldend op mezelf"'. The revese happened as well, by the way. Kaas, *Buchenwald*, 73
45: Woltz, 'Trip naar "42"', 7-6-1969
46: Heil, 'Drugs wekken emotie in Zürich', 16-1-1970
47: Verburgh, 'Prof Bastiaans in conflict met Leidse universiteit', 27-1-1983; Van Heerden, 'Het onduidelijke KZ-syndroom', 3-2-1983

6. The Working Group Camp Syndrome

1: 'Het post-concentratiekampsyndroom', 25-9-1970
2: Ibidem; Withuis, *Erkenning*, 93; Withuis, Mooij, 'From totalitarianism to trauma', 203
3: Withuis, *Erkenning*, 30
4: 'Het post-concentratiekampsyndroom', 25-9-1970
5: Van der Wild, 'Kamerlid H.J.L. Vonhoff', 9-12-1970
6: Ibidem
7: 'Werkgroep onderzoekt post-concentratiekampsyndroom', 23-12-1970; Mooij, 'De langste schaduw', 277
8: 'Werkgroep voor behandeling concentratiekampslachtoffers', 15-1-1971; 'Installatie werkgroep kampsyndroom', 15-1-1971; 'Werkgroep onderzoekt concentratiekampsyndroom', 16-1-1971
9: 'Werkgroep onderzoekt concentratiekampsyndroom', 16-1-1971
10: 'Installatie werkgroep kampsyndroom', 15-1-1971; 'Installatie van commissie voor kamp-syndroom', 16-1-1971

11: Also: 'Protesten tegen vrijlating "Drie"', 23-2-1972; Withuis, *Erkenning*, 40-41
12: Ruyter, 'Mr van de Poel', 30-3-1971
13: Ibidem
14: Ibidem
15: Ibidem
16: Ibidem; Withuis, Mooij, 'From totalitarianism to trauma', 205-6
17: Van Bossum, 'Ons recht, de slachtoffers en de drie', 28-2-1972
18: Cohen, 'Vechten om ziek te mogen zijn', 13-3-1971
19: Ibidem
20: Ibidem
21: Ibidem
22: Ibidem. Also: Van Bergen, *De Zwaargewonden Eerst?*; Grüter, *Kwesties van Leven en Dood*
23: Cohen, 'Vechten om ziek te mogen zijn', 13-3-1971

7. The advent of the Post Concentration Camp Syndrome Clinic

1: 'Nog duizenden lijden aan naweeën oorlog', 21-4-1971
2: Ibidem; Hieselaar, 'Na 26 jaar kliniek voor slachtoffers concentratiekampen', 29-5-1971; Enning, *De Oorlog van Bastiaans*, 106; Piersma, *De Drie van Breda*, 142
3: Jansen, 'Gesprek met goede vriend leert', 26-6-1971; 'KZ-syndroom kliniek wordt enige ter wereld', 2-3-1972
4: Hieselaar, 'Na 26 jaar kliniek voor slachtoffers concentratiekampen', 29-5-1971
5: Ibidem
6: Enning, *De Oorlog van Bastiaans*, 24-32
7: Hieselaar, 'Na 26 jaar kliniek voor slachtoffers concentratiekampen', 29-5-1971

8. The Breda Three

1: Bodewes, 'Emoties uit het verleden', 9-3-1972
2: Peereboom, 'Pensioen zou helpen bij behandeling KZ-syndroom', 18-3-1972
3: Kuin, '"Voor slachtoffers is tot nu toe erg weinig gedaan"', 11-3-1972; For the debate on the Breda Three and the role of psychotrauma and Bastiaans, also see: Enning, *De Oorlog van Bastiaans*, 132-146
4: 'Ik zie het zo', 25-9-1971

5: Withuis, Mooij, ‘From totalitarianism to trauma’, 206-8
6: Godschalk, ‘Het Blow-up effect van de televisie informatie’, 11-3-1972
7: Ibidem
8: ‘Kamer wankelt onder protest tegen gratie’, 23-2-1972
9: ‘Minister en Kamerleden zagen kampsyndroomfilm’, 24-2-1972; ‘Minister ziet film over syndroom’, 24-2-1972
10: ‘“Begrijpt u nu waarom ik huil?” op VARA-tv’, 25-2-1972; ‘Debat over Bredase “3” direct op televisie’, 26-2-1972; ‘“Begrijpt u nu waarom ik huil?” vandaag voor tv’, 26-2-1972
11: Van Hoof, ‘Prof. dr. J. Bastiaans: “Drie van Breda”’, 19-2-1972
12: ‘De “Drie” stuk voor stuk vrij’, 28-2-1972
13: ‘De drie voelen zich veilig in Breda’, 24-2-1972
14: Kat, ‘Vrijlating van de “drie van Breda” zou een aanval in de rug van voormalig verzet zijn’, 23-2-1972
15: Ibidem
16: Hofhuizen, ‘Gezien’, 23-2-1972; Scheepmaker, ‘Collin Welland’, 23-2-1972; ‘Uit de Gooise lucht gegrepen’, 23-2-1972
17: ‘Achteraf bekeken’, 23-2-1972. Also: ‘Steeds meer aandacht voor Nazi-slachtoffers’, 23-2-1972; ‘Televisienieuws’, 23-2-1972
18: ‘Prof. Bastiaans waarschuwt voor acute ziekteverergering’, 23-2-1972
19: Kuin, ‘Prof. J. Bastiaans “tendeert naar vrijlating”’, 24-2-1972; ‘Hoogleraren voor en tegen gratie’, 23-2-1972
20: ‘Prof. Bastiaans waarschuwt voor acute ziekteverergering’, 23-2-1972; ‘Protesten tegen vrijlating “Drie”’, 23-2-1972
21: ‘Prof. Bastiaans waarschuwt voor acute ziekteverergering’, 23-2-1972; ‘Protesten tegen vrijlating “Drie”’, 23-2-1972
22: ‘Kamerleden zien film over kamp-syndroom’, 24-2-1972; Eiselin, ‘Levenslang is discriminatie’, 24-2-1972
23: ‘Minister ziet film over syndroom’, 24-2-1972
24: ‘Minister en Kamerleden zagen kampsyndroomfilm’, 24-2-1972; ‘Bij Kamerleden meer twijfels over de “Drie”’, 24-2-1972; Kuin, ‘Prof. J. Bastiaans “tendeert naar vrijlating”’, 24-2-1972
25: ‘Twijfel wint terrein’, 24-2-1972; Kuin, ‘Prof. J. Bastiaans “tendeert naar vrijlating”’, 24-2-1972
26: Enning, *De Oorlog van Bastiaans*, 144
27: ‘Minister ziet film over syndroom’, 24-2-1972
28: Ibidem
29: Boas, ‘Een afwijkende mening over de “drie van Breda”’, 24-2-1972
30: Herzberg, ‘Laat, om onzentwil, de Drie van Breda vrij’, 27-1-1976
31: Boas, ‘Drie van Breda (4)’, 4-2-1976

32: 'Israël: laat drie niet vrij', 29-2-1972; 'Abba Eban: geen gratie voor "drie"', 1-3-1972; Van Damme, 'Veertig jaar geleden'
33: '"Drie" niet vrij bij verzet Kamer', 24-2-1972
34: 'Emoties maken veel indruk op Van Agt', 24-2-1972
35: Ibidem; 'Bij Kamerleden meer twijfels over de "Drie"', 24-2-1972
36: Kuin, 'Prof. J. Bastiaans "tendeert naar vrijlating"', 24-2-1972; Piersma, *De Drie van Breda*, 120
37: 'Emoties maken veel indruk op Van Agt', 24-2-1972
38: 'Protest van vele honderden in Amersfoort', 24-2-1972
39: 'Hoorzitting over "Drie" begint in gespannen sfeer', 24-2-1972; Mooij, 'De langste schaduw', 279; Piersma, *De Drie van Breda*, 121
40: 'Groot aantal meldingen voor hearing', 22-2-1972; 'Kamerleden herzien mening over gratie', 23-2-1972; Van Hoof, 'Prof. dr. J. Bastiaans: "Drie van Breda"', 19-2-1972
41: 'Spanning en emotie tijdens hoorzitting', 25-2-1972; 'Veel emoties op hoorzitting "drie" Breda', 25-2-1972; 'Regering houdt nog vast aan gratie', 25-2-1972; 'Voorstanders vrijlating door luid geschreeuw onderbroken', 25-2-1972
42: 'Verhouding stemmen in kamer nog onduidelijk', 25-2-1972
43: Look, 'De Drie van Breda', 29-2-1972
44: 'Veel emoties op hoorzitting "drie" Breda', 25-2-1972; 'Regering houdt nog vast aan gratie', 25-2-1972; Piersma, *De Drie van Breda*, 121-122
45: 'Voorstanders door anonymi bestookt', 25-2-1972; 'Regering houdt nog vast aan gratie', 25-2-1972; Fahrenfort, 'Van Agt's aftreden ondanks geestelijke terreur nog net voorkomen', 4-3-1972; 'Kamermeerderheid is tegen collectieve vrijlating', 29-2-1972; 'Kabinet beslist misschien zelf', 25-2-1972; Scheepmaker, 'Kastje Kijken', 28-2-1972; 'Bomalarm in VARA-studio', 28-2-1972
46: Scheepmaker, 'Kastje Kijken', 28-2-1972; 'Bomalarm in VARA-studio', 28-2-1972; 'Minister heeft vertoning film niet verboden', 28-2-1972
47: 'Prof. Weijel hekelt "bot beleid" regering', 28-2-1972
48: 'Kabinet beslist misschien zelf', 25-2-1972; 'Emoties op de hoorzitting niet in bedwang te houden', 25-2-1972. Also: 'Regering zou willen afzien van Kamerdebat', 25-2-1972; 'Kabinet beslist misschien zelf', 25-2-1972
49: 'Kabinet wil toch gratie', 26-2-1972
50: 'Gratiebesluit staat vast', 26-2-1972
51: 'Spanning en emotie tijdens hoorzitting', 25-2-1972; 'Prof. Weijel hekelt "bot beleid" regering', 28-2-1972

52: ‘Spanning en emotie tijdens hoorzitting’, 25-2-1972; ‘Verhouding stemmen in kamer nog onduidelijk’, 25-2-1972; ‘Prof. Weijel hekelt “bot beleid” regering’, 28-2-1972
53: ‘Gratiedebat onzeker’, 25-2-1972; Piersma, *De Drie van Breda*, 104
54: ‘Emoties op de hoorzitting niet in bedwang te houden’, 25-2-1972
55: ‘Regering houdt nog vast aan gratie’, 25-2-1972
56: Ibidem
57: ‘Ruime meerderheid is tegen vrijlating’, 29-2-1972
58: Geurtsen, ‘Waarom ik “om” ging’, 29-2-1972; ‘Kamerlid Geurtsen ging “om” door losgeslagen emoties’, 29-2-1972
59: Geurtsen, ‘Waarom ik “om” ging’, 29-2-1972; ‘Kamerlid Geurtsen ging “om” door losgeslagen emoties’, 29-2-1972
60: Geurtsen, ‘Waarom ik “om” ging’, 29-2-1972
61: ‘Kamermeerderheid is tegen collectieve vrijlating’, 29-2-1972
62: ‘Meerderheid laat belang slachtoffers prevaleren’, 1-3-1972; ‘Bundel informatie over oorlogsleed’, 8-3-1972
63: ‘Snelle publikatie over KZ-syndroom’, 8-3-1972
64: Hulsman, ‘Gratie van de drie van Breda minste van twee kwaden’, 28-2-1972
65: Van Bossum, ‘Ons recht, de slachtoffers en de drie’, 28-2-1972
66: Duynstee, ‘Tweede Kamer heeft ernstig gefaald…’, 29-2-1972
67: Ibidem
68: ‘Nog eens “de drie van Breda”’, 3-6-1972; Withuis, *Erkenning*, 45; Enning, *De oorlog van Bastiaans*, 139; Piersma, *De Drie van Breda*, 120-121
69: ‘Politici menen na 85 stemmen tegen’, 1-3-1972
70: ‘Na kabinetsbesluit over drie van Breda’, 6-3-1972; ‘Reacties verdeeld’, 6-3-1972; ‘Regeringsbesluit over de Drie verdeeld ontvangen’, 6-3-1972
71: ‘“Begrijpt u nu waarom ik huil?” voor VARA-tv’, 25-2-1972; ‘Debat over Bredase “3” direct op televisie’, 26-2-1972; ‘“Begrijpt u nu waarom ik huil?” vandaag voor tv’, 26-2-1972; Withuis, *Erkenning*, 43; Bossenbroek, *De Meelstreep*, 435

9. The TV broadcast of *Do you now understand why I cry…*

1: Bank, ‘KZ-slachtoffers “herontdekt” op televisie’, 26-2-1972
2: Ibidem; For the broadcast and the reactions, see: Enning, *De Oorlog van Bastiaans*, 139-145
3: Bank, ‘KZ-slachtoffers “herondekt” op televisie’, 26-2-1972

4: 'Film over KZ-syndroom vanavond op tv', 26-2-1972; 'Film over behandeling kamp-syndroom vanavond uitgezonden', 26-2-1972
5: 'Film', 28-2-1972; 'Film KZ-syndroom roept veel positieve reacties op', 28-2-1972; 'Film KZ-syndroom: veel reacties', 28-2-1972; 'Slachtoffers van KZ-syndroom komen nu los', 28-2-1972; 'Minister heeft vertoning film niet verboden', 28-2-1972; Withuis, *Erkenning*, 114; Withuis, Mooij, 'From totalitarianism to trauma', 196-7
6: 'Beroep op begrip', 28-2-1972
7: 'Minister Engels was tegen uitzending', 28-2-1972; 'Honderden reacties op omstreden film', 28-2-1972; Scheepmaker, 'Kastje Kijken', 28-2-1972; 'Syndroomfilm: 800 reacties', 28-2-1972; 'Film KZ-syndroom roept veel positieve reacties op', 28-2-1972; 'Minister heeft vertoning film niet verboden', 28-2-1972. For Aalders see: http://www.stolpersteine-dordrecht.nl/het_voorbije_joodse_dordrecht_mr_charlie_aalders.html (seen: 14-9-2021)
8: 'Expogé-voorzitter C. (sic) Aalders overleden', 28-2-1972; 'Mr. Aalders van Expogé overleden', 28-2-1972
9: 'Stuyt: "Begrijpt u nu…" op televisie was onjuist', 12-4-1972; 'Stuyt veroordeelt vertoning film over KZ-syndroom', 12-4-1972; 'Voor milieu gevaarlijke produkten belast', 12-4-1972; 'Twijfels over film', 12-4-1972; 'Stuyt twijfelt aan medische ethiek bij film KZ-syndroom', 12-4-1972; 'Vragen over film KZ-syndroom', 12-4-1972
10: 'Prof. Bastiaans contra Stuyt', 19-4-1972; 'Prof. Bastiaans vindt uitlating minister Stuyt onbegrijpelijk', 19-4-1972; 'Prof Bastiaans vindt uitlating minister Stuyt "onbegrijpelijk"', 19-4-1972; 'Bastiaans tegen Stuyt over filmvertoning', 19-4-1972. For a recapitulation, see: Van den Berg, De Lange, 'De zaak-Rost past in beeld van affaire "drie van Breda"', 24-11-1986
11: 'Slachtoffers van KZ-syndroom komen nu los', 28-2-1972
12: De Vreede, 'Echtpaar uit syndroomfilm zat gespannen te kijken', 29-2-1972
13: De Vreede, 'Na dertig jaar nog niet vrij', 3-5-1975
14: 'Honderden reacties op omstreden film', 28-2-1972; Scheepmaker, 'Kastje kijken', 28-2-1972; 'Minister Engels was tegen uitzending', 28-2-1972; 'Film KZ-syndroom: veel reacties', 28-2-1972
15: Van Tijn, 'Film terecht uitgezonden', 28-2-1972
16: Jungman, 'Zwaar geschut en polarisatie', 28-2-1972
17: 'Prof. Weijel hekelt "bot beleid" regering', 28-2-1972
18: Ibidem; Withuis, *Erkenning*, 46-47
19: 'Honderden reacties op omstreden film', 28-2-1972; 'Syndroomfilm: 800 reacties', 28-2-1972; 'Film KZ-syndroom: veel reacties', 28-2-1972;

'Slachtoffers van KZ-syndroom komen nu los', 28-2-1972; 'Conclusie informatiebundel', 4-3-1972; 'Louis van Gasteren: "Dat Europa, dat is toch iets"', 29-6-1972; Hieselaar, 'Psychiater Bastiaans', 3-3-1973
20: 'Slachtoffers van KZ-syndroom komen nu los', 28-2-1972
21: Los, 'Leven na een oorlog', 6-4-1972
22: 'Honderden reacties op omstreden film', 28-2-1972; 'Syndroomfilm: 800 reacties', 28-2-1972; Van Tijn, 'Leven na een oorlog', 24-3-1972; 'Film KZ-syndroom: veel reacties', 28-2-1972; 'Slachtoffers van KZ-syndroom komen nu los', 28-2-1972; 'Conclusie informatiebundel', 4-3-1972
23: Scheepmaker, 'Kastje Kijken', 28-2-1972; Scheepmaker, 'Standbeeld voor gefolterde mens van twintigste eeuw', 28-2-1972; Scheepmaker, 'Achteraf bekeken', 28-2-1972
24: 'Slachtoffers van KZ-syndroom komen nu los', 28-2-1972
25: Scheepmaker, 'Kastje Kijken', 28-2-1972; Scheepmaker, 'Standbeeld voor gefolterde mens van twintigste eeuw', 28-2-1972; 'Achteraf bekeken', 28-2-1972
26: Scheepmaker, 'Kastje Kijken', 28-2-1972; Hofhuizen, 'Gezien. Huiveringwekkend', 28-2-1972; 'Uit de Gooise lucht gegrepen', 28-2-1972
27: 'Film', 28-2-1972
28: Duynstee, 'Tweede Kamer heeft ernstig gefaald…', 29-2-1972
29: Hofhuizen, 'Gezien. Huiveringwekkend', 28-2-1972
30: Ibidem
31: Jungman, 'Zwaar geschut en polarisatie', 28-2-1972
32: Ibidem
33: 'Vrouwen van de Drie zijn verdwenen', 29-2-1972; 'Nationaal centrum volksgezondheid geeft boekje uit', 3-3-1972; 'Brochure over KZ-syndroom', 4-3-1972
34: Bloch, 'Het post-concentratiekampsyndroom'; Enning, *De oorlog van Bastiaans*, 105
35: Van Tijn, 'Leven na een oorlog', 24-3-1972; 'Informatiebundel over verwerken van oorlogsleed', 29-2-1972; 'Vrouwen van de Drie zijn verdwenen', 29-2-1972; 'Nationaal centrum volksgezondheid geeft boekje uit', 3-3-1972; 'Conclusie informatiebundel', 4-3-1972; 'Leven na een oorlog', 4-3-1972; 'Brochure over KZ-syndroom', 4-3-1972; '"Leven na een oorlog" gebundeld', 7-3-1972; 'Snelle publikatie over KZ-syndroom', 8-3-1972; 'Bundel informatie over oorlogsleed', 8-3-1972; 'Bundel informatie over oorlogsleed', 8-3-1972; Bodewes, 'Emoties uit het verleden', 9-3-1972; 'KZ-syndroom: "Iedereen kan helpen"', 4-3-1972
36: Bastiaans et al., *Leven na een Oorlog*, Amsterdam 1972

37: Los, 'Leven na een oorlog', 6-4-1972; Snelders, *LSD en de Psychiatrie in Nederland*, 105
38: 'Prof. Bastiaans pleit voor een centraal behandelingsapparaat oorlogsslachtoffers', 8-3-1972
39: 'Drie niet gelijktijdig vrij', 17-3-1972; 'Minister van Agt: Geen programma voor vrijlating Drie van Breda', 17-3-1972; 'Boek over kampsyndroom in voorbereiding', 17-3-1972; 'Sociologisch onderzoek reacties op KZ-syndroom', 17-3-1972; 'Boek over KZ-syndroom', 20-3-1972

10. The influence of the Breda Three discussion

1: Ruyter, 'De verlate belangstelling voor de kampslachtoffers', 12-5-1973
2: Eiselin-Hoon, 'Kliniek', 3-3-1972
3: 'KZ-syndroom kliniek wordt enige ter wereld', 2-3-1972
4: Jansen, 'Speciale kliniek opgezet', 23-2-1972
5: 'KZ-syndroom kliniek wordt enige ter wereld', 2-3-1972
6: Ibidem
7: 'Oorlogsslachtoffers krijgen meer hulp', 7-3-1972
8: Ibidem
9: Kuin, '"Voor slachtoffers is tot nu toe erg weinig gedaan"', 11-3-1972
10: Neyenhuys, 'Oorlogsslachtoffers nog geen uitstervende groep', 18-12-1976
11: Kuin, '"Voor slachtoffers is tot nu toe erg weinig gedaan"', 11-3-1972
12 Ibidem; Kat, 'De schaduwen van het kamp zullen blijven', 13-3-1972; Peereboom, 'Pensioen zou helpen bij behandeling KZ-syndroom', 18-3-1972; Van Tijn, 'Leven na een oorlog', 24-3-1972
13: Kuin, '"Voor slachtoffers is tot nu toe erg weinig gedaan"', 11-3-1972; Kat, 'De schaduwen van het kamp zullen blijven', 13-3-1972; Peereboom, 'Pensioen zou helpen bij behandeling KZ-syndroom', 18-3-1972; Van Tijn, 'Leven na een oorlog', 24-3-1972
14: Kuin, '"Voor slachtoffers is tot nu toe erg weinig gedaan"', 11-3-1972
15: Ibidem
16: Peereboom, 'De straf voor verzetswerk', 31-3-1972
17: Ibidem
18: Kalk, 'Het verzet "loont" niet', 1-4-1972
19: Ibidem

11. The construction of the Post Concentration Camp Syndrome Clinic

1: 'Deze maand begint bouw KZ-paviljoen', 1-4-1972
2: 'Eerste paal van centrum aan lijders KZ-syndroom', 18-4-1972; 'Tehuis voor lijders aan KZ-syndroom', 18-4-1972; 'Eerste paal voor KZ-syndroomkliniek', 18-4-1972
3: 'Deze maand begint bouw KZ-paviljoen', 1-4-1972; Ruyter, 'De verlate belangstelling voor de kampslachtoffers', 12-5-1973
4: 'Deze maand begint bouw KZ-paviljoen', 1-4-1972; 'Controverse nasleep affaire-Dennendal', 1-6-1972; Gonggrijp, 'Prof. Speyer is uitgekeken op de universiteit', 9-6-1972; Enning, *De oorlog van Bastiaans*, 152
5: 'Deze maand begint bouw KZ-paviljoen', 1-4-1972; 'Prins bij begin bouw kliniek: Bouw KZ-centrum "ere-verplichting"', 18-4-1972; 'Prins sloeg paal voor z'n vrinden', 18-4-1972; Ruyter, 'De verlate belangstelling voor de kampslachtoffers', 12-5-1973
6: 'Deze maand begint bouw KZ-paviljoen', 1-4-1972; 'Prins bij begin bouw kliniek: Bouw KZ-centrum "ere-verplichting"', 18-4-1972; 'Prins sloeg paal voor z'n vrinden', 18-4-1972
7: 'Prins bij begin bouw kliniek', 18-4-1972
8: 'In centrum KZ-syndroom staat openheid voorop', 18-4-1972; Driever, *De Onderlinge Belofte*, 210
9: 'In centrum KZ-syndroom staat openheid voorop', 18-4-1972; Huib Goudriaan, 'Noodzaak van K.Z.-kliniek laat ingezien', 22-4-1972; Driever, *De Onderlinge Belofte,* 7; Mooij, 'De langste schaduw', 288; https://www.st4045.nl/wie-zijn-wij (seen: 4-6-2021)
10: 'Prins bij begin bouw kliniek', 18-4-1972
11: Ibidem; 'Eerste paal van centrum lijders KZ-syndroom', 18-4-1972
12: 'Eerste paal voor KZ-syndroomkliniek', 18-4-1972
13: 'Prins bij begin bouw kliniek', 18-4-1972
14: Goudriaan, 'Noodzaak van K.Z.-kliniek laat ingezien', 22-4-1972
15: F.i.: De Mari, 'Verwoest naar Oegstgeest', 11-3-1981
16: Withuis, *Erkenning*, 64-65
17: Herbergs, 'Terug naar Oegstgeest', 23-6-1973
18: Ruyter, 'De verlate belangstelling voor de kampslachtoffers', 12-5-1973
19: Goudriaan, 'Noodzaak van K.Z.-kliniek laat ingezien', 22-4-1972
20: 'Bij het slaan van een eerste paal', 22-4-1972
21: 'Prins bij begin bouw kliniek', 18-4-1972
22: 'Bij het slaan van een eerste paal', 22-4-1972
23: Ibidem

24: Ibidem
25: Ibidem
26: 'Deze maand begint bouw KZ-paviljoen', 1-4-1972
27: 'Stichting '40-'45 blij met laat begrip voor oorlogsslachtoffers', 6-10-1972
28: 'Leidse psychiatrie blijkt ernstig ziek', 20-10-1972; Enning, *De Oorlog van Bastiaans*, 149-154; Rooijmans, *99 Jaar tussen Wal en Schip*, 102-106
29: 'Centrum '45 start zonder staf', 2-3-1973
30: 'Prijs voor prof. Bastiaans', 9-2-1973; 'Mensen', 10-2-1973; 'Personalia', 10-2-1973; 'Foresterprijs uitgereikt aan prof. Bastiaans', 27-2-1973; 'Prijs prof. Bastiaans', 27-2-1973; 'Nieuws. Prijs', 27-2-1973; Pam, 'Ordinaire smartlap', 28-2-1973
31: 'Na dertig jaar eigen "thuis" voor oorlogsslachtoffers', 2-3-1973
32: 'Kliniek voor oorlogsslachtoffers', 2-3-1973; Ruyter, 'De verlate belangstelling voor de kampslachtoffers', 12-5-1973; 'Centrum '45 voor verzetsslachtoffers nu gereed', 2-3-1973
33: Mooij, 'De langste schaduw', 277
34: 'Kliniek voor oorlogsslachtoffers', 2-3-1973; Van Gasteren, 'Begrijpt U?...', 16-5-1984
35: 'Kliniek voor oorlogsslachtoffers', 2-3-1973. For Arendsen Hein see: Snelders, *LSD en de Psychiatrie in Nederland*, 80-97
36: 'Centrum '45 start zonder staf', 2-3-1973; 'Senator wil onderzoek bij Centrum '45', 18-5-1973
37: 'Centrum '45 voor verzetsslachtoffers nu gereed', 2-3-1973; 'Na dertig jaar eigen "thuis" voor oorlogsslachtoffers', 2-3-1973
38: 'Centrum '45 voor verzetsslachtoffers nu gereed', 2-3-1973; 'Na dertig jaar eigen "thuis" voor oorlogsslachtoffers', 2-3-1973
39: 'Centrum '45 voor verzetsslachtoffers nu gereed', 2-3-1973; 'Na dertig jaar eigen "thuis" voor oorlogsslachtoffers', 2-3-1973
40: 'Na dertig jaar eigen "thuis" voor oorlogsslachtoffers', 2-3-1973
41: F.i.: Herzberg, *Kroniek der Jodenvervolging*, 178-181, 261-280; Grüter, *Een Fantast schrijft Geschiedenis*
42: 'Na dertig jaar eigen "thuis" voor oorlogsslachtoffers', 2-3-1973
43: Ibidem
44: Ibidem
45: 'Centrum '45 start zonder staf', 2-3-1973
46: Ibidem
47: Ibidem
48: 'Koningin opende Centrum '45', 17-5-1973
49: 'Koningin opent vandaag kliniek Centrum '45', 16-5-1973
50: Hieselaar, 'Psychiater Bastiaans', 3-3-1973

51: Ibidem
52: Ibidem
53: Ibidem
54: Ibidem

12. The opening of Centre '45

1: 'Koningin opent vandaag kliniek Centrum '45', 16-5-1973; 'Centrum voor behandeling KZ-syndroom officieel geopend', 16-5-1973; Katz, 'Kliniek "Het Centrum" voor oorlogsslachtoffers geopend', 18-5-1973; Rooijmans, *99 Jaar tussen Wal en Schip*, 106-109
2: Van Overeem, 'Oorlog duurt voort in Centrum '45', 14-5-1973; Waltmans, 'Overeem'
3: Helversteijn, 'Kliniek voor slachtoffers van syndroom', 5-5-1973; Goudriaan, 'Koningin opent kliniek voor oorlogsslachtoffers, 5-5-1973
4: Ruyter, 'De verlate belangstelling voor de kampslachtoffers', 12-5-1973
5: Ibidem
6: Van Dam thought, that, even if you didn't agree with them, people like Bastiaans were above criticism. Enning, *De Oorlog van Bastiaans*, 197
7: Helversteijn, 'Kliniek voor slachtoffers van syndroom', 5-5-1973
8: Ibidem
9: Withuis, *Erkenning*, 59-60
10: Helversteijn, 'Kliniek voor slachtoffers van syndroom', 5-5-1973
11: Ibidem
12: Ibidem
13: Ibidem
14: Ruyter, 'De verlate belangstelling voor de kampslachtoffers', 12-5-1973
15: Herbergs, 'Terug naar Oegstgeest', 23-6-1973
16: Ruyter, 'De verlate belangstelling voor de kampslachtoffers', 12-5-1973; Van Overeem, 'Oorlog duurt voort in Centrum '45', 14-5-1973
17: Herbergs, 'Terug naar Oegstgeest', 23-6-1973
18: Helversteijn, 'Kliniek voor slachtoffers van syndroom', 5-5-1973
19: 'Centrum '45 geopend', 16-5-1973; 'Koningin opent Centrum '45', 16-5-1973; 'Centrum '45 geopend door Koningin', 16-5-1973; 'Meedogenloze machtsstrijd schakelt prof. Bastiaans uit', 17-5-1973; Piersma, *De Drie van Breda*, 117
20: Eiselin, 'Centrum '45 start met conflict', 17-5-1973; Gonggrijp, 'Incident bij opening van "Centrum '45"', 17-5-1973
21: 'Centrum '45 is geopend', 17-5-1973; 'Binnenland', 17-5-1973
22: Eiselin, 'Centrum '45 start met conflict', 17-5-1973
23: 'Meedogenloze machtsstrijd schakelt prof. Bastiaans uit', 17-5-1973

24: 'Koningin opent Centrum '45', 16-5-1973; 'Professor Bastiaans slachtoffer van de universitaire machtsstrijd', 16-5-1973
25: 'Conflict ontsiert opening "Centrum '45"', 16-5-1973
26: 'Professor Bastiaans slachtoffer van de universitaire machtsstrijd', 16-5-1973; 'Meedogenloze machtsstrijd schakelt prof. Bastiaans uit', 17-5-1973; Enning, *De Oorlog van Bastiaans*, 167, 182
27: 'Professor Bastiaans slachtoffer van de universitaire machtsstrijd', 16-5-1973; 'Meedogenloze machtsstrijd schakelt prof. Bastiaans uit', 17-5-1973. Also: 'Prof. Bastiaans teleurgesteld over centrum lijders KZ-syndroom', 17-5-1973; 'Ruzie bij opening van nieuwe oorlogsslachtoffers-kliniek', 17-5-1973; Eiselin, 'Centrum '45 start met conflict', 17-5-1973
28: 'Prof. Bastiaans over conflict Centrum '45', 19-05-1973; Enning, *De oorlog van Bastiaans*, 152
29: 'Professor Bastiaans slachtoffer van de universitaire machtsstrijd', 16-5-1973; 'Meedogenloze machtsstrijd schakelt prof. Bastiaans uit', 17-5-1973
30: 'Centrum '45 is geopend', 17-5-1973
31: 'Conflict ontsiert opening "Centrum '45"', 16-5-1973; Rooijmans, *99 Jaar tussen Wal en Schip*, 94-95
32: 'Conflict ontsiert opening "Centrum '45"', 16-5-1973
33: Ibidem
34: 'Meedogenloze machtsstrijd schakelt prof. Bastiaans uit', 17-3-1973
35: 'Centrum '45 is geopend', 17-5-1973; 'Prof. Bastiaans teleurgesteld over centrum lijders KZ-syndroom', 17-5-1973; Eiselin, 'Centrum '45 start met conflict', 17-5-1973; Gonggrijp, 'Incident bij opening van "Centrum '45"', 17-5-1973; 'Prof. J. Bastiaans, "Bemanning Centrum '45 onvoldoende"', 17-5-1973
36: 'Prof. J. Bastiaans, "Bemanning Centrum '45 onvoldoende"', 17-5-1973; Eiselin, 'Centrum '45 start met conflict', 17-5-1973; 'Prof. Bastiaans teleurgesteld over centrum lijders KZ-syndroom', 17-5-1973; 'Ruzie bij opening van nieuwe oorlogsslachtoffers-kliniek', 17-5-1973; 'Centrum '45 door koningin geopend', 17-5-1973; 'Binnenland', 17-5-1973; Katz, 'Kliniek "Het Centrum" voor oorlogsslachtoffers geopend', 18-5-1973; Enning, *De oorlog van Bastiaans*, 152
37: Baan, 'J. Bastiaans'
38: Eiselin, 'Centrum '45 start met conflict', 17-5-1973; 'Prof. Bastiaans teleurgesteld over centrum lijders KZ-syndroom', 17-5-1973; 'Ruzie bij opening van nieuwe oorlogsslachtoffers-kliniek', 17-5-1973; 'Centrum '45 door koningin geopend', 17-5-1973; 'Binnenland', 17-5-1973; 'Prof. Bastiaans over conflict Centrum '45', 19-5-1973; Enning, *De oorlog van Bastiaans*, 152

39: 'Meedogenloze machtsstrijd schakelt prof. Bastiaans uit', 17-5-1973
40: Eiselin, 'Centrum '45 start met conflict', 17-5-1973; Katz, 'Kliniek "Het Centrum" voor oorlogsslachtoffers geopend', 18-5-1973
41: 'Meedogenloze machtsstrijd schakelt prof. Bastiaans uit', 17-5-1973
42: Katz, 'Kliniek "Het Centrum" voor oorlogsslachtoffers geopend', 18-5-1973
43: 'Weekbladen', 16-7-1987; Fortuin, '"Wat worden wij daar nou wijzer van, papa Bas?"', 31-10-1987
44: Katz, 'Kliniek "Het Centrum" voor oorlogsslachtoffers geopend', 18-5-1973
45: 'Ernstige moeilijkheden rond nieuwe kliniek van prof. Bastiaans', 19-5-1973
46: Boer, 'Centrum '45', 18-5-1973
47: Ibidem
48: Enning, *De Oorlog van Bastiaans*, 121; Piersma, *Jaap le Poole*, 87-88
49: 'Ernstige moeilijkheden rond nieuwe kliniek van prof. Bastiaans', 19-5-1973. It wouldn't be the last time Bastiaans mistakenly was called the head of Centre '45. Also: 'Overval consulaat "spontaan" plan', 22-12-1975
50: '"Experts twijfelen aan methode Bastiaans"', 19-5-1973; Piersma, *Jaap le Poole*, 88-89
51: '"Experts twijfelen aan methode Bastiaans"', 19-5-1973
52: Piersma, *Jaap le Poole*, 89
53: Koopmans, 'Prof. Bastiaans', 24-5-1973; Terwindt, 'Bastiaans', 25-5-1973; Enning, *De Oorlog van Bastiaans*, 163, 231-236
54: 'Prof. Bastiaans over conflict Centrum '45', 19-05-1973
55: Ibidem
56: Ibidem
57: Ibidem
58: Ibidem
59: Ibidem
60: 'Onderscheiding aan ziekbed', 28-4-1973
61: 'Kamerlid wil onderzoek naar conflicten rond Centrum '45', 18-5-1973; 'Vragen over Centrum '45', 18-5-1973; 'Eibert Meester vraagt minister over beleid rond Centrum '45', 18-5-1973; 'Onderzoek gevraagd naar de gang van zaken rond Centrum '45 in Oegstgeest', 18-5-1973; 'Onderzoek gevraagd naar Centrum '45', 18-5-1973; 'Senator wil onderzoek bij Centrum '45', 18-5-1973; 'Onderzoek naar conflict bij Centrum '45 gevraagd', 18-5-1973; 'Onderzoek gevraagd naar passeren prof. Bastiaans', 18-5-1973
62: 'Onderzoek naar Centrum '45', 25-5-1973; 'Onderzoek naar conflict over Centrum '40-'45', 25-5-1973; 'Prof. Bastiaans: Samenwerking goed

met staf Centrum '45', 25-5-1973; 'Prof Bastiaans verduidelijkt kritiek op Centrum '45', 25-5-1973; 'Prof. Bastiaans: goede samenwerking met staf van Centrum '45', 25-5-1973; 'Prof. Bastiaans: geen sprake van ruzie', 26-5-1973; 'Overleg over positie van prof. Bastiaans', 6-6-1973

63: Herbergs, 'Terug naar Oegstgeest', 23-6-1973

64: 'Voorstel Bastiaans over Centrum '45', 25-5-1973; 'Prof. Bastiaans in brief aan prof. Muntendam', 25-5-1973

65: 'Onderzoek naar Centrum '45', 25-5-1973; 'Onderzoek naar conflict over Centrum '40-'45', 25-5-1973; 'Prof. Bastiaans: goede samenwerking met staf van Centrum '45', 25-5-1973; 'Prof. Bastiaans: samenwerking met staf Centrum '45 goed', 25-5-1973; 'Conflict rondom prof. Bastiaans', 26-5-1973; 'Prof Bastiaans verduidelijkt kritiek op Centrum '45', 25-5-1973; 'Onderzoek naar Centrum '45', 4-6-1973

66: 'Centrum', 1-6-1973

67: 'Problemen rond Centrum '45 lijken opgelost', 6-6-1973; 'Centrum '45 over samenwerking met prof. Bastiaans', 6-6-1973; 'Problemen Centrum '45 worden uitgepraat', 6-6-1973; 'Overleg over positie van prof. Bastiaans', 6-6-1973

68: 'Weekbladen van week tot week', 2-5-1975

69: Meijer, *Brief aan mijn Moeder*; Welgraven, 'Wat 25 jaar na zijn dood vooral beklijft: Ischa Meijer schond de norm dat je oorlogsslachtoffers ontziet.', 29-1-2020; Withuis, *Erkenning*, 135.

13. The war syndrome and LSD's medical use both criticised and praised

1: 'Brits leger tussen twee vuren', 18-5-1974; 'Prof. Bastiaans werkt mee aan rapport', 28-7-1973

2: For this see: Scagliola, *Last van de Oorlog*, 108-110, 295-321

3: '…in een doolhof', 22-11-1973; '"Leven in een doolhof"', 22-11-1973; Scheepmaker, '"En wij, wij leven voort in een doolhof…"', 23-11-1973; Scheepmaker, 'Kastje kijken', 23-11-1973; Jungman, 'Een oorlog en zijn nasleep', 23-11-1973; 'Achteraf bekeken', 23-11-1973; Scheepmaker, '"Wij leven voort" was in vreemde vorm gegoten', 21-12-1973; Scheepmaker, 'Kastje Kijken', 21-12-1973; 'Achteraf bekeken', 21-12-1973

4: 'Zware keus vanavond', 22-11-1973;

5: Van Vonderen, 'Brief van oud-vrijwilliger basis voor documentaire', 22-11-1973

6: Ris, 'Gat in Avenue-stijl', 21-12-1973

7: Scheepmaker, '"Wij leven voort" was in vreemde vorm gegoten', 21-12-1973; Scheepmaker, 'Kastje Kijken', 21-12-1973; 'Achteraf bekeken', 21-12-1973
8: Scheepmaker, '"Wij leven voort" was in vreemde vorm gegoten', 21-12-1973; Scheepmaker, 'Kastje Kijken', 21-12-1973; 'Achteraf bekeken', 21-12-1973
9: Kopuit, 'Jom Kippoeroorlog vergt nog jaren slachtoffers', 18-1-1974; 'Jom-Kipoer-oorlog eiste erg veel psychische slachtoffers', 21-2-1974; 'Oktober-oorlog eiste veel psychische slachtoffers onder militairen Israël', 22-2-1974
10: 'Dr. H. Milikowski over het omgekeerde KZ-syndroom', 9-2-1974
11: 'Bundel opstellen van Milikowski', 1-12-1973
12: 'Gebruik van LSDin psychiatrie blijft uiterst discutabel', 15-11-1975; Milikowski, 'Het KZ-syndroom', 92; Withuis, *Erkenning*, 94-96
13: 'De strijd, die niet ophield', 9-2-1974; Withuis, *Erkenning*, 95
14: 'De strijd, die niet ophield', 9-2-1974; Milikowski, 'Het KZ-syndroom', 97
15: 'De strijd, die niet ophield', 9-2-1974; Withuis, *Erkenning*, 95
16: Enning, *De Oorlog van Bastiaans*, 160
17: Wennekes, *Allemaal rottigheid*, 5
18: 'Ontsnapping KZ-syndroom met LSD kuur', 21-3-1975; 'Zes verslagen LSD therapieën', 21-3-1975
19: 'Ontsnapping KZ-syndroom met LSD kuur', 21-3-1975; 'Zes verslagen LSD therapieën', 21-3-1975; 'Weekbladen van week tot week', 27-3-1975; 'Weekbladen', 27-3-1975; De Leeuw, 'Oud-verzetsman in kliniek terug naar oorlogsjaren', 7-4-1975; Peereboom, 'Waardevol boek over KZ-syndroom', 3-5-1975; De Vreede, 'Na dertig jaar nog niet vrij', 3-5-1975
20: 'Ontsnapping KZ-syndroom met LSD kuur', 21-3-1975; 'LSD hulp voor KZ-patiënten', 21-3-1975; Rondagh, 'LSD gesprekken met verzetsman', 28-3-1975; De Leeuw, 'Oud-verzetsman in kliniek terug naar oorlogsjaren', 7-4-1975
21: 'Ontsnapping KZ-syndroom met LSD kuur', 21-3-1975; 'LSD hulp voor KZ-patiënten', 21-3-1975; Rondagh, 'LSD gesprekken met verzetsman', 28-3-1975
22: 'Ontsnapping KZ-syndroom met LSD kuur', 21-3-1975; 'LSD hulp voor KZ-patiënten', 21-3-1975; De Leeuw, 'Oud-verzetsman in kliniek terug naar oorlogsjaren', 7-4-1975
23: 'LSD hulp voor KZ-patiënten', 21-3-1975
24: 'Gebruik van LSDin psychiatrie blijft uiterst discutabel', 15-11-1975
25: Ibidem

14. The first Moluccan hostage-takings: Wijster and Amsterdam

1: www.allesopeenrij.nl/macht/recht-criminaliteit/gijzelingen-in-nederland (seen: 30-5-2021)
2: 'Rust voor vrijgelaten gegijzelden het belangrijkst', 9-12-1975
3: Ibidem
4: Ibidem
5: Ibidem
6: 'Onderzoek naar langdurige begeleiding van gegijzelden', 15-12-1975; 'Gijzelaars krijgen ook op lange termijn begeleiding', 15-12-1975; 'Den Uyl onder de indruk van woorden van prof. Bastiaans', 15-12-1975
7[1] 'Onderzoek naar langdurige begeleiding van gegijzelden', 15-12-1975; Jungman, 'Van Klinkklaar naar Beilen', 15-12-1975; 'Ir. Manusama acht nieuwe harde acties niet uitgesloten', 15-12-1975; 'Gijzelaars krijgen ook op lange termijn begeleiding', 15-12-1975; Hydra, 'Vreemde dag', 15-12-1975; 'Den Uyl onder de indruk van woorden van prof. Bastiaans', 15-12-1975; 'Bij nazorg gijzelaars huisarts betrekken', 20-12-1975; 'Gesprekken Hendriks-Bastiaans', 20-12-1975; 'Toezegging van gesprek maakt eind aan gijzeling', 20-12-1975; 'Den Uyl over gesprek met Zuidmolukkers', 20-12-1975; 'Overval consulaat "spontaan" plan', 22-12-1975; 'Malik: "Acties tegen Indonesië hard aanpakken"', 22-12-1975
8: 'Prof. Bastiaans over drama bij Wijster', 20-12-1975
9: Ibidem; 'Gijzelaars kregen hersenspoeling', 20-12-1975. For alexithymia see: Van der Ploeg, Weerts, *Veteranen in Nederland*, 80-81
10: 'Prof. Bastiaans over drama bij Wijster', 20-12-1975
11: Ibidem
12: 'Speciaal opvangteam', 22-12-1975; 'Overval consulaat "spontaan" plan', 22-12-1975; 'Overval op consulaat was niet gepland', 22-12-1975; 'Malik: "Acties tegen Indonesië hard aanpakken"', 22-12-1975; 'Amsterdamse actie na "Wijster" gepland', 22-12-1975
13: Boer, 'De echte kater komt nog', 18-6-1977
14: 'Prof. Bastiaans over drama bij Wijster', 20-12-1975; 'Gijzelaars kregen hersenspoeling', 20-12-1975
15: Peereboom, 'Kapers en gijzelaars als één groep', 17-12-1975; Van Overeem, 'Nietes-welles', 18-12-1975
16: 'Tien jaar na Wijster', 30-11-1985; 'De echo van dertien bange en barre dagen', 30-11-1985; 'Wrok maar ook begrip', 7-12-1985
17: 'Gijzelaars kregen hersenspoeling', 20-12-1975
18: 'Prof. Bastiaans over drama bij Wijster', 20-12-1975
19: Ibidem

20: Ibidem
21: Rondagh, 'Vermoeden psycholoog', 15-12-1975
22: Van Dam, 'Zelf doen', 27-12-1975
23: Ibidem
24: Ibidem
25: 'Staatssecretaris installeert projectgroep', 15-1-1976
26: 'Helpers Ex-Gijzelaars', 15-1-1976
27: 'Projectgroep gijzelaars begint', 14-1-1976; 'Projectgroep nazorg van ex-gijzelaars kan aan het werk', 14-1-1976; 'Installatie van projectgroep nazorg van ex-gijzelaars', 14-1-1976; 'Nazorg-groep ex-gijzelaars samengesteld', 14-1-1976; 'Staatssecretaris installeert projectgroep', 15-1-1976; 'Projectgroep nazorg gijzelaars ingesteld', 15-1-1976; 'Helpers Ex-Gijzelaars', 15-1-1976
28: 'Ex-gijzelaar vindt begeleiding "te ambtelijk"', 12-2-1976; 'Ernstige kritiek van ex-gijzelaars op nazorg', 13-2-1976; Also: Kuipers, 'Ex-gegijzelde Ger Vaders', 29-11-1980
29: 'Ex-gijzelaar vindt begeleiding "te ambtelijk"', 12-2-1976; 'Ernstige kritiek van ex-gijzelaars op nazorg', 13-2-1976
30: 'Ex-gijzelaar vindt begeleiding "te ambtelijk"', 12-2-1976
31: 'Nieuwe poging van Agt', 17-3-1976
32: Hydra, 'Natuurlijk', 17-3-1976; 'Afwijzende reacties op pleidooi om drie van Breda weg te zenden', 17-3-1976; 'Ex-gevangenen verzetten zich tegen vrijlating Drie van Breda', 17-3-1976; 'Vrijlaten "drie" nog steeds onhaalbaar', 17-3-1976
33: Sprenger, 'Drie van Breda', 27-3-1976

15. A first dent in the image

1: Jungman, 'Pratend over Colditz', 21-4-1975
2: Piët, 'In een geur van braadvlees', 9-9-1976
3: Withuis, *Erkenning*, 54; Voor een portret van Meester: Enning, *De Oorlog van Bastiaans*, 170-175
4: 'Kamerlid in opspraak', 1-4-1976; 'Verleden kamerlid onder de loep', 2-4-1976
5: 'Spoedig uitslag over pensioen E. Meester', 3-4-1976
6: Lulofs, 'Zootje', 21-8-1976
7: Schumacher, 'De oorlog duurt voort…', 10-7-1976; Enning, *De oorlog van Bastiaans*, 174
8: Schumacher, 'De oorlog duurt voort…', 10-7-1976; Enning, *De oorlog van Bastiaans*, 174
9: Kleyn, 'Verzetsverleden steeds moeilijker na te gaan', 14-8-1976

10: 'Verzetsgroepen in actie tegen Stichting '40-'45', 18-2-1984; Pijper, 'Meertens bemiddelde bij prins voor schimmige sjeik', 23-2-1984; Polak, 'Verzetsgroepen in actie tegen Stichting '40-'45', 23-2-1984; Buijze, 'Niet alleen verzet Meertens roept vragen op', 23-2-1984
11: Schumacher, 'De oorlog duurt voort…', 10-7-1976
12: Derksen, 'Op zicht. Het grote zwijgen (1)', 1-12-1982
13: 'Meester stapt op', 2-8-1976; 'Eibert Meester om gezondheidsredenen uit Eerste Kamer', 2-8-1976; 'Meester uit Kamer', 2-8-1976; 'Eibert Meester', 2-8-1976; 'Eibert Meester uit Senaat', 2-8-1976; 'Eibert Meester treedt terug', 2-8-1976; 'Eibert Meester uit Eerste Kamer', 2-8-1976
14: Lulofs, 'Zootje', 21-8-1976
15: Enning, *De oorlog van Bastiaans*, 174
16: '*Vrij Nederland*: zwarte handel', 9-9-1976
17: Kleisen, 'Openbare diagnoses?', 11-1-1977; Bossenbroek, *De Meelstreep*, 497. For likewise criticism, see: Van Duijn, 'Moffenhoer?', 16-4-2016
18: 'Weekbladen', 22-12-1976; Piët, 'Uit de weekbladen', 23-12-1976; 'HP deze week', 22-12-1976
19: 'Weekbladen van week tot week', 23-12-1976
20: Enning, *De oorlog van Bastiaans*, 175; Van der Ploeg, 'LSD in de psychiatrie', 16-6-2000; Van der Steen, 'Uithuilen aan de borst van papa Bas', 4-4-2009
21: 'Twee verzetslieden eisen vervolging van oud-kamerlid', 11-1-1978; 'PSP-Kamerlid', 11-1-1978; 'Oud-verzetslieden in beroep tegen beslissing van officier', 11-1-1978
22: Peereboom, '"Van oorlogsslachtoffer werd problematiek niet begrepen"', 26-3-1977; Mooij, 'De langste schaduw', 277; Van der Hart et al., 'Psychotraumatologie', 49; Bossenbroek, *De Meelstreep*, 435
23: Peereboom, '"Van oorlogsslachtoffer werd problematiek niet begrepen"', 26-3-1977; Bastiaans, 'De Behandeling van oorlogsslachtoffers', 9
24: Peereboom, '"Van oorlogsslachtoffer werd problematiek niet begrepen"', 26-3-1977

16. 4 May 1977: commemorating the dead

1: Gisolf, 'Er gebeurde iets vreemds met de ex-mariniers', 4-5-1977
2: Gisolf, 'Kind uit het verzet', 4-5-1977
3: Gisolf, 'Na de oorlog geboren, soms toch "oorlogservaring"', 4-5-1976
4: Gisolf, 'Het kampsyndroom', 4-5-1977
5: Ibidem
6: Ibidem

7: Ibidem
8: Hers, *Stress*, 3
9: Peereboom, 'De oorlog werkt bij velen nog diep na', 4-5-1977
10: Van Loon, '800 Vergeten oorlogshelden wachten op een gebaar van Den Haag', 22-7-1977
11: Peereboom, 'De oorlog werkt bij velen nog diep na', 4-5-1977
12: Ibidem; Van Loon, '800 Vergeten oorlogshelden wachten op een gebaar van Den Haag', 22-7-1977; Piersma, *De Drie van Breda*, 142-143

17. Two more Moluccan hijackings: Bovensmilde and De Punt

1: Jansma, 'Bovensmilde ultimatum', 25-5-1977; Glimmerveen, 'Psychiatrie van de mollegang', 6-10-1981
2: Jansma, 'Opvang al optimaal geregeld', 25-5-1977
3: Van Overeem, 'Hulpverleners, bemoei je er niet mee', 28-5-1977
4: Herbergs, 'De hulpverleners belagen de gegijzelden', 4-6-1977
5: 'Veel extra leed oorlogsslachtoffers', 1-6-1977; 'Prof. dr. J. Bastiaans: 14% gegijzelden', 16-6-1977
6: 'Veel extra leed oorlogsslachtoffers', 1-6-1977
7: 'Beeldspraak', 8-6-1977; 'Speciaal vandaag', 7-6-1977
8: 'Prof. dr. J. Bastiaans: 14% gegijzelden', 16-6-1977
9: Ibidem; Boer, 'De echte kater komt nog', 18-6-1977
10: 'Prof. dr. J. Bastiaans: 14% gegijzelden', 16-6-1977
11: Boer, 'De echte kater komt nog', 18-6-1977
12: 'Prof. dr. J. Bastiaans: 14% gegijzelden', 16-6-1977
13: Ibidem
14: Ibidem
15: Ibidem
16: Ibidem
17: Woltz, 'Buitenlandse deskundigen', 18-6-1977
18: Boer, 'De echte kater komt nog', 18-6-1977
19: Ibidem
20: Ibidem
21: Ibidem
22: 'Huisarts moet ex-gegijzelde direct helpen', 22-6-1979; 'Beoordeling van daders "neutraal"', 22-6-1979
23: Heil, 'De betrokkene', 10-7-1979
24: Boer, 'De echte kater komt nog', 18-6-1977
25: Ibidem; Melkman, 'Psychische invloed van vervolging op symposium', 11-11-1977

26: Rosenthal, 'Psychiater Mulder in Israël', 19-10-1977; 'Nazorg voor àlle slachtoffers van geweld en rampen', 31-12-1977; 'Huisarts moet ex-gegijzelde direct helpen', 22-6-1979
27: Rosenthal, 'Psychiater Mulder in Israël', 19-10-1977
28: 'Er komt geen anti-terreurgroep onder ministerie van defensie', 21-10-1977
29: nl.wikipedia.org/wiki/Bijzondere_Bijstandseenheid (seen: 29-8-2021)
30: Van der Ploeg, 'Preludium'
31: 'Laat men bezwaren brengen waar ze horen', 6-8-1977
32: Ibidem
33: Ibidem
34: 'Nazorg voor àlle slachtoffers van geweld en rampen', 31-12-1977
35: Herbergs, 'Een half jaar nazorg aan ex-gegijzelden', 31-12-1977
36: Ibidem; 'We hebben 't juist uitstekend gedaan', 31-12-1977
37: Herbergs, 'Een half jaar nazorg aan ex-gegijzelden', 31-12-1977
38: Ibidem
39: Ibidem
40: Ibidem

18. Right and wrong

1: 'Nieuwe medicijnen beïnvloeden chemische hersenwerking', 6-2-1978
2: Ibidem
3: Ibidem
4: Ibidem; Snelders, *LSD en de Psychiatrie in Nederland*, 29, 32-34
5: Goulooze, 'Lijdensweg voor politieke gevangenen in Sowjet-Unie', 18-11-1975; 'Verontrusting over lot van psychiaters in de Sovjet-Unie', 18-4-1978
6: 'Verontrusting over lot van psychiaters in de Sovjet-Unie', 18-4-1978; 'Psychiatrie met politieke bijsmaak in Sowjet-Unie', 25-8-1978; 'Misbruik psychiatrie op grote schaal in Rusland', 14-10-1978
7: Gisolf, 'Oorlog is weer actueel', 3-5-1978
8: Ibidem
9: Ibidem
10: Ibidem; Gisolf, 'Twee levens', 3-5-1978
11: Gisolf, 'De behandeling', 3-5-1978
12: Knoop, 'Nieuwe kans voor historie', 2-6-1978
13: 'Joop Wolff verwijt justitie gebrek aan wil', 31-7-1978
14: 'Prof. dr. J. Bastiaans heeft liever meer hulp voor hun slachtoffers', 12-8-1978
15: 'Joop Wolff verwijt justitie gebrek aan wil', 31-7-1978

16: Van Schie, 'Hoe ziek zijn zij die om vervolging roepen?', 12-8-1978
17: Ibidem
18: Ibidem
19: Ibidem
20: 'Uitvlucht', 18-8-1975
21: 'Het syndroom van "maatschappelijke begeleiders"', 23-8-1978
22: Ibidem
23: 'Aanvallen op onderzoek-Aantjes', 10-11-1978
24: 'Aantjes werd voor de wolven gegooid', 9-11-1978; 'Prof. Bastiaans in Leiden', 9-11-1978; 'Prof Bastiaans: "Behandeling van Aantjes onmenselijk"', 10-11-1978; 'Prof Bastiaans: Aantjes publiekelijk gegijzeld', 10-11-1978; 'Veel kritiek op procedure Aantjes', *Limburgsch Dagblad*, 10-11-1978
25: 'Prof. Bastiaans in Leiden', 9-11-1978; 'Prof. dr. J. Bastiaans over affaire-Aantjes', 10-11-1978
26: 'Prof. dr. J. Bastiaans over affaire-Aantjes', 10-11-1978
27: Hofstede, 'De media en Aantjes', 18-11-1987
28: Wigbold, 'De hoofd- en bijzaken in de affaire-Aantjes', 10-11-1978; Hofstede, 'De media en Aantjes', 18-11-1987; For Foudraine see: Blok, *Baas in eigen Brein*
29: 'De verstokte', 16-2-1981
30: Enning, *De Oorlog van Bastiaans*, 211-213
31: Koopman, 'Belangstelling voor Tweede Wereldoorlog leeft in 1978 plotseling weer fel op', 2-12-1978; 'Veel slachtoffers verkeren nu in uitputtingsfase', 13-12-1978
32: 'Dossier-Wijster is nog niet afgesloten', 16-12-1978
33: Van Dijk, 'Signalement van een onmogelijkheid', 14-12-1978
34: 'Mevrouw Donker', 6-12-1978; 'Weduwe Donker ontkent handeltje met Menten', 7-12-1978

19. The Holocaust TV series TV series

1: Kleyn, 'Elke dag krijg je wel een flits van het concentratiekamp', 11-1-1986
2: Van Overeem, 'Ervaring voor Joodse wezen les voor alle traumata', 22-2-1979; Boltendal, 'Keilsons proefschrift tevens kroniek van menselijk leven en lijden', 20-7-1979; Van der Hart et al., 'Psychotraumatologie', 50-51; Aarts, 'De geschiedenis', 25; Groen-Prakken, 'Trauma en ontwikkelingsinterferentie'
3: De Mari, 'Oude oorlogshelden bestoken elkaar met grof geschut', 24-2-1979
4: Van der Put, 'Maar deze mug blijft doorgaan', 6-1-1979

5: 'Minister stelt richtlijnen voor', 3-2-1979; 'Richtlijnen van CRM voor uitzendingen over oorlog', 9-2-1979; 'Gevoelens', 9-2-1979
6: 'Richtlijnen van CRM voor uitzendingen over oorlog', 9-2-1979. For a critique on the terminology, f.i. see: De Swaan, 'Het onvermogen om te luisteren', 3-5-1980; Schütz, 'Memory Unbound, Unfounded Memory?', 79; Van Os, *Liever dier dan mens*, 246
7: 'Laatste deel Englandspiel vanavond op het TV scherm', 1-2-1979; Hydra, 'Er knaagt iets aan de helden zonder glorie', 1-2-1979; 'Gedenkteken slachtoffers Englandspiel', 12-5-1979; 'Alsnog gedenkteken voor slachtoffers Englandspiel', 15-5-1979
8: 'Richtlijnen van CRM voor uitzendingen over oorlog', 9-2-1979
9: 'Gevoelens', 9-2-1979
10: Ibidem
11: Ibidem
12: 'Problemen oorlogsslachtoffers worden nog steeds onderschat', 17-2-1979; 'Nieuwe instelling voor oorlogsslachtoffers', 21-2-1979; Van den Houten, 'Landelijk centrum geeft informatie aan oorlogsgetroffenen', 23-2-1979; Alink, 'Recht & slecht. Schreeuw om hulp', 21-7-1979; Withuis, *Weest manlijk*, 311
13: 'Problemen oorlogsslachtoffers worden nog steeds onderschat', 17-2-1979
14: Ibidem
15: Van den Houten, 'Landelijk centrum geeft informatie aan oorlogsgetroffenen', 23-2-1979
16: De Groot, 'Bevrijding… spreekkamers zullen volstromen', 1-4-1985
17: 'Hulpverlening oorlogsgetroffenen is veel te laat', 6-4-1979; *Immateriële Hulpverlening aan Oorlogsgetroffenen*
18: 'Hulpverlening oorlogsgetroffenen is veel te laat', 6-4-1979
19: Ibidem; Enning, *De Oorlog van Bastiaans*, 198-199
20: *Immateriële Hulpverlening aan Oorlogsgetroffenen*, 6
21: 'Henk Leliefeld, algemeen medicus', 6-4-1979; De Leeuw, 'Reacties op Holocaust zijn nauwelijks te voorspellen', 21-4-1979
22: 'Henk Leliefeld, algemeen medicus', 6-4-1979; De Leeuw, 'Reacties op Holocaust zijn nauwelijks te voorspellen', 21-4-1979
23: Jungman, 'De kijk van Jungman', 22-1-1979
24: Ibidem
25: 'Aanslagen tegen "Holocaust" op Duitse tv', 20-1-1979; 'TROS bereidt zich voor op reacties TV serie Holocaust', 30-1-1979; Hofstede, 'Tros brengt Holocaust', 6-2-1979; 'Nederlands Auschwitz Comité vindt Holocaust "goede" film', 10-2-1979; 'Auschwitz Comité vindt Holocaust goede film', 8-2-1979; 'Uit de weekbladen', 1-2-1979; 'Tros brengt

"Holocaust"', 20-1-1979; 'Beslissing', 6-2-1979; Derksen, 'Zes miljoen doden op de toonbank', 31-3-1979; Vaders, 'Moet dat nou, Holocaust', 6-4-1979; 'Weekbladeren', 12-4-1979; 'Jodenvervolging als TV spel', 17-4-1979; Abrahams, 'Discussie ook hier noodzakelijk', 18-4-1979; 'Tros' informatie gaat aan te veel voorbij', 21-4-1979; Van de Poel, 'Zo mag ik 't zien', 24-4-79; Herzberg, 'Holocaust verzwakt de werkelijkheid', 30-4-1979

26: 'Richtlijnen van CRM voor uitzendingen over oorlog', 9-2-1979; 'TROS dringt terecht aan op begeleiding van "Holocaust"', 7-3-1979

27: See: Müller-Bauseneik, 'Die US-Fernsehserie "Holocaust"'; Wilke, 'Die Fernsehserie "Holocaust" als Medienereignis'

28: 'Neo-nazi's van aanslag op TV masten verdacht', 20-1-1979; 'Aanslagen tegen "Holocaust" op Duitse tv', 20-1-1979; 'Neo-nazi's willen meer acties tegen TV serie Holocaust', 22-1-1979; 'TROS bereidt zich voor op reacties TV serie Holocaust', 30-1-1979

29: 'Dr. A. Sunier', 6-4-1979

30: 'Kijken naar Holocaust afgeraden', 23-4-1979

31: 'Kijk niet', 20-4-1979

32: Ibidem

33: Loonstein, 'Joods Nederland bekeek Holocaustserie nauwelijks', 27-4-1979

34: 'Centrum '45: "TROS moet Holocaust uitstellen"', 7-2-1979; 'Opvang en begeleiding tijdens Holocaust-serie', 8-2-1979; 'Holocaust begeleid door radioserie', 8-2-1979; 'Verzoek van Centrum '45 aan TROS', 8-2-1979; 'TROS zal de serie Holocaust niet uitstellen', 8-2-1979; 'Nederlands Auschwitz Comité vindt Holocaust "goede" film', 10-2-1979; 'Intensieve begeleiding "Holocaust" in Nederland', 8-2-1979; 'Gevoelens', 9-2-1979; 'Holocaust, huiveringwekkend stuk geschiedenis, op tv', 2-4-1979

35: 'Holocaust toch in Duitse versie', 8-2-1979; 'Holocaust begeleid door radioserie', 8-2-1979

36: 'TROS bereidt zich voor op reacties TV serie Holocaust', 30-1-1979; Hofstede, 'Tros brengt Holocaust', 6-2-1979; 'Opvang en begeleiding tijdens Holocaust-serie', 8-2-1979; 'Holocaust begeleid door radioserie', 8-2-1979; 'Nederlands Auschwitz Comité vindt Holocaust "goede" film', 10-2-1979; 'Auschwitz Comité niet gekend in voorlichting over Holocaust', 16-2-1979; 'Expoge biedt Tros hulp bij nazorg', 16-2-1979; 'Henk Leliefeld, algemeen medicus', 6-4-1979; 'TROS dringt terecht aan op begeleiding van "Holocaust"', 7-3-1979; Sant, 'Holocaust wordt nú al begeleid door de TROS', 26-3-1979; 'Holocaust vertoond voor Friese hulpverleners', 4-4-1979; De Leeuw, 'Reacties op Holocaust zijn

nauwelijks te voorspellen', 21-4-1979; Withuis, Mooij, 'From totalitarianism to trauma', 197
37: Hofstede, 'Tros brengt Holocaust', 6-2-1979
38: 'Holocaust, huiveringwekkend stuk geschiedenis, op tv', 2-4-1979
39: 'Holocaust op Nederlandse tv', 7-4-1979
40: 'Holocaust, huiveringwekkend stuk geschiedenis, op tv', 2-4-1979; 'Dr. A. Sunier', 6-4-1979; 'Holocaust op Nederlandse tv', 7-4-1979
41: 'Holocaust, huiveringwekkend stuk geschiedenis, op tv', 2-4-1979; 'Holocaust op Nederlandse tv', 7-4-1979
42: Haveman, 'Ze kunnen De Waarheid nooit vertellen, nooit', 21-4-1979
43: 'Holocaust: nog niet erg veel heftige emoties', 24-4-1979; 'Bommeldingen na eerste uitzending Holocaust', 24-4-1979; 'Nederland ontvangt Holocaust beheerst', 24-4-1979; 'Na Holocaust 400 tot 500 telefoontjes', 24-4-1979; Langerak, 'Wisselende reacties op Holocaust', 25-4-1979; 'Hulpdienst verwerkte 500 reacties na Holocaust', 27-4-1979
44: 'Holocaust: nog niet erg veel heftige emoties', 24-4-1979; 'Bommeldingen na eerste uitzending Holocaust', 24-4-1979; 'Nederland ontvangt Holocaust beheerst', 24-4-1979; 'Na Holocaust 400 tot 500 telefoontjes', 24-4-1979; Langerak, 'Wisselende reacties op Holocaust', 25-4-1979; 'Hulpdienst verwerkte 500 reacties na Holocaust', 27-4-1979
45: 'Holocaust: nog niet erg veel heftige emoties', 24-4-1979
46: Ibidem; 'Bommeldingen na eerste uitzending Holocaust', 24-4-1979; 'Nederland ontvangt Holocaust beheerst', 24-4-1979; 'Na Holocaust 400 tot 500 telefoontjes', 24-4-1979
47: Langerak, 'Wisselende reacties op Holocaust', 25-4-1979
48: 'Telefoon roodgloeiend na derde deel Holocaust', 30-4-1979; 'Holocaust: weer vele reacties', 30-4-1979; Abel Herzberg, 'Holocaust verzwakt de werkelijkheid', 30-4-1979
49: 'Telefoon al tijdens uitzending Holocaust roodgloeiend', 4-5-1979; Gnirrep, 'Holocaust – de niet te bevatten werkelijkheid', 5-5-1979
50: Sereny, *De Duisternis Tegemoet*
51: Van Zweden, 'Dodenkamp Sobibor aan de vergetelheid ontrukt', 24-4-1979
52: 'Prof. Bastiaans bij presentatie boek van Cohen', 24-4-1979; Kamphuis, 'De negentien treinen naar Sobibor', 21-4-1979
53: Kamphuis, 'De negentien treinen naar Sobibor', 21-4-1979
54: Ibidem; Van der Hart et al., 'Psychotraumatologie', 49

20. The caregiving criticised

1: 'Bij bijna alle slachtoffers van gijzelingen nadelige gevolgen', 22-6-1979
2: 'Rapport roept op tot actieve hulpverlening', 22-6-1979
3: 'Rapport roept op tot actieve hulpverlening', 22-6-1979; 'Huisarts moet ex-gegijzelde direct helpen', 22-6-1979; 'Gijzelaars willen spontane hulp', 22-6-1979; 'Gijzelaars willen spontane hulp', 22-6-1979; De Groot, 'Gijzelingenrapport', 22-6-1979; 'Gegijzelden houden nog lang klachten', 22-6-1979; 'Gijzeling heeft soms ook positief gevolg', 22-6-1979; 'Gijzeling laat doorgaans lange tijd sporen na', 22-6-1979
4: 'Rapport roept op tot actieve hulpverlening', 22-6-1979
5: Ibidem; 'Gijzelaars willen spontane hulp', 22-6-1979; 'Gijzelingen werkten positief uit op slachtoffers', 22-6-1979; De Groot, 'Gijzelingenrapport', 22-6-1979; 'Gegijzelden houden nog lang klachten', 22-6-1979; 'Bij bijna alle slachtoffers van gijzelingen nadelige gevolgen', 22-6-1979; 'Rapport Leidse onderzoekers', 22-6-1979; 'Ex-gegijzelden hebben kritiek op autoriteiten', 22-6-1979; 'Beoordeling van daders "neutraal"', 22-6-1979; 'Helft slachtoffers positief over eigen rol', 22-6-1979; 'Gijzeling laat doorgaans lange tijd sporen na', 22-6-1979
6: 'Terug naar Alfaques om afstand te kunnen nemen', 14-7-1979
7: Ibidem
8: 'Gegijzelden zijn soms te diep in de put gedrukt', 31-7-1979
9: Van der Ploeg, 'Preludium'
10: Snelders, *LSD en de Psychiatrie in Nederland*, 96-97
11: 'Klacht tegen Bastiaans na behandeling', 7-9-1979; 'Directeur kliniek aangeklaagd voor LSD behandeling', 7-9-1979; 'Klacht tegen professor Bastiaans', 7-9-1979; 'Klacht na toediening LSD door hoogleraar', 7-9-1979; 'Artsen beticht van ingreep in hersenen', 7-9-1979; 'Scientology-sekte klaagt LSD kuur in psychiatrie aan', 19-2-1980; Nietsch, 'Bastiaans', 5-2-1983
12: Gonggrijp, 'Sciëntologen krijgen ongelijk van het Medisch Tuchtcollege', 8-10-1980; 'Tuchtcollege pleit psychiater vrij', 8-10-1980; 'Psychiater door Tuchtcollege vrijgesproken', 8-10-1980; 'Klacht over psychiater afgewezen', 8-10-1980
13: Van der Hooff, 'Ik heb de gijzeling positief uitgebuit…', 10-10-1979
14: Ibidem
15: 'Nazorg, ja, maar zó mag het nooit meer', 10-10-1979
16: Ibidem
17: 'Post-Abortussyndroom onderwerp bijeenkomst Nederl. Artsenverbond', 25-10-1979; Van Overeem, 'De druppel die de emmer doet overlopen', 29-10-1979

18: 'Hoogleraren pleiten voor andere abortuswetgeving', 5-6-1976; 'Artsen roepen op tot aanpassing abortuswet', 5-6-1976
19: 'Syndroom', 3-11-1979
20: Van Overeem, 'De druppel die de emmer doet overlopen', 29-10-1979; 'Syndroom', 3-11-1979
21: Van Overeem, 'De druppel die de emmer doet overlopen', 29-10-1979
22: 'Syndroom', 3-11-1979
23: Spanjer, 'Bastiaans', 31-10-1979; 'Vertoont het post-abortus-syndroom overeenkomst met het KZ-syndroom?', 1-11-1979
24: 'Vertoont het post-abortus-syndroom overeenkomst met het KZ-syndroom?', 1-11-1979
25: 'Syndroom', 3-11-1979

21. The story continues

1: Frequin, *Ga Maar Rustig Slapen*, 5-6
2: De Swaan, 'Het onvermogen om te luisteren', 3-5-1980
3: Ibidem; Enning, *De Oorlog van Bastiaans*, 17-19, 169. For De Swaan's vision also see: Withuis, 'Het concentratiekampsyndroom'; Citroen, *U wordt door Niemand Verwacht*, 153-154; Hondius, *Terugkeer*, 171; Piersma, *De Drie van Breda*, 195
4: Alink, 'Gevolgen van de oorlog zijn nog lang niet opgevangen', 10-5-1980
5: 'Oorlogsslachtoffers nog steeds in het verdomhoekje', 3-12-1979
6: Ibidem
7: 'Nederlanders over hun "rampen"-syndroom', 9-4-1980; Diepstraten, 'Nuttige discussie over oorlogsjaren', 9-4-1980; Van Dijk, 'Aart C. Gisolf en 't "rampen-syndroom"', 9-4-1980; 'Onvoltooid verleden', 10-4-1980; '"Rampen-syndroom" in Artsenij', 10-4-1980; '"Artsenij" ontrafelt het "rampensyndroom"', 10-4-1980
8: Nijkamp-van Doornik, '"Onvoltooid verleden" – NS-documentaire over rampen-syndroom', 10-4-1980
9: 'Nederlanders over hun "rampen"-syndroom', 9-4-1980; Diepstraten, 'Nuttige discussie over oorlogsjaren', 9-4-1980; Van Dijk, 'Aart C. Gisolf en 't "rampen-syndroom"', 9-4-1980; 'Onvoltooid verleden', 10-4-1980; '"Rampen-syndroom" in Artsenij', 10-4-1980; Nijkamp-van Doornik, '"Onvoltooid verleden" – NS-documentaire over rampen-syndroom', 10-4-1980
10: 'Onvoltooid verleden', 10-4-1980; '"Artsenij" ontrafelt het "rampensyndroom"', 10-4-1980

11: Van den Houten, ‘Belevingsboeken over oorlog meer dan naakt feitenmateriaal’, 2-5-1980
12: Van de Poel, ‘Zo mag ik ’t zien’, 11-4-1980
13: Diepstraten, ‘Nuttige discussie over oorlogsjaren’, 9-4-1980
14: Peereboom, ‘Littekens gijzeling blijven’, 5-1-1980; ‘Prof. Bastiaans over gegijzelden in Teheran’, 11-4-1980; ‘Prof. Bastiaans over gijzelaars in Teheran’, 14-4-1980; ‘Prof.dr. J. Bastiaans over toestand gegijzelden in Teheran’, 16-4-1980
15: Peereboom, ‘Littekens gijzeling blijven’, 5-1-1980
16: Ibidem
17: Ibidem
18: Ibidem
19: Ibidem
20: ‘Scientology-sekte klaagt LSD kuur in psychiatrie aan’, 19-2-1980
21: Ibidem
22: Grijpma, ‘Na 35 jaar weerzien met Auschwitz’, 25-6-1980
23: Withuis, *Erkenning*, 241
24: ‘Herdenking einde van oorlog 1945’, 10-7-1980; ‘Herdenking eind tweede wereldoorlog’, 14-7-1980

22. The East Indies Camp syndrome

1: Bossenbroek, *De Meelstreep*, 534
2: Hulst, ‘Indisch oorlogsleed en Nederlands onbegrip’, 25-8-1979
3: Ibidem
4: Kousbroek, ‘Terug naar Negri Panerkomst 20’; Bekkering, ‘De Japanse kampen’.
5: Kousbroek, ‘Terug naar Negri Panerkomst 20’;
6: Ibidem
7: Kousbroek, ‘Terug naar Negri Panerkomst 21’
8: Kuipers-De Haan, ‘Kampsyndroom’; Stout, ‘Kampsyndroom’
9: Dikkers, ‘Echte dromen’
10: Engelbrecht, ‘Het Indische kampsyndroom’
11: ‘Leed in Jappenkampen lange tijd verdrongen’, 27-8-1983; Kreutzer, ‘Lange tijd is leed in Jappenkampen verdrongen’, 29-8-1983
12: Engelbrecht, ‘Gevangenen van de vrede’, 23-7-1980; Buijze, ‘Vergeten kampslachtoffers’, 9-8-1980
13: Buijze, ‘Vergeten kampslachtoffers’, 9-8-1980
14: Engelbrecht, ‘Gevangenen van de vrede’, 23-7-1980
15: Ibidem
16: Ibidem

17: Engelbrecht spoke of "the three standard works". He meant: D. van Velden, *De Japanse burgerkampen*, E. van Witsen, *Krijgsgevangenen in de Pacific-oorlog* and I.J. Brugmans, *Nederlands-Indië onder Japanse bezetting*
18: Engelbrecht. 'Gevangenen van de vrede', 23-7-1980
19: F.i.: 'Ir. G.S. Vrijburg: "Echt bevrijd zijn wij niet"', 9-8-1980; Van der Put, 'Wim des Celles al jarenlang ondergedoken in zijn "vaderland"', 9-8-1980
20: Buijze, 'Vergeten kampslachtoffers', 9-8-1980
21: Ibidem
22: 'Einde van oorlog herdacht', 16-8-1980
23: 'Slachtoffers in Ned.-Indië herdacht', 15-8-1980; 'Japanse overgave herdacht', 16-8-1980
24: 'Einde van oorlog herdacht', 16-8-1980
25: 'Sfeervolle herdenking van Japanse capitulatie in 1945', 16-8-1980
26: Bastiaans, *Isolement en Bevrijding*
27: 'Slachtoffers in Ned.-Indië herdacht', 15-8-1980; 'Japanse overgave herdacht', 16-8-1980; '"Zij zijn erg eenzaam"', 14-8-1982
28: 'Japanse overgave herdacht', 16-8-1980; 'Sfeervolle herdenking van Japanse capitulatie in 1945', 16-8-1980; 'Einde van oorlog herdacht', 16-8-1980
29: Buijze, 'Vergeten kampslachtoffers', 9-8-1980. Also: 'Syndroom', 22-11-1986

23. The aftercare under fire and the hostage-taking in Tehran

1: 'Televizier-Magazine over jaar gijzelaars in Iran', 24-10-1980; 'Televizier', 24-10-1980
2: Voituron, 'Gijzelaars bedreigd door kampsyndroom', 29-10-1980
3: Ibidem
4: Ibidem
5: Kuipers, 'Ex-gegijzelde Ger Vaders', 29-11-1980
6: Ibidem
7: Ibidem
8: Vaders, 'Prof. Bastiaans', 12-2-1986
9: Kuipers, 'Ex-gegijzelde Ger Vaders', 29-11-1980
10: Ibidem
11: Wiese, 'Te veel publiciteit?', 29-11-1980
12: Kuipers, 'Ex-gegijzelde mevrouw Giessen', 29-11-1980
13: Ibidem

14: Van der Hoek, 'Prof. Bastiaans over "Teheran"', 20-1-1981
15: Ibidem
16: Kuipers, 'Nederlandse psychiaters adviseren bij hulp aan Amerikaanse gijzelaars', 20-1-1981. Also: Van Loon, 'Vier geleerden schreven boek over gijzelingen', 29-9-1981
17: 'Prof. Bastiaans: Voldoende hulp voor gijzelaars', 21-1-1981
18: Spaan, 'Goede raad is duur', 21-1-1981
19: 'Gardeniers is voor monument in Westerbork', 29-1-1981
20: 'Groeiende nood onder oorlogsslachtoffers', 29-1-1981
21: Ibidem
22: Ibidem
23: '"Verbijsterend wat kinderen van NSB'ers na de oorlog is aangedaan"', 13-1-1983; 'Kind van NSB'er klaagt zijn nood', 13-1-1983; 'NSB-kinderen: "Niet de schuld, wel de straf"', 13-1-1983; 'Boek over leed NSB-kinderen', 13-1-1981; 'Kinderen van NSB'ers komen nu in de problemen', 14-1-1983; '"Leed van kinderen van NSB'ers vaak onderschat"', 14-1-1983; 'NSB-kinderen: niet de schuld, wel de straf', 14-1-1983; Lulofs, 'Taboe', 5-2-1983
24: Benders, 'Een gijzeling en de nazorg', 7-2-1981
25: Ibidem
26: Ibidem
27: Ibidem
28: Ibidem
29: Ibidem

24. Financial and medical worries

1: Rooijmans, *99 Jaar tussen Wal en Schip*, hfdst. 5 en 6
2: 'Professor Bastiaans: "Behandeling van oorlogsslachtoffers naar dieptepunt"', 16-7-1981
3: Ibidem; 'Professor Bastiaans over oorlogsslachtoffers', 17-7-1981
4: De Groot, 'Bevrijding… spreekkamers zullen volstromen', 1-4-1985
5: Heijmans, 'Dit was een Jappenkamp', 14-1982
6: Dikkers, 'Uitkering aan Indische ex-kampmensen een afvalrace', 15-8-1981
7: Hagers, 'Spanningen tussen medewerkers', 31-7-1981; Bruinsma, 'Pionierswerk Centrum '40-'45 zeker zinvol', 24-1-1984
8: Bruinsma, 'Pionierswerk Centrum '40-'45 zeker zinvol', 24-1-1984
9: Buijze, '"Je moet opnieuw door de hel, maar ik wil het nu afmaken"', 17-3-1984

25. The book *People at Hostage-takings*

1: Bastiaans, Mulder, Van Dijk, Van der Ploeg, *Mensen bij Gijzelingen*
2: Van Loon, 'Vier geleerden schreven boek over gijzelingen', 29-9-1981; 'Premier Van Agt ontvangt boek "Mensen bij gijzelingen"', 29-9-1981; 'Boek over de gevolgen van gijzelingen', 29-9-1981
3: Boltendal, 'Mensen bij Gijzelingen', 21-8-1982
4: Van der Hoek, 'Mensen bij gijzelingen', 1-10-1981
5: 'Psychiater verwacht sterke uitbreiding terrorisme', 28-9-1981; 'Terroristen zoeken naar nieuwe vormen van actie', 28-9-1981; 'Psychiater D. Mulder in boek "Mensen bij gijzelingen": "Terrorisme"', 29-9-1981; 'Psychiater D. Mulder in boek "Mensen bij gijzelingen": Terrorisme', 29-9-1981
6: 'Psychiater verwacht sterke uitbreiding terrorisme', 28-9-1981; 'Terroristen zoeken naar nieuwe vormen van actie', 28-9-1981; 'Psychiater D. Mulder in boek "Mensen bij gijzelingen": "Terrorisme"', 29-9-1981; 'Psychiater D. Mulder in boek "Mensen bij gijzelingen": Terrorisme', 29-9-1981
7: 'Psychiater verwacht sterke uitbreiding terrorisme', 28-9-1981
8: 'Snel intensieve hulp voor ex-gijzelaars', 28-9-1981; Bagijn, 'Gijzelaars hebben nog lang angst', 29-9-1981
9: 'Snel intensieve hulp voor ex-gijzelaars', 28-9-1981; Van Loon, 'Vier geleerden schreven boek over gijzelingen', 29-9-1981
10: Bagijn, 'Gijzelaars hebben nog lang angst', 29-9-1981
11: Ibidem
12: Van Loon, 'Vier geleerden schreven boek over gijzelingen', 29-9-1981
13: Van der Hoek, 'Mensen bij gijzelingen', 1-10-1981
14: 'Ervaringen geleerden in boek gepubliceerd', 30-9-1981
15: Klinkenberg, 'Hannie Schafts ideologie is in film verdoezeld', 1-10-1981
16: Boltendal, 'Mensen bij Gijzelingen', 21-8-1982
17: Glimmerveen, 'Psychiatrie van de mollegang', 6-10-1981
18: Ibidem
19: Boltendal, 'Mensen bij Gijzelingen', 21-8-1982
20: Vaders, 'Einde van een illusie', 29-9-1981
21: Nieboer, 'Terrorisme niet los te zien van publieke norm-ondergraving', 14-6-1982
22: Van der Hoek, 'Mensen bij gijzelingen', 1-10-1981
23: Peereboom, 'Het trauma van de gegijzelde mens', 17-10-1981
24: Koolbergen, 'Kernwapens en pudding', 8-10-1981

26. The endgame

1: 'Hoogleraar weigert verhuizing patiënten', 21-9-1982; 'Bastiaans wil niet verhuizen', 21-9-1982; 'Bastiaans', 29-10-1982; 'Prijs', 30-10-1982
2: Thomassen, 'Universiteit van Leiden ontslaat directeur kliniek', 19-1-1983
3: 'Prof. Bastiaans wil functie niet neerleggen', 20-1-1983; Nietsch, 'Bastiaans', 5-2-1983
4: 'Patiënten op de bres voor "hun" Bastiaans', 26-1-1983
5: Ibidem
6: Ibidem
7: Verburgh, 'Professor Bastiaans in conflict met Leidse universiteit', 27-1-1983; Nietsch, 'Bastiaans', 5-2-1983
8: Komrij, 'Een en ander', 2-2-1983
9: Enning, *De Oorlog van Bastiaans*, 230-231; Piersma, *De Drie van Breda*, 108, 126
10: 'Brieven', 14-2-1983; Scheepmaker, 'Trijfel', 21-2-1983; Enning, *De Oorlog van Bastiaans*, 233-234; Piersma, *De Drie van Breda*, 108
11: Verburgh, 'Professor Bastiaans in conflict met Leidse universiteit', 27-1-1983
12: 'Bastiaans mag tot in 1985 behandelen', 5-2-1983; 'Conflict opgelost', 7-2-1983; 'Prof. Bastiaans mag behandeling oorlogssyndroom voortzetten', 7-2-1983; 'Prof. Bastiaans kan doorgaan', 7-2-1983; 'Prof. Bastiaans blijft nog tot 1985 werken', 7-2-1983; 'Prof. Bastiaans zet werk voort', 7-2-1983; 'Prof. Bastiaans kan oorlogsslachtoffers blijven behandelen', 8-2-1983; 'Bastiaans blijft bij Jelgersmakliniek', 8-2-1983; 'Prof. Bastiaans blijft werken onder oorlogsslachtoffers', 8-2-1983
13: Gisolf, 'Bastiaans: bewonderd en gehaat', 14-2-1983
14: 'Prof. Bastiaans mag patiënten niet toelaten tot collegezaal', 26-4-1983; 'Patiënten prof. Bastiaans mogen college niet meer in', 26-4-1983; 'Universiteit wil na 1 juni van hoogleraar af', 29-3-1985; Rooijmans, 'Bastiaans', 6-4-1985; Enning, *De Oorlog van Bastiaans*, 238-241, 248
15: 'Werkgroep wil voortzetting van therapie prof. Bastiaans', 30-1-1984; Hagers, 'Oorlogssyndroom neemt toe', 4-5-1984; Terwindt, 'Syndroom', 9-5-1984; 'Kamerleden bezorgd over vertrek van prof. Bastiaans', 5-7-1984; 'Weekbladeren', 2-8-1984; 'Aanblijven professor Bastiaans bepleit', 27-2-1985; 'Verzet bepleit voortzetting van therapie Bastiaans', 27-2-1985; Van den Berg, 'Slachtoffers van oorlog bepleiten bij Kamer voortzetting therapie-Bastiaans', 27-2-1985; 'Prof. Bastiaans mag van Kamer behandeling nog even voortzetten', 27-2-1985; 'Bastiaans mag slachtoffers oorlog blijven behandelen', 27-2-1985; 'Bewindsman streeft ernaar werk

Bastiaans te redden', 28-2-1985; 'Kort', 28-2-1985; '"Methode Bastiaans handhaven"', 28-2-1985; Buijze, 'Bastiaans verliest', 28-2-1985; 'Van der Reijden weigert garantie aanblijven prof. Bastiaans', 28-2-1985; 'Voortzetting van therapie Bastiaans is nog onzeker', 28-2-1985; 'Van der Reijden (WVC)', 28-3-1985; 'Kamer: werk van Bastiaans moet doorgaan', 29-3-1985; 'Kamer: werk prof. Bastiaans moet voortgezet', 29-3-1985; De Groot, 'Patiënt van prof. Bastiaans', 2-4-1985; Pons, 'Mei geen jubelmaand voor ex-verzetsmensen', 4-4-1985/11-4-1985; 'Weekbladen', 11-4-1985; 'Stichting voor slachtoffers van oorlog en geweld', 20-6-1985; Jacobus, 'Stichting opgericht voor slachtoffers van geweld', 28-6-1985

16: 'Tweede kliniek Centrum '45', 20-6-1985; 'Staatssecretaris reikt Centrum '45 helpende hand', 21-6-1985; 'Van der Reijden bereid Centrum '45 uit te breiden', 21-6-1985; 'Hulp slachtoffers oorlog uitgebreid', 21-6-1985

17: '"Psychische gevolgen van oorlogservaringen veel te laat ontdekt"', 8-5-1985

18: 'Bewindsman beziet of opvolger Bastiaans met LSD mag werken', 12-9-1984; 'Na vertrek van Bastiaans toepassing LSD niet toegestaan', 12-9-1984; 'Van der Reijden: voortzetting werk Bastiaans onzeker', 28-2-1985; Roy Buijze, 'Bastiaans verliest', 28-2-1985; 'Van der Reijden voor methode van Bastiaans', 28-2-1985; 'Staatssecretaris Van der Reijden weigert toezegging', 28-2-1985; 'Bewindsman wil Bastiaans behouden, dat wel', 1-3-1985; 'Kamer wil therapie Bastiaans behouden', 1-3-1985; 'Bewindsman steunt Bastiaans in voortzetten hulp oorlogsvervolgden', 28-3-1985; 'Universiteit wil na 1 juni van hoogleraar af', 29-3-1985; 'Werk Bastiaans zal worden voortgezet', 5-4-1985; 'Centrum '45 neemt hulp oorlogsslachtoffers van prof. Bastiaans over', 20-6-1985; 'Verzet is ongerust over trage behandeling werk van professor Bastiaans', 13-12-1985; 'Overleg opgeschort over Centrum '45', 18-12-1985

19: 'Bastiaans bij afscheid: onzekerheid leidt tot isolement', 29-6-1985; 'Bastiaans neemt afscheid van universiteit', 29-6-1985; 'Prof. Bastiaans neemt afscheid als hoogleraar', 29-6-1985. Also: Bastiaans, *Isolement en Bevrijding*, 9-17

20: Huijskens, 'Degradatie prof. Bastiaans wekt alom bevreemding', 23-1-1986

21: Huygen, 'Prof Bastiaans kijkt terug bij emeritaat', 3-7-1985

22: 'Prof. Bastiaans kan doorgaan met behandeling', 9-5-1985; 'Bastiaans kan oorlogsslachtoffers blijven behandelen', 9-5-1985; 'Ruimte voor oorlogspatiënten aangeboden', 11-5-1985; 'Prof. Bastiaans krijgt ruimte op Endegeest', 11-5-1985; 'Aanbod Endegeest voor voor opvang patiënten Bastiaans', 11-5-1985; 'Psychiatrisch centrum wil doorgaan met opvang van oorlogsslachtoffers', 11-5-1985; 'Pleidooi heropenen van kliniek Bastiaans', 21-5-1985; 'Commissie ziet kansen voor continueren werk Bastiaans', 22-5-1985; 'Oplossing voor werk Bastiaans', 22-5-1985; 'Oplossing nabij voor patiënten van Bastiaans', 22-5-1985; 'Bastiaans', 23-5-1985; 'Oplossing voor patiënten prof. Bastiaans in zicht', 23-5-1985; 'Centrum '45 zet werk van prof. J. Bastiaans voort', 20-6-1985; 'Oorlogsslachtoffers moeten tijdelijk ondergebracht', 14-4-1987; 'Bastiaans zoekt tijdelijk onderdak', 14-4-1987; 'Bastiaans', 16-4-1987; 'Bastiaans', 18-6-1987; 'Hulp blijft voor oorlogsslachtoffers', 18-6-1987; Enning, *De Oorlog van Bastiaans*, 246

23: Withuis, *Erkenning*, 83

24: Van der Ploeg, 'Stress en psychotrauma's', 6

25: 'Van der Reijden regelt opvolgen Bastiaans niet', 13-2-1986; 'Twee psychiaters moeten Bastiaans opvolgen', 13-2-1986; 'Voor opvolging prof. Bastiaans 2 kandidaten', 13-2-1986; 'Bewindsman bemoeit zich niet met opvolging dr. J. Bastiaans', 13-2-1986; Luirink, 'Methode Bastiaans dreigt te verdwijnen', 12-5-1987; 'Kamer wil snel opvolger Bastiaans', 18-6-1987; 'Bastiaans krijgt half jaar voor regelen opvolger', 18-6-1987; 'Centrum '45 accepteert de methode-Bastiaans', 18-6-1987; 'Prof. Bastiaans werkt opvolgers in', 11-7-1987; 'Prof. Bastiaans werkt zelf zijn drie opvolgers in', 11-7-1987; 'Bastiaans (bijna 70) werkt drie opvolgers in', 21-8-1987; 'Drie artsen "leren" methode Bastiaans', 22-8-1987; 'Slachtoffers geweld in de kou', 18-9-1987; 'Drie artsen opvolgers van psychiater Bastiaans', 20-11-1987; 'Bastiaans opgevolgd door drie man bij Centrum 45', 21-11-1987; 'Oorlogsslachtoffers klagen arts van Centrum '45 aan', 30-11-1987

26: 'Sluiting dreigt voor kliniek van Bastiaans', 13-4-1987; 'Prof. Bastiaans moet stoppen met kliniek', 13-4-1987; 'Prof. Bastiaans dreigt dakloos te worden', 14-4-1987; 'Kliniek Bastiaans tijdelijk dakloos', 14-4-1987; 'Patiënten Bastiaans tijdelijk dakloos', 14-4-1987

27: 'Behandelploeg Bastiaans rond', 23-1-1986

28: Bruinsma, 'Inspectie kritiseert therapie Bastiaans', 23-1-1986; 'Onderzoek naar gebruik LSD in therapie Bastiaans', 23-1-1986; 'Pentothal-behandeling Bastiaans onderzocht', 23-1-1986; 'Onderzoek naar werkmethoden van professor J. Bastiaans', 24-1-1986; 'Onderzoek naar methode Bastiaans', 24-1-1986

29: 'Prof. Bastiaans', 6-2-1986; Musaph, 'LSD wordt steeds minder gebruikt', 7-2-1986; Boer, 'Slechts weinig onderzoek gedaan', 7-2-1986; Van Amsterdam, 'LSD: onberekenbaar medicijn', 8-2-1986; Van Dijk, 'LSD: Van alles gaan de helften uiteen', 8-2-1986; 'De methode-Bastiaans', 8-2-1986; Van der Hoek, 'Hebt u onder de bom gezeten dan?', 3-3-1986;

Fortuin, '"Wat worden wij daar nou wijzer van, papa Bas?"', 31-10-1987; 'Maar meneer', 12-11-1987; Bolle, 'Bastiaans', 3-12-1987

30: Van der Hooff, 'Jan Bastiaans en het contactisolement', 10-6-1985/13-6-1985

31: 'Bastiaans komt tegemoet aan eisen inspecteur', 24-1-1986

32: 'Nieuw conflict over methode Bastiaans', 1-2-1986; 'Prof Bastiaans mag bij nieuwe patiënten geen LSD gebruiken', 3-2-1986; 'Prof Bastiaans voorziet weinig problemen na verbod gebruik LSD', 3-2-1986; 'Geen nieuwe patiënten voor artsen met opiumverlof', 4-2-1986; 'Toediening LSD bij behandelen patiënten voorlopig verboden', 4-2-1986; 'Nieuwe behandelingen met LSD verboden', 4-2-1986; 'Verbod op kuren met hallucinerende middelen', 4-2-1986; '"Behandeling nieuwe patiënten met LSD voorlopig verbieden"', 5-2-1986

33: 'Bastiaans mag LSD methode blijven toepassen', 6-2-1986; Huijskens, 'Professor Bastiaans mag LSD therapie blijven toepassen', 6-2-1986; 'Bastiaans mag LSD blijven toepassen', 6-2-1986; 'LSD therapie voortgezet', 6-2-1986; 'Bastiaans mag met LSD blijven werken', 6-2-1986; 'Bastiaans mag LSD gebruiken', 6-2-1986; 'Prof Bastiaans mag therapie voortzetten', 6-2-1986; 'Voorwaarden aan LSD therapie', 6-2-1986; Huijskens, 'Weer aan het werk en nog subsidie ook', 8-2-1986

34: Vroon, 'LSD', 1-2-1986

35: Vroon, 'Geurtjes', 4-5-1985; Vroon, 'LSD', 1-2-1986; Vroon, 'Liegen', 8-2-1986. Also: Eeraerts, 'LSD', 30-5-1985

36: Vroon, 'Geurtjes', 4-5-1985

37: Van Hoorn, 'De vergelijking tussen de methodes van Bastiaans en Freud is misplaatst', 20-2-1986

38: 'Holocaust-hallucinaties tijdens Leidse LSD kuur te boek gesteld', 29-5-1987; 'Weekbladeren', 4-9-1987; Ka-Tzetnik 135633, *Shivitti*; Snelders, *LSD en de Psychiatrie in Nederland*, 111, 119-121

39: Polak, 'Van Meekren, waarom?', 29-11-1986

40: 'Bastiaans: bestraffen oorlogsmisdadiger "dwaas"', 16-11-1987; Fortuin, 'De deskundigheid van prof. J. Bastiaans lijkt grenzeloos', 26-11-1987; Wolff, 'Bastiaans', 3-12-1987

41: Metz, 'Bastiaans', 5-12-1986

42: Nanninga, 'Oud-consul moet boeten voor fraude', 7-2-1987; Metz, 'Ton boete, geen cel geëist tegen oud-consul', 7-2-1987

43: Haveman, 'En dan ga je naar de beul', 16-3-1985; '"Geen korting geld oorlogsslachtoffers"', 28-3-1985; 'Kamer steunt zuinig kabinet in kwestie oorlogsslachtoffers', 29-3-1985; 'Aandacht voor vergeten veteranen', 15-5-1985; 'Stichting '40-'45 "is nog lang niet klaar met werk"', 11-5-1985

44: De Lange, 'Ben Polak vreest voor oorlogsgetroffenen', 2-9-1985; Bruinsma, '"Sluiten wetten slachtoffers oorlog aantasting ereschuld"', 3-9-1985; Soetendorp, 'Blijf kinderen van slachtoffers oorlog helpen!', 1-4-1986; Van der Hooff, 'De barre lijdensweg van kandidaten voor een uitkering voor oorlogsslachtoffers', 10-7-1986; '"Uitkering burgeroorlogsslachtoffers een lijdensweg"', 25-10-1986. For the ideas of Polak also see the 1989 book from ICODO *Oorlogstrauma's na 45 jaar?* Engelsman, *Oorlogstrauma's*, 105-112. His minority view is listed on 111-112. In the preface (7-8) Lou de Jong make a stand in favour of pensions.
45: 'Rapport haalt basis van recht oorlogsslachtoffer op een uitkering weg', 19-3-1987; 'Aanvragers oorlogsuitkering vrezen verzwaring bewijslast', 23-3-1987; Van Oosten, 'Het verzet en het onbegrip van twee psychiaters', 4-5-1987; 'Oorlogsgetroffenen vragen Brinkman duidelijkheid', 13-5-1987; Mooij, 'De langste schaduw', 282; Enning, *De Oorlog van Bastiaans*, 277-278; Withuis, *Erkenning*, 80-83; Van der Hart et al., 'Psychotraumatologie', 49; Hafkenscheid, 'Het (on)gewone in de diagnostiek'; Bossenbroek, *De Meelstreep*, 455
46: 'Brieven', 16-4-1987; Pennewaard, 'Na veertig jaar', 4-5-1987
47: Heertje, 'Een rapport dat maar geheim moet blijven', 21-3-1987
48: 'Prof. Bastiaans: LSD kan het slot openen', 14-12-1987; Mooij, 'De langste schaduw', 282-283; Bossenbroek, *De Meelstreep*, 456
49: Bruinsma, '"Buitenwereld maakt van Bastiaans soort goeroe"', 12-12-1987. Also: Hers, *Stress*, 173: 'Every disease of unknown origin that develops in an individual who was a victim of the war or participated in the resistance can, may and indeed must be ascribed to the war or the resistance, because proof of the opposite cannot be given.'
50: 'Conclusies psychiaters zouden kabinet goed uitkomen', 7-4-1987; De Wind, 'De onvoorspelbaarheid van het late optreden van oorlogstrauma's', 22-4-1987. The book *Oorlogstrauma's na 45 jaar?* (War Trauma's after 45 years?) opend by asking: 'Is it possible to get invalidated in 1989 because of traumatic events experienced in 1943?' The answer was: 'It not only is possible, it even happens quite frequently.' Engelsman, *Oorlogstrauma's*, 9
51: Boer, 'Oorlogsslachtoffers en literatuuronderzoek', 9-4-1987
52: '"Oorlogsslachtoffers hebben vooral behoefte aan rust"', 23-3-1987
53: 'Kenmerk besteedt aandacht aan werk prof. Bastiaans', 21-7-1987
54: Van der Ploeg, *Onderzoek naar de Behandeling van Oorlogsslachtoffers*
55: Willems, 'Prof. Bastiaans (70) staakt met tegenzin zijn controversiële werkwijze', 31-10-1987; Van den Berg, 'Prof. Bastiaans moet nu echt stoppen', 31-10-1987; 'Onderzoek naar resultaten therapie is mislukt', 6-11-1987; 'Onderzoek naar gevolg LSD behandeling Bastiaans mislukt', 6-11-1987; 'Gegevens ontbreken voor onderzoek Bastiaans', 6-11-1987; 'Te

weinig gegevens voor onderzoek van resultaten methode prof. Bastiaans', 6-11-1987; 'Onderzoek methode-Bastiaans mislukt', 6-11-1987; 'Studie methode-Bastiaans mislukt', 6-11-1987; Van den Berg, 'Bastiaans tuimelt van voetstuk', 14-11-87; 'Onderzoek naar methode Bastiaans is mislukking', 6-11-1987; 'Onderzoek methode-Bastiaans mislukt', 7-11-1987; Enning, *De Oorlog van Bastiaans*, 258-261; Rooijmans, *99 Jaar tussen Wal en Schip*, 127-129

56: Van der Ploeg, 'LSD in de psychiatrie', 16-6-2000

57: Memelink, 'Toen voelde ik dat mijn bevrijding voltooid was', 14-11-1987; 'Patiëntenactie voor aanblijven Bastiaans', 2-12-1987; 'Patiënten bezorgd over toekomst methode-Bastiaans', 3-12-1987; 'Patiënten bezorgd over voortbestaan methode-Bastiaans', 3-12-1987; 'Patiënten dringen aan op aanblijven prof. Bastiaans bij centrum', 3-12-1987; 'Bastiaans laat een onzekere toekomst achter', 3-12-1987; Snelders, *LSD en de Psychiatrie in Nederland*, 191-194

58: Van den Berg, 'Bastiaans tuimelt van voetstuk', 14-11-87

59: 'Geen voortzetting van LSD therapie', 21-12-1987; 'Opvolger Bastiaans vraagt toestemming voor gebruik LSD', 22-12-1987; Enning, *De Oorlog van Bastiaans*, 267

60: 'Behandelaar van oorlogstrauma's Bastiaans overleden', 1-11-1997

61: Garschagen, 'Therapeut', 31-12-1987

62: Bruinsma, 'Buitenwereld maakt van Bastiaans soort goeroe', 12-12-1987; 'Behandelaar van oorlogstrauma's Bastiaans overleden', 1-11-1997; For the status Bastiaans had, see: Enning, *De Oorlog van Bastiaans*, 169

63: Veltkamp, 'Kan prof. Bastiaans echt niet weg?', 27-3-1985; Enning, *De Oorlog van Bastiaans*, 226, 234; Rooijmans, *99 Jaar tussen Wal en Schip*, 119-131

64: Enning, *De Oorlog van Bastiaans*, 226

65: Lulofs, 'Ontslag', 9-3-1985

66: Willems, 'Prof. Bastiaans (70) staakt met tegenzin zijn controversiële werkwijze', 31-10-1987

67: Bastiaans, 'Hollands dagboek', 6-4-1985

68: 'Behandeling patiënten met oorlogstrauma in gevaar', 28-2-1987

69: Vaders, 'Vaders' visie: Prof. Bastiaans', 12-2-1986

70: Stein-Olman, 'Isolement en bevrijding voor de medische boekenkast', 27-3-1987

71: Bastiaans, *Isolement en Bevrijding*, 2

72: Fortuin, '"Wat worden wij daar nou wijzer van, papa Bas?"', 31-10-1987

73: Los, 'Prof. Bastiaans helpt vernielde mensen', 6-2-1987

74: Terwindt, 'Bastiaans', 15-3-1985; Du Chatenier, 'Leemte', 9-3-1985; Alons, 'Prof. Bastiaans', 13-3-1985; Aker, 'Prof. Bastiaans', 28-1-1986; Rep, 'Trix Terwindt', 9-4-1987; 'Voormalig verzetsstrijdster Trix Terwindt overleden', 10-4-1987; Croes-de Groot, 'Prof. Bastiaans', 22-8-1987; nl.wikipedia.org/wiki/Trix_Terwindt (seen: 25-10-2021)

75: Fortuin, 'De deskundigheid van prof. J. Bastiaans lijkt grenzeloos', 26-11-1987; Bruinsma, '"Buitenwereld maakt van Bastiaans soort goeroe"', 12-12-1987. Also: Wilschut, *Tussen Psychiatrie en Filosofie*, 294-295: noot 8

76: Gisolf, 'Bastiaans: bewonderd en gehaat', 14-2-1983

77: Willems, 'Libanon-syndroom na gewelddadige ervaringen', 25-10-1986. For the psychological effects of so-called peacemissions, see: Bramsen et al., *Deelname aan Vredesmissies*

78: '"Slechte opvang van militairen uit Indonesië leidt nu tot trauma's"', 22-5-1987

79: Goudriaan, 'Dertig jaar na "Korea". Het ergste komt later', 8-10-1983; Van Meurs, *Over de Gevechtsuitputting*

80: Goudriaan, 'Oud Indonesiëgangers', 24-4-1985; '"Slechte opvang van militairen uit Indonesië leidt nu tot trauma's"', 22-5-1987; For the problems of Indonesia veterans see: Scagliola, *Last van de Oorlog,* and for the Second World War and Korea as well, see: Van der Ploeg, Weerts, *Veteranen in Nederland*

81: De Groot, 'De mensen voor wie de oorlog telkens weer begint', 4-4-1985

82: Pennewaard, 'Na veertig jaar', 4-5-1987; Willems, 'Prof. Bastiaans (70) staakt met tegenzin zijn controversiële werkwijze', 31-10-1987

83: Fortuin, 'De deskundigheid van prof. J. Bastiaans lijkt grenzeloos', 26-11-1987

84: Van Heerden, 'Het onduidelijke KZ-syndroom', 3-2-1983; Pannekoek, *Memoires*, 134-135; Enning, *De oorlog van Bastiaans*, 143

85: F.i. Kaas was anything but a fan of solitary confinement. Kaas, *Buchenwald*, 27-29

86: Pannekoek, *Memoires*, 85; Cohen, *Het Duitse Concentratiekamp*, 108-109

87: Pannekoek, *Memoires*, 135; Aarts, 'De geschiedenis', 22

88: Van Heerden, 'Het onduidelijke KZ-syndroom', 3-2-1983

89: Ibidem

90: Ibidem

91: Van der Hooff, 'Jan Bastiaans en het contactisolement. "Ook een rotjeugd kan leiden tot een soort KZ-situatie"', 10-6-1985/13-6-1985

92: Historianet.nl/oorlog/tweede-wereldoorlog/hitler/had-hitler-maar-een-testikel (seen: 30-10-2021)

Closing remarks

1: Withuis, *Erkenning*, 85-98
2: Ibidem, 79
3: F.i.: De Ridder, Withuis, '"Scheldend op mezelf"'
4: Van der Hart et al., 'Psychotraumatologie', 47
5: Shorter, *A History of Psychiatry*, 303-305; Dean, *Shook over Hell*, chs. 1, 5; Young, *Harmony of Illusions*
6: Shorter, *A History of Psychiatry*, 304-305; Lifton, *Home from the War*; Lifton, Nazi-*doctors*; Fortuin, 'De deskundigheid van prof. J. Bastiaans lijkt grenzeloos', 26-11-1987; Withuis, *Erkenning*, 227-228; Van der Hart, Broeze, 'Posttraumatische stress', 34-35; Van der Hart et al., 'Psychotraumatologie', 52-53; Babington, *Shell-Shock*, 167-169; Hovens, Van der Ploeg, 'Hoe het trauma het gewone leven binnendrong', 803; McManners, *The Scars of War*, 12
7: Van der Hart, Broeze, 'Posttraumatische stress', 33
8: Acton, Potter, *Working in a World of Hurt*; McManners, *The Scars of War*, 305
9: Young, *The Harmony of Illusions*; Summerfield, 'The invention'; Rosen, Lilienfeld, 'Posttraumatic Stress Disorder'; Shorter, *A History of Psychiatry*, 303; Withuis, *Erkenning*, 216-219; Binneveld, *Om de Geest van Jan Soldaat*, 239-241; Montgomery, *The Invisible Injured*, 215; Shepard, *A War of Nerves*, 390-391, 396. For an abstract om the PTSD-discussion, see: Gersons, 'Traumaspectrumstoornissen'. Especially on Summerfield: 69-70. Quote: 76
10: Hovens, Van der Ploeg, 'Hoe het trauma het gewone leven binnendrong', 809; Withuis, Mooij, 'From totalitarianism to trauma', 212
11: Binneveld, *Om de Geest van Jan Soldaat*, 241-242; Montgomery, *The Invisible Injured*, 178-215; Van der Hart et al., 'Psychotraumatologie', 49; Gersons, 'Traumaspectrumstoornissen'
12: Andere Tijden, 'Bastiaans'
13: 'Executie van een onverwerkt verleden' (bron onbekend. Kopie in bezit auteur); Bastiaans, 'Executie'; Hagers, '"Joegoslavië roept oorlogsherinneringen op"'; Mooij, 'De langste schaduw', 274
14: 'Prof. Jan Bastiaans (1917-1997), 3-11-1997
15: Schreuder, 'In memoriam prof.dr. J. Bastiaans', 13-12-1997, 2479
16: Ibidem

17: F.i.: Van Bergen, *Van Genezen in Geloof*, Deel II, hfdst 6; Brabers, *Hippocrates op Heyendaal*, Hfdst. 3 en 4; Klein, *Verlangen naar Verbetering*, hfdst. 7
18: Withuis, *Erkenning*, 12, 244; Withuis, 'De opmars van het slachtoffer'; Shepard, *A War of Nerves*, 385-399
19: Also: Enning, *De Oorlog van Bastiaans*, 191-194
20: Snelders, Pieters, 'De opkomst, val en mogelijke opkomst van LSD', 709; Enning, *De Oorlog van Bastiaans*, 46

INDEX OF PERSONS

Aalders, Gerhard Charles 81-2
Aantjes, Willem 168-71
Agt, Dries van 14, 52, 67-70, 72, 74, 77-8, 98, 139, 144, 167, 213, 223
Amsberg, Claus von 9, 209
Arendsen Hein, Wil 102, 191

Baan, Pieter 115-6, 122
Barnhoorn, Johannes 25-6
Baruch, Jacques 91
Bastiaans, Jan passim
Beatrix, princess/Queen 9, 209
Beenen, Folkert 217
Beets, Nicolaas 209
Benders, Henri 217-9, 225
Bernhard, Prince 58, 65, 68, 95-96, 98, 112, 117, 121, 128
Bertina, Bob 50-54
Bhagwan Shree Rajneesh 169, 240
Biesheuvel, Barend 74, 76, 83, 91, 98, 100
Binneveld, Hans 14
Blijham, Harmannus 192, 194-5
Boas, Henriette 71-2, 248-9
Boellaard, Pim 176
Boer, E.J. 117-8, 121
Booij, Jan 47-8
Borghart, C. 211
Borssum Waalkes, Jan van 233
Brauw, Mauk de 100
Breuer, Josef 234
Bueren, Peter van 49, 128

Ceha, Karel 221
Cohen, David 219
Cohen, Elie Aron 17, 21, 30-1, 33, 35, 37, 42, 57-9, 61-4, 71, 80, 116, 186, 187, 248-9, 257

Dam, G.G. van 137
Dam, R. van 109, *332*
Dantzig, Andries van 22
Dedem, Godert Willem Baron van 92-3, 95
Derksen, Leo 143, 179
Diepenhorst, Isaac 82
Dijk, Wybo Kuno van 150, 152-3, 160-1, 192, 214-6, 218, 223-5
De-Nur, Yehiel (Ka-Tsetnik) 234
Doorn, Harry van 121
Dorsman, Jacob 122
Duynstee, Frans 77, 85

Eban, Abba 72
Eitinger, Leo 1, 31
Eleveld, W. 220
Elsberg, Daniel 130
Elsen, Hans van der 182-3
Elsen, Joop van 93
Emde Boas, Coen van 44-7, 71
Engelbrecht, Corina 205-8
Engels, Piet 81-2, 90
Es, Adri van 93

Fanggidaej, Benjamin 138
Fischer, Franz 13, 28, 67
Flapper, George 191-2
Fortuin, Johanna 241
Foudraine, Jan 169-70
Frequin, Louis 196
Fünten, Ferdinand aus der 13, 28, 62, 67
Furth-Halverstad, Eva 111-2

Gardeniers, Til 173-6, 184, 216
Gasteren, Louis van 44-6, 48, 50-4, 57, 61-2, 77, 74, 81, 87-8, 116, 118, 120, 127-8, 199

Gersons, Berthold 253
Geurtsen, Aart 76-8
Giesen-Rosenhart, Truus van der 214
Gisolf, Aart 147-8, 164-5, 198-200, 231, 240
Glimmerveen, Henk 227
Godschalk, Jan 68-9
Goudsmit, Anneke 77, 80
Grant, Cary 9
Grobin, Wulf 33, 35
Grosheide, Hans 68

Hamburger, Max 73
Hearst, Patricia 155
Heertje, Arnold 236
Heijermans, Herman Louis 40
Heil, Piet 155
Hemert, E. van 115
Hendriks, Jo 134-6, 138, 156
Heringa, Gerard Carel 30
Hers, Hans 148-9, 158
Herzberg, Abel 71, 103, 185
Heusinger, Adolf 29
Hoek, Sietse van der 223, 226, 228
Hofhuizen, Herman 85-6
Hofman, Karel 55
Hofstede, Peter 169
Hoorn, Willem van 234
Hugenholtz, Paul Theodore 26, 83, 123, 164-5
Hulsman, Louk 74, 77
Hustinx, A. 13, 108, 194
Huygen, Frans 138

Illich, Ivan 218

Jong, Lou de 38-9, 43, 166, 168-70, 179, 208, 235 ,*356*
Jong, Piet de 44, 58, 91, 93, 100
Juliana, Queen 44, 58, 95, 102, 111-2, 132, 230
Jungman, Wim 85-6, 178

Kaas, Andries 22-3, 35, 55, 257
Kater, Joseph 1-4, 21, 30, 33
Keilson, Hans 172
Kleerekoper, Joseph 101
Klompé, Marga 44, 46
Knoop, Hans 165
Kolk, Bessel van der 8
Komrij, Gerrit 18-9, 230-1
Kossman, Ernst Heinrich 232
Kotalla, Joseph 13, 28, 67
Kousbroek, Rudy 16-9, 205-6, 242
Kraaijeveld-Wouters, Jeltien 175-6, 220
Kroef, Cees van der 163
Kruisinga, Roelof 44, 59, 64-5, 95-6, 121
Krumperman, A. 238

Ladee, George 177
Lages, Willy 28, 61
Langebent, Ad 141
Lanschot, Willem-Bib van 172
Leeuw, André de 13
Leeuw, Hans van der 170
Leliefeld, Henk 177-8, 181-3
Lemaire, W.C. 204
Loggem, Manuel van 27
Londen, Joop van 138-9, 154-6, 158
Londo, Gerard 235
Los, Pieter Leendert 87-8, 240
Lubbers, Rob 150, 160
Lulofs, Bart 142, 239
Lumeij, Jan 78

Maliepaard, Piet 65, 100, 103, 112-3, 116-7, 247
Manusama, Johan 223
Matussek, Paul 26
McAnelly, Henry 105
Meekren, Jaap van 235
Meerendonk, Huub van de 142
Meerloo, Joost 21
Meester, Eibert (Willem van Salland) 19, 121-2, 129, 141-5, 158, 234,
Meijer, Ischa 123
Meijer, Wim 142, 156, 206

Meijering, W.L. 95-6, 98, 101-5, 108-111, 113-6, 118-21, 123, 174, 180, 221
Menten, Pieter 143, 165, 170-1, 197, 235
Milikowski, Herman 52-3, 126-7, 129-30, 132, 168, 248
Mochel, Henk 124
Montessori, Mario 217
Mooij, Annette 13, 23, *145*
Mulder, Dirk 138, 150, 153-4, 156-7, 160, 215, 223-4, 226-8
Muntendam, Piet 65, 96-9, 102-3, 111, 116, 119, 122
Musaph, Herman 26-7, 75, 78, 84, 107, 232, 237

Namen, Arie van 158-9
Noordhoek Hegt, Pim 25-6, 41-2, 58-9, 64

Ochberg, Frank M. 154, 160
Oldenborgh, Ineke van 176
Overeem, Bob van 59, 98
Overeem, Emmy van 108, 136, 172, 193-5

Pannekoek, Yvo (Frits Dekking) 142
Peereboom, Klaas 47-8, 201, 228
Pepplinkhuizen, Lolke 236
Ploeg, Henk van der 190, 192, 220, 223-5, 237, 256
Poel, Cor van de 199
Poel, Hein van de 60-1
Polak, Ben 223, 235-6
Polak, Carel 61, 67, 77
Poole, Jaap le 118-9
Praag, At van 36, 38, 44
Praag, Jaap P. van 156, 181
Presser, Jacques 38, 39, 103

Reagan, Ronald 214
Reemst, Theo van 27-8
Reijden, Joop van der 229, 232-3
Rijke, Rien de 235
Rooijmans, Harry 220, 231, 239
Ross, Thomas Arthur 2-3
Rost van Tonningen, Florrie 235
Rost van Tonningen, Meinoud 235
Rümke, Cornelis 154
Rümke, Henricus Cornelius 21, 35, 154

Schaft, Hannie 226
Schakel, Maarten 165
Scheepmaker, Nico 84-5, 125
Schudel, Willem Joost 236
Sereny, Gitta 186
Seyss-Inquart, Arthur 128
Slagter, Jos 69
Snelders, Stephen 1, 9-10
Soetendorp, Avraham 68, 70, 72
Speidel, Hans 29
Speijer, Nico 36, 44, 59, 65, 95-6, 100, 113, 115, 120, 156
Sprenger, Wim 140
Streep, Meryl 173
Stuyt, Louis 82
Summerfield, Derek 252-3
Sunier, Armand 73, 75, 179
Swaan, Abram de 19, 196-7, 237, 248-9
Szasz, Thomas 191

Tas, Eva 98, 111
Tas, Jacques 21, 30, 33, 48, 257
Teengs Gerritsen, Hans 65, 68-9, 73, 89-90, 112, 116-7
Telling, Joop 102, 104, 118
Terwindt, Trix 119, 174, 230, 240
Theodorakis, Mikis 125
Thygesen, Paul 24
Tol, Dick van 44, 83-4, 86-8, 101, 147

Udink, Be 44
Uyl, Joop den 121, 134, 142-3

Vaal, Otto de 51
Vaders, Ger 138-9, 189, 212-4, 227, 239

Veder-Smit, Els 188
Virchow, Rudolf 31
Vogt, Joop 144
Vogt, Tini 141-2, 144
Vonhoff, Henk 58, 92
Voogd, Joop 59-60, 89, 91-2, 221
Vorrink, Irene 121-2
Vredeling, Henk 139
Vrijburg, Gerhard Sietse 209
Vroom, Merinus 21
Vroon, Piet 234

Wallagh, Constant 50
Wangh, Martin 35-6
Wayne, John 52
Weegen, Maartje van 200
Weetering, Irene van de 49
Weijel, Jacques 77, 83-7
Weinreb, Friedrich 103-4, 143
Wennekes, Wim 128, 130, 141, 143, 196
Westerman Holstijn, Toon 26
Wibaut, Frank Peter 25-6
Wiegel, Hans 221
Wiesenthal, Simon 5
Wigbold, Herman 169-70
Wilbrink, Willem 5
Wind, Eddy de 5, 22-3, 33-5, 37, 43, 60, 116, 187, 216, 232, 237, 257
Withuis, Jolande 13-4, 246, 255
Wolff, Joop 165, 167

Young, Allan 252